The one-stop healthcare book that no home should be without

THE COMPLETE GUIDE TO FAMILY HEALTH

DR NIGHAT ARIF

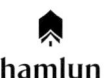
hamlyn

To my husband and my boys, for bearing with me through my difficult second album.

hamlyn

First published in Great Britain in 2026 by Hamlyn, an imprint of Octopus Publishing Group Ltd
Carmelite House
50 Victoria Embankment
London EC4Y 0DZ
www.octopusbooks.co.uk

An Hachette UK Company
www.hachette.co.uk

The authorized representative in the EEA is Hachette Ireland, 8 Castlecourt Centre, Dublin 15, D15 XTP3, Ireland (email: info@hbgi.ie)

Text copyright © Dr Nighat Arif 2026
Design and layout copyright © Octopus Publishing Group 2026

Distributed in the US by
Hachette Book Group
1290 Avenue of the Americas,
4th and 5th Floors
New York, NY 10104

Distributed in Canada by
Canadian Manda Group
664 Annette St., Toronto,
Ontario, Canada M6S 2C8

All rights reserved. No part of this work may be reproduced or utilised in any form or by any means, electronic or mechanical, including photocopying, recording or by any information storage and retrieval system, without the prior written permission of the publisher.

Dr Nighat Arif has asserted their right under the Copyright, Designs and Patents Act 1988 to be identified as the author of this work.

ISBN: 978-1-78325-643-3
eISBN: 978-1-78325-644-0

A CIP catalogue record for this book is available from the British Library.

Printed and bound in China.

10 9 8 7 6 5 4 3 2 1

Publisher: Kate Fox
Senior Developmental Editor:
    Pauline Bache
Art Director: Jaz Bahra
Editorial Consultant: Liz Marvin
Illustrator: Liliana Rasmussen
Picture Research Manager:
    Jennifer Veall
Copy Editor: Emma Bastow
Assistant Production Manager:
    Lisa Pinnell

All reasonable care has been taken in the preparation of this book but the information it contains is not intended to take the place, where appropriate, of in-person examination and treatment by a qualified medical practitioner.

CONTENTS

Introduction 4

THE WHOLE BODY
The Musculoskeletal System 28
The Skin 48
The Blood 62
The Immune System 70
The Endocrine System 86

THE HEAD & NECK
The Brain & Nerve Network 100
The Eyes 136
The Ears, Nose & Throat 146

THE UPPER & LOWER BODY
The Respiratory System 164
The Cardiovascular System 176
The Digestive System 190
The Urinary System 212
The Female Reproductive System 222
The Male Reproductive System 240

Glossary 250
Resources 252
Index 253
Acknowledgements 256

Introduction

Welcome to *The Complete Guide to Family Health*. I have written this book to be a friendly and reassuring source of clear information about your health and the things that can go wrong with it, so that it will live helpfully on your shelf for many years to come, ready for whenever you need it.

First port of call

We have access to a lot of information online, which is wonderful in many ways, but the reality is that much of it is confusing, conflicting and may be inaccurate. This book contains no complex technical information and no medical jargon; just straightforward, simple explanations of symptoms, causes, diagnosis and possible treatments. It's no substitute for a consultation from a medical professional – because no book can be – but it's the perfect first port of call when you have health concerns and need advice. My hope and intention is that it will help you feel confident in dealing with the day-to-day issues of your family's health.

You know yourself best

No one knows your body like you do – only you know how you feel and what's normal for you. The first, most important part of living a healthy life is to empower yourself with knowledge – such as about eating well and the importance of good sleep and exercise – to give yourself the best chance of an active, happy older age. Our bodies and our minds are unique, and we all need to take charge of our own health.

We will all fall ill at some point; it's unavoidable. For most of us, most of the time, this will be a cold, the flu or a minor injury. But sometimes it will be something more serious. The sobering statistic is that half of us will be diagnosed with some kind of cancer in our lifetime. But cancers and many other diseases are much more likely to be successfully treated if they are caught early, so by knowing your own body, understanding the signs and getting anything unusual checked, you can make a big difference to the outcome if you do have a serious illness.

- 🔴 **Contagious**
- ⚫ **Transmissable**
- 🟢 **Non-contagious**
- 🟢 **Genetic**

A note on labels

Some conditions are particularly dangerous because they can spread so quickly from infected people before they even know they are infected. Throughout the book you will see these Contagious alerts to flag where infections are contagious (either airborne or through food and non-close contact). Transmissable flags highlight infections that can be passed from person to person, or animal to person, but through closer contact, either via blood or sexual contact. On the flip side, some people with certain conditions can find themselves stigmatised due to incorrectly held beliefs that their condition is contagious. Because of this, I have included notes in the SKIN, THE IMMUNE SYSTEM and THE RESPIRATORY SYSTEM chapters for all conditions, to make it clear where a condition is not contagious, or is genetic (or inherited as a hereditary disease).

How to use this book

I have included as many common health conditions as possible in these pages, as well as some of the rarer ones which, although I may not see them often in my surgery, are worth being aware of.

You will find that the entries are grouped together in the chapters based on a system or area of the body – for example, conditions affecting the skin, the digestive system or respiratory system can all be found in the same section. This is to make it easier to browse through connected or similar conditions. Some illnesses affect more than one part of our bodies, of course, although they usually originate from one area, and many conditions have similar symptoms. To avoid repeating information, I have used a cross-reference system – text that looks LIKE THIS indicates another entry elsewhere that it's worth you taking a look at. You can also use the index on pages 253–5 to find specific conditions.

When do I need to get medical help?

It can be difficult to determine the difference between emergency and urgent symptoms and when an issue can be managed at home. Often, certain types of pain or discomfort are actually normal bodily responses; ways in which we would expect the body to react within the normal parameters to protect itself. For these, I advise at-home treatments to ease your discomfort.

Other symptoms or pain are not immediate cause for alarm but should be monitored closely and medical help sought from a professional if they persist, worsen or cause concern (gut instinct is a wonderful thing!). For these the next course of action is to call your GP surgery or 111 for advice.

Finally, throughout the book I have listed red flag symptoms, which can be a sign of something seriously wrong. Where I note these, it is important to seek urgent medical attention. In the case of babies and small children, go to your nearest hospital or call an ambulance.

> ### Red flags
> Knowing when to seek attention from a medical professional can be difficult to determine. The short answer is that if you are very worried, call your doctor, call 111 (in the UK) or go to A&E. I would rather someone come in to see me than suffering in silence with something that needs prescription medication or to be checked out with tests.
>
> I do see a lot of minor ailments that could have been treated with over-the-counter medication on the advice of a pharmacist, rather than the person waiting a week to see me, worrying and feeling uncomfortable. And there are things that your GP just can't help with – if you have broken a bone, for example, you will need to go to hospital for an X-ray and possibly to have it set.
>
> So, with this in mind, I have included a 'red flag' section where relevant to indicate when you should definitely see a doctor or, in more extreme cases, call an ambulance. This of course isn't – and could never be – a comprehensive, fail-safe guide. Always use your own common sense and judgement, and trust your intuition.

Medical professionals

Most people know what a GP does. Here are some other healthcare professionals who you might see in primary care or when you need a particular type of treatment.

Allied health professionals

In the UK and some other countries, this refers to a group of medical professionals who are highly trained in their specialities, but are not doctors. This group includes paramedics, speech therapists, radiographers and dieticians. They provide essential care and support to patients, for example:

Chiropractor: Treats issues around the movement of the spine. They may be able to help with shoulder or neck pain and HEADACHES that come from this area, too.

Osteopath: An expert in the musculoskeletal system. They look for causes of pain throughout the body and treat the issue with massage, manipulation of joints and stretching.

Physiotherapist: Uses exercise and movement to help people affected by injury and some illnesses to get back to mobility and health.

Occupational therapist: Helps people work out how to carry out day-to-day activities when they have been affected by illness or injury.

Dietician: An expert on food and nutrition who will offer advice to help with particular medical conditions to manage symptoms and complement medical treatment.

Physician associate: Trained to support GPs, physician associates undertake a two-year postgraduate degree and can give patient consultations, undertake physical exams and develop treatment plans.

Community midwife & health visitor: Those with a low-risk pregnancy can self-refer to the community midwife for antenatal care. When your baby is born, they will be under the care of a health visitor for all their regular check-ups and health support until the age of five.

District nurse: A qualified nurse who provides care for patients at home and in residential care.

Community mental health nurse: A specialist mental health nurse who provides care and support at home and in residential care.

Community paramedics: A specialist offering treatment at home or in a healthcare setting.

Nurse practitioner: A highly experienced nurse who can make some diagnoses, write prescriptions and carry out HRT reviews.

Practice nurse: A qualified nurse working in a GP surgery. They can carry out many different tasks, including blood tests, vaccinations, changing dressings and giving advice on a range of topics, from CONTRACEPTION to stopping smoking.

Pharmacy first

Most pharmacists train for five years to achieve a Masters of Pharmacy degree and can often advise on straightforward problems. If they have any concerns, they can trigger a referral to your GP. Otherwise, they recommend over-the-counter medicines, antibiotics or antivirals.

The seven conditions you should consult a pharmacist about, rather than waiting to see a doctor, are: SORE THROAT, EARACHE, INFECTED INSECT BITE, IMPETIGO, SHINGLES, SINUSITIS AND uncomplicated URINARY TRACT INFECTION in women between the ages of 16 and 64. Pharmacists also have a 'serious shortage protocol' – if there is a shortage of a particular drug they can replace your prescription with the most appropriate substitute.

First Aid Kit

First aid can mean either being the first responder to an accident (see page 16) or the treatment of minor ailments, for which it's good to be prepared with a simple first aid kit.

It's a good idea to have a larger first aid kit for home and a smaller one for the car or for carrying with you. What you put in it will depend on the size and needs of your family, but below are the basics – don't forget to check expiry dates regularly.

- Sterile gauze pads and adhesive tape or dressings in various sizes for wounds.
- Plasters.
- Antiseptic wipes or solution to clean wounds.
- Tweezers for removing splinters or ticks, etc.
- Scissors for cutting bandages.
- Digital thermometer.
- Burn spray.
- Eyewash solution.
- Gentle laxatives to treat constipation.

An instant cold pack for SPRAINS, injuries, etc. is useful for the car – at home you can use a bag of frozen vegetables wrapped in a tea towel. You might also want to include an emergency foil blanket for when you are out and about.

Over-the-counter treatments for common illnesses

It can be difficult to know which over-the-counter medications you should take for common pains and illnesses. There are children's versions of all these medications (except aspirin) available too. Always ensure you stick within the recommended doses and, if you are taking multiple medications, check that the active ingredient is not repeated. Here are some general guidelines:

Paracetamol should be your first port of call for fever and pain.

Ibuprofen can be taken if a fever is not coming down after paracetamol. It is also an anti-inflammatory so works well to reduce swelling and pain from inflammation. Ibuprofen can irritate the stomach so should be taken with food. You should not take ibuprofen if you have ASTHMA, kidney- or stomach-related problems, and it should not be given to children under the age of 16 who have a rash. Seek advice from your GP if you are unsure.

Aspirin works in a similar way to ibuprofen so the two should not be taken together without medical guidance. It is an anti-inflammatory and also works as a blood thinner. Aspirin should not be given to children under the age of 16.

Antihistamines are used to relieve rash and sinus-related symptoms of allergic reactions, such as HAY FEVER, insect bites or HIVES. Some antihistamines can make you drowsy so avoid driving or operating heavy machinery when using them and ensure that children avoid climbing, cycling or being alone after having taken antihistamines. Check with your GP if you or your child have chronic LIVER DISEASE before using antihistamines. You should also check with your GP if you are taking antidepressants or medication for stomach issues. Antihistamines are available to take orally, through nasal sprays or via the skin.

Living a healthy life

In order to have healthy bodies and minds, and to give us the best possible chance for staying healthy and active in older age, we need to consider our diets, exercise and sleep as well as our emotional wellbeing.

Healthy eating

Eating well is a fundamental pillar of achieving and maintaining good health. High-calorie, low-nutrition foods are everywhere, often more affordable than healthier options. This can lead to us viewing sugary, fatty foods as a 'treat', so we feel we are depriving ourselves if we try to avoid them.

The reality is that, while it's absolutely fine to have a piece of cake occasionally, we are really not 'treating' ourselves when we overindulge. We need the right vitamins and minerals to be healthy, and if we become overweight or OBESE, we are drastically increasing our chances of developing TYPE 2 DIABETES, heart conditions and many other debilitating, life-changing, and potentially life-shortening conditions. And there are further consequences. For example, if you become sick, there may be fewer treatment options available if you are overweight or have other health conditions. In addition, the majority of health conditions will see at least some improvement if you achieve and maintain a healthy weight through a good diet and adequate movement.

Healthy eating habits

- **Eat lots of fruit and vegetables** – at least five portions per day; 'eat the rainbow'.
- **Eat protein** – try to include a palm-sized portion of protein with each meal.
- **Eat fibre** – this is important for good digestion and to keep you regular!
- **Eat wholegrains** – like oats, brown or wild rice, barley, quinoa and bulgar. Among other benefits, they help with regulating blood sugar and digestive health.
- **Avoid ultra processed foods (UPFs)** – such as shop-bought cakes, sweetened cereals, fast food, energy drinks and processed meat like chicken nuggets and some deli meats.
- **Drink at least 2 litres (7fl oz) of water a day** – 'drink water' might be the most boring advice there is, but I promise that good hydration is very important and underpins so much of what is going on in our bodies.
- **Plan your meals** and have *tasty* healthy options in your home. You are far more likely to pick up a ready-meal or takeaway if there's nothing in the fridge. Think about what your week will look like and make a meal plan.

Exercise

Our bodies are built to move – the sitting still that modern life encourages is so bad for us. Of course some health conditions make exercise more challenging, but for almost all of us, finding a way to exercise that works for our own bodies is crucial. We know that regular exercise: reduces stress levels, increases levels of dopamine (the 'feelgood' hormone), improves sleep, increases energy levels, helps manage blood sugar levels and metabolism, keeps our heart healthy, makes our joints and muscles stronger and more mobile, aids recovery from illness and injury, and increases our chances of having a healthy, independent older age.

Good exercise habits

- **At least 30 minutes' movement/day** – is the aim if you are aged 19-64 . Walking counts so think about times when you can walk somewhere rather than drive or get the bus.
- **Moderate-to-intense exercise at least two times/week** – this should make you feel out of breath.
- **Strength/resistance exercises at least two times/week** – these are where you use some weight (including your own body weight) or force (like a resistance band) to strengthen muscles. It also builds bone and joint strength – great for all of us and especially important for women as they age.
- **Find what works for you** – either with a group, a friend or by yourself. The main goal is to identify a form of exercise you actually want to do and keep doing it!

Sleep

Most adults need between six and eight hours of good quality, uninterrupted, restorative sleep a night. It's fundamental to our health and wellbeing and yet so often we take it for granted. It's just as essential as exercise and good nutrition. Studies have linked a lack of sleep with an increased risk of developing ALZHEIMER'S DISEASE and as well as increased levels of the hormones that make you want to eat. Getting enough sleep allows our brains to process information, is essential for memory, slows down our metabolism, helps us manage stress and bolsters our immune system – it's when we are asleep that the body can repair itself.

See page 135 for more on lifestyle changes to encourage good sleep hygiene.

Relationships & emotional wellbeing

As a doctor, I see first-hand how important feeling comfortable in our minds and happy in our relationships is to our overall health. Life will throw difficult things at all of us, but knowing how to look after our wellbeing, turn to people we trust for help and comfort, value what's good in our lives and feel we have the power to make changes is what gets us through and keeps us healthy in the broadest sense of the word.

Habits to support emotional wellbeing

- **Play** – research shows it's important to make time to play, whether that's a sport or activities you loved when you were younger. Exploring new hobbies is also valuable, keeping our minds sharp and reducing stress.
- **Spend time in nature** – even a walk around the block will help your wellbeing.
- **Be in touch with your emotions** – being able to process our feelings is an ongoing skill. Journalling for just five minutes a day can help.
- **Spirituality** – this means something different to us all; whether it's faith, a practice like yoga, meditation or mindfulness, or being in nature, ensure you make space for it in your life. Spiritual connection has a big impact on cortisol levels and helps manage stress.
- **Connection and community** – studies show that the people who live longest are those with strong human connections. Social media has many advantages, but it's no replacement for time with people face to face. Nurture relationships: make time for family and friends, join a club, volunteer or participate in community events.

Alcohol, smoking & drugs

We all have our weaknesses – mine is chocolate – but it's important to ensure they don't interfere with our best efforts at healthy living.

Alcohol

The recommended maximum you should drink is 14 units a week, spread over at least three days. A unit is calculated based on the alcoholic strength of the drink and how much of it you are drinking. While most of us aren't going to get our calculators out if we want to have a drink, here's how to work out the number of units: **strength (ABV percentage) x volume (in ml) ÷ 1,000 = units**

Drinking is bad for BLOOD PRESSURE and therefore heart health, as well as for our livers, but there are many other benefits of limiting our alcohol intake to below the recommended level, including:

- Better sleep.
- Clearer skin and easier weight management.
- More energy.
- Improved mood and memory.
- Setting a good example to young people in our lives.

If you choose to cut down, the first step is to be honest about how much you are drinking, use an app to help you track this and motivate you towards achieving your goal. Some people find doing this with someone – a partner or friend – can be helpful, so you can encourage each other. Avoid binge drinking and aim to have at least three alcohol-free days every week.

Smoking

Many smokers find it difficult to imagine a life without cigarettes, but it is always possible to quit, with help and support. The NHS Stop Smoking programme is a great first port of call if you are in the UK. They may be able to offer nicotine replacement therapy on prescription too.

Even if you didn't smoke much, you'll be amazed how much better (and financially better off!) you will feel when you quit. If you are a heavy smoker, quitting will be genuinely life-changing – as well as most likely life-prolonging.

Vapes have been shown to help people to quit, but children and nonsmokers should never vape.

Recreational drugs

Unlike alcohol, which is a legal drug and carefully regulated, you have no idea what is in an illegal substance; it passes through many hands before it gets to the end user and there is no label telling you how strong it is. Illegal drugs have many health risks, including but not limited to:

- HEART ATTACK.
- Seizure (see EPILEPSY).
- STROKE.
- Mental and emotional disorders (paranoia, DEPRESSION, ANXIETY, lack of motivation).
- Sexual dysfunction.

Over time, a drug user's body adapts and needs more and more of a substance to experience the same effects. The worrying psychological effects will often build up gradually, with the user unaware of the damage to their mental and physical health. If you take illicit drugs, educate yourself on the risks and long-term effects of what you are taking, and what to do in an emergency.

There is a lot of information online about how to talk to children about drug use. It's always best to have open conversations. The websites Talk to Frank (www.talktofrank.com) and Barnardos's Alcohol and Drug Misuse pages are really useful resources in the UK.

Regular health checks for adults

The NHS offers health checks and screening programmes for people at different ages to identify health conditions. A health check is more general whereas a screening programme looks for specific illnesses.

It's up to you if you want them, but I would always recommend taking up the offer of any health checks or screenings that are available to you. The following is a general guide to what is available in the UK on the NHS at time of writing but should be a useful indication wherever you live.

If you already know you have a certain health condition, such as DIABETES or HEART DISEASE, you will be offered more specific checks to monitor this and other conditions you are more likely to develop. Make sure you know what is available to you – check the NHS website or speak to your GP.

NHS Health Check

This is a general check-up of your overall health available to people aged 40 to 74, every five years. The following will be checked:

- Your height, weight and waist measurement.
- Your BLOOD PRESSURE.
- Your CHOLESTEROL level.
- Possibly your blood sugar level.

You will be asked about your medical history and your family history, as well as lifestyle questions. You will be advised on your likelihood of developing TYPE 2 DIABETES, problems with your heart or circulation, or having a STROKE.

Eye exams & hearing tests

It's recommended that you have your eyes tested at an opticians every two years (some people are eligible for free eye tests).

There are free online hearing tests available from organisations such as RNI:D. Many opticians and some pharmacies offer this too.

See pages 139 and 152 for more on sight and hearing tests.

Sexual health

If you are sexually active with more than one partner, you should ideally have an STI check every year, or more often if you regularly have sex with more than one partner and do not use a condom. It's very easy to do – you can go to a sexual health clinic in complete confidentiality or get a free at-home test through the post. Go to www.sh.uk in the UK and see page 220 for more on sexual health.

The NHS screening programme

National screening programmes mean that issues can be detected early. This is the NHS programme but other countries may have their own versions for you to attend.

For men

Type of screening	Screens for	Age when you are eligible	How often
Abdominal aortic aneurysm (AAA)	Swelling and weakening in the aorta – the major blood vessel from the heart	65	Once, unless an issue is found

For women

Type of screening	Screens for	Ages when you are eligible	How often
Cervical screening	HPV (the cause of CERVICAL CANCER)	25–64	Every three years ages 25–49; every five years 50–64
Breast screening/ mammogram	BREAST CANCER	50–71	Every three years

For everyone

Type of screening	Screens for	Ages when you are eligible	How often
FIT kit (at-home test)	BOWEL CANCER	50–74 (opt-in for ages 75 and over)	Every two years

Private screening

There are an increasing number of companies offering private screening, such as full-body MRI scans and online genetic testing. This may be suitable for some people but it's important to do your research, as there is some evidence that the harms can outweigh the benefits. For example, you may be told you have an increased chance of getting a certain illness, which could still be relatively low, but could cause stress and anxiety.

The NHS vaccination programme

The national vaccination programme helps protect against fatal diseases.

The groups who should have vaccinations are:
- Babies and children.
- Adults aged over 65.
- People who are travelling to certain countries (see page 19).
- Those with health conditions (such as immunodeficiency) that places them in an at-risk group.
- Pregnant women.

Adult Vaccination Programmes

Age	Vaccine	Protects against
65 years and over	Flu vaccine	Certain types of influenza virus (given annually)
65 years	Shingles	Shingles (single dose)
65 years	Pneumococcal	Several serious bacterial infections, including pneumonia and meningitis (single dose)
75 to 79 years old	RSV	Respiratory syncytial virus
75 years and over	Covid-19	Covid-19, every year in spring and winter

If you are pregnant

You will usually be offered vaccinations against FLU, whooping cough and respiratory syncytial virus (RSV).

If you think you are in an at-risk group
Speak to your GP as you may be eligible for different vaccines or early vaccination.

What to do if you miss a vaccination
If you think you have missed a vaccination, speak to your GP. It's often still possible – and advisable – to have it.

Child development checks & children's health

From birth to the age of two, babies in the UK are offered regular checks from a health visitor to reassure you that their development is what we would expect to see and that there aren't any issues that need to be investigated. Child development checks include:

- Shortly after birth, babies are weighed, given a check-up and hearing test.
- A few days after birth, babies are given a blood spot test/heel prick test. This checks for rare diseases like SICKLE CELL DISEASE and CYSTIC FIBROSIS.
- In the first 10 to 14 days, a health visitor will check in. They can give advice on looking after the baby and sleeping, as well as explaining vaccinations and how often your baby should be weighed (usually once a month for the first six months and then every two or three months).
- At six to eight weeks your baby will be offered another check-up, usually at a clinic or the doctor's surgery.
- When your baby is nine to twelve months, you will be given a questionnaire to fill in about their development. The health visitor can help with this, and you'll be able to discuss any concerns.
- At two or two-and-a-half years, you'll complete another questionnaire and there will be another appointment to check your child's health and development.

In addition to these checks, your child will be offered the NHS vaccination schedule. This gives them enhanced protection against a range of illnesses, such as MEASLES, MENINGITIS, SEPSIS, polio and tetanus. Many of these illnesesses can be extremely serious or even fatal. Childhood vaccination is the unsung hero in healthcare and has contributed to dramatically reducing deaths and serious illness over the past decades.

As well as protecting individuals, when a large portion of a population is vaccinated it achieves 'herd immunity', so that instances of the disease become so low that even individuals who have not been vaccinated are somewhat protected, as they are less likely to come across the disease in the first place. So I cannot emphasise enough how lucky we are to have access to these resources and how much I recommend taking advantage of them. Vaccines save lives!

Your baby's red book

In the UK, shortly after your baby's birth, you'll be given a book in which to record your child's personal health information. This is often called the 'red book'. You can also add your child's development milestones yourself – like when they first sleep through the night, sit up unaided, etc. It's very, very useful and it's important to take it to every appointment if you can.

The NHS vaccination programme

Babies & children

Age	Vaccine	Protects against
8 weeks old	6-in-1 (first dose)	Diphtheria, tetanus, pertussis (whooping cough), polio, Haemophilus influenzae type b (Hib) and hepatitis B
	MenB (first dose)	Several serious bacterial infections, including meningitis and sepsis
	Rotavirus (first dose)	Rotavirus
12 weeks oldw	6-in-1 (second dose)	Diphtheria, tetanus, pertussis, polio, Hib and hepatitis B
	Rotavirus (second dose)	Rotavirus
	Pneumococcal (first dose)	Several serious bacterial infections
16 weeks old	6-in-1 (third dose)	Diphtheria, tetanus, pertussis, polio, Hib and hepatitis B
	MenB (second dose)	Several serious bacterial infections, including meningitis and sepsis
1 year old	Hib/MenC vaccine (first dose)	Hib and a certain type of meningitis
	MMR and chickenpox (first dose)	Measles, mumps, rubella and chickenpox
	Pneumococcal (second dose)	Several serious bacterial infections
	MenB (third dose)	Several serious bacterial infections, including meningitis and sepsis
2 to 15 years old	Flu vaccine	Some types of the influenza virus
3 years and 4 months old	MMR and chickenpox (second dose)	Measles, mumps, rubella and chickenpox
	4-in-1 pre-school booster	Diphtheria, polio, tetanus, whooping cough
12 to 13 years old	HPV	Human papillomavirus (linked to certain cancers, such as cervical cancer)
14 years old	3-in-1 teenage booster	Tetanus, diphtheria and polio
	MenACWY vaccine	Serious bacterial infections, including some types of meningitis

Emergency first aid

It's such a good idea to have a working knowledge of emergency first aid. Knowing what to do in an emergency will make you feel calmer and you may even save a life. A study commissioned by the Red Cross found that nearly two out of three people who died from an injury may have survived if they'd received effective first aid treatment before an ambulance arrived, while statistically women are less likely to receive chest compressions than men in an emergency.

Watching videos or attending a course are the best ways to learn first aid – the Red Cross has lots of videos on their website (www.redcross.org.uk). They also offer online courses and you can download their app which has simple, clear first aid advice.

If someone is hurt and appears to be unconscious:

▼

Check for **danger** – what has hurt them and could it hurt you?

▼

Check for **responsiveness** – can they hear you? Ask a bystander for help if you can.

▼

If they are unresponsive, open their airway – tilt their head back by pushing lightly on their forehead. Look at their chest and put your face over their mouth for 10 seconds to see if you can hear or feel breathing.

▼

If they are not breathing, start chest compressions – call 999 and the operator will talk you through this. If a bystander is available to help, get them to call 999.

▼

If they are breathing normally or irregularly, put them in the recovery position (see below), with their head on their hand, leg bent to prop them slightly forwards, and airway open.

Call 999 if they are unresponsive or their injuries cannot be treated by first aid. Call 111 if the situation is not an emergency but you need urgent advice for further treatment.

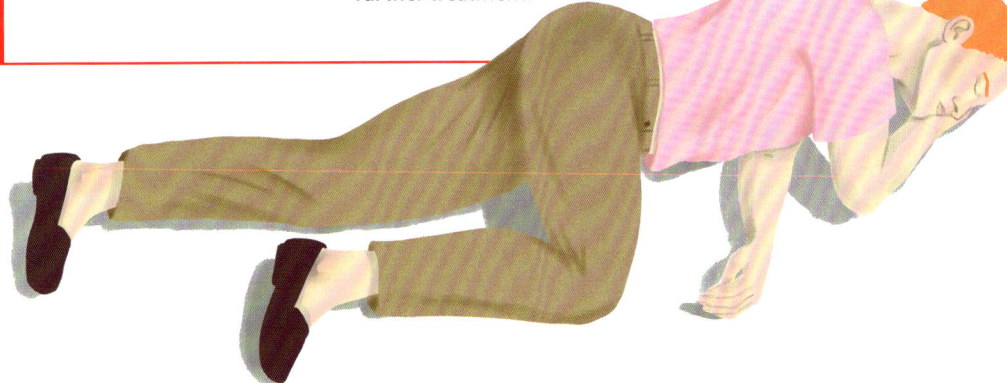

> **Red flag – first aid**
>
> Most public places or care settings will have defibrillators (a device that uses electrical shocks to restore a normal heartbeat when someone is in a cardiac arrest), which include instructions to follow. They can be used in emergency situations where you do not know what the unresponsive person is suffering as, if the defibrillator doesn't detect an irregular heartbeat, it will remain inactive.
>
> For more information about specific emergency situations, see:
> - HEART ATTACK on page 180.
> - STROKE on page 126.
> - ASTHMA ATTACK on page 168.
> - SEPSIS on page 27.
> - FRACTURES on page 40.
> - SPRAINS and STRAINS on page 32.

Be prepared

No one wants to dwell on the possibility of accidents or illness, or enjoys having difficult conversations about what they want to happen if they are unable to make decisions for themselves. It might feel like we are tempting fate by discussing such situations, but if something does go wrong you and your family will be grateful that you were prepared.

In case of emergency

In an emergency situation where you are unable to speak for yourself, first responders and medical professionals will need to be able to access information that will help them know how to treat you, particularly if you have any underlying health conditions.

Medical bracelets & necklaces

Consider wearing one if you have a condition that may affect how you are treated. If you would tell a medical professional about this condition or medication (for example, if you have a serious ALLERGY or take blood-thinning medication), the same information also needs to be relayed if you are unable to communicate for some reason. First responders are trained to check for medical bracelets and necklaces if a patient is unresponsive.

Medical ID

Most mobile phones have a medical ID function, where you can add details about your emergency contacts, allergies, medications you are taking and more. You can select for this to be available for medical professionals to read even if your phone is locked, so if you are unconscious, medical professionals will still be able to access crucial information about you.

Family information

Not everyone feels comfortable sharing their medical information with their family and our natural inclination is often to respect people's privacy and not push. However, knowing what medication your loved ones take and any health conditions they have – or at least having access to this information – can be useful in a situation where they cannot advocate for themselves.

Pins and passwords

You may choose to give a couple of trusted people your phone pin and other key passwords, so if you are incapacitated they can access information that may be helpful. Of course, it's important to be mindful of the security of sensitive information.

Power of attorney

It's worth considering who you would want to make medical decisions for you if you are unable to make decisions for yourself in the future. This is called 'lasting power of attorney' and more information can be found on the NHS website under End of Life Care/Planning Ahead.

Organ transplants

In the UK, we have an 'opt out' system for organ transplants, which means that everyone over the age of 18 will be considered a donor in the event of their death if transplant is possible, unless they have actively opted out via the NHS Organ Donation Register, they are in certain protected groups or their family objects.

Next of kin will always be consulted, which is why it's important to share your wishes with those closest to you. Note that a will isn't usually read immediately after someone dies, so putting your wishes in your will and not communicating them to anyone is unlikely to be effective.

The 'opt out' system only covers what is known as routine transplants, which includes heart, lungs, kidneys, liver, corneas, pancreas, small bowel and tissue. Anything more unusual still requires specific consent.

Travel

As exciting as it is to go on holiday, accidents and illnesses can happen regardless of how old you are, your medical background and general health. Therefore it's important to be prepared to ensure you have the best experience on your holiday.

Ten weeks before you travel

- Check to see if you need any vaccinations or if MALARIA tablets are required or recommended for your travel destination. The NHS Fit For Travel website (www.fitfortravel.nhs.uk/destinations) is a good resource.
- Check if the country you are visiting requires you to show proof of vaccination.
- Bear in mind that some vaccines take a while to work in your body, so you need them well in advance.
- Get a prescription for MALARIA tablets, if needed, or they are available over the counter. You need to start taking them some time before you travel for them to be effective.

Two to three weeks before you travel

- Make sure you have the right travel insurance so you are covered for all the activities you want to do.
- Check you have enough prescription medication to last your trip (including CONTRACEPTION) with some spare. Make sure you have a copy of your prescription with you in case you are asked to prove what it is and that it's for your personal use.

One week before you travel

- Consider packing a small first aid kit (see page 7).
- Stock up on things like painkillers, hand sanitiser and over-the-counter diarrhoea relief. Even if you can easily buy these things where you are going, it's good to have it with you in case you suddenly feel unwell.
- Ensure you know the emergency number for the country you are visiting and whether it's safe to drink the water (you may want to take water purification tablets). Parents may want to research local healthcare, too.

UK Global Health Insurance Card (GHIC)

If you are a resident of the UK, you can apply for this before you travel. It works in the European Economic Area (EEA) and some other countries, and it means you can get access to the same state-provided healthcare as a resident of the country, when it's medically necessary. This is not a substitute for travel insurance, though, and everyone (even children) needs their own card.

See: www.nhs.uk/using-the-nhs/healthcare-abroad/apply-for-a-free-uk-global-health-insurance-card-ghic

Safeguarding

The role of a GP extends beyond medical practice to psycho-social care and ensuring public safety, as the GP surgery is a hub for the health of the community.

Safeguarding is a term we use to mean institutions and organisations that ensure there is protection for those at higher risk of neglect or abuse, particularly if they find it difficult to speak up. So, for example, children and adolescents, people who have been victims of domestic violence, and adults with learning disabilities or other challenges that mean they are more at risk. We use this word a lot in the NHS, partly because of the personal and intimate nature of healthcare, although the principles are important in many other areas, such as care homes and schools.

GPs (and other surgery staff) are known as 'primary care providers' – usually the first point of contact someone has with the health service. This means that we can be uniquely placed to recognise that someone is at risk or needs help. We undergo training to help us spot the signs of abuse, or that someone is in an unsafe situation. If we see these signs, we have a responsibility to act.
Remember: abuse takes many forms and you can always speak to your GP if you are concerned.

The six principles of safeguarding

These were included in the Care Act – government legislation introduced in 2014. They apply in different ways in different settings, but this is how they work in the context of a GP practice.

- **Protection** – healthcare professionals have a duty to look out for those at risk of harm.
- **Prevention** – we receive training to recognise the signs when something isn't right; it is always better to do something than wait for a situation to become more serious.
- **Accountability** – if you tell us something that indicates someone might be suffering abuse, by law we have to report it, and be open with you that this is the case.
- **Empowerment** – it's crucial the person feels that they are in control of what's happening; they should feel supported at all times.
- **Proportionality** – we have to report our concerns in a way that matches how serious the situation is. There are lots of rules and guidelines that we have to be trained in.
- **Partnership** – all health and social care professionals should work together to detect signs of abuse and act to help.

If you think someone is suffering abuse or neglect

Try to reassuringly talk to them in private if you can, letting them know that it is safe for them to talk to you. They might feel reluctant to share what is happening, so you need to be patient. Don't act on their behalf unless you think they are in danger.

Local authorities have adult safeguarding co-ordinators who can help and advise. Anyone can call the local authority (social care section) of the person who is suffering abuse or neglect, or see Resources (page 252) for charities who can help. Speak to the police if you think a crime has been committed, and always call 999 if you or someone else is in immediate danger.

Trans health

While reports suggest that there have been improvements in NHS healthcare for trans people, there are still barriers to overcome and steps that need to be taken to make sure we have a health service that's fully inclusive of everyone.

Gender identity & medical care

Anyone can change their name and gender at their doctor's surgery, and let the practice know what pronouns they prefer. There should be a form you can fill in – ask the receptionist. This means the GP will already know to call you by your preferred name and pronouns every time you go in for an appointment.

Note that when this happens, you may be issued with a new NHS number. Make sure your health records have been updated and all your information moved across.

Attending screenings as a trans person

The screenings you are invited to will be based on the sex you were assigned at birth. For example, a man with a uterus should still have a CERVICAL SCREENING TEST every three or five years. Some trans men who have had top surgery will not need a routine mammogram, whereas others who still have breast tissue might. Talk to your GP about your needs and concerns, as they should be aware that attending screenings based on sex assigned at birth can be traumatic for trans people. Most surgeries have a trans health policy, and some will have a practitioner who has a specialist training.

Gender dysphoria

This means that someone is experiencing distress because their sex assigned at birth does not match how they want to live. It's important to note that it is not a mental illness, but the stress it causes can lead to DEPRESSION, ANXIETY and other MENTAL HEALTH CONDITIONS.

Many young people question or want to explore their gender identity at some point. This is completely normal and doesn't necessarily mean they will choose a different gender for themselves (although some may well). In an ideal world, young people would be given the space and encouragement to figure it out for themselves in their own time, changing their minds as many times as they wish, without stigma, pressure or shame.

Some people will want to be referred to a gender identity or gender dysphoria clinic (GDC), or to access gender-specific counselling, medical or surgical affirming therapy, or hormone therapy. This situation requires specialist care; patients should expect to be treated with dignity and respect while the options available to them and how they access them are clearly explained.

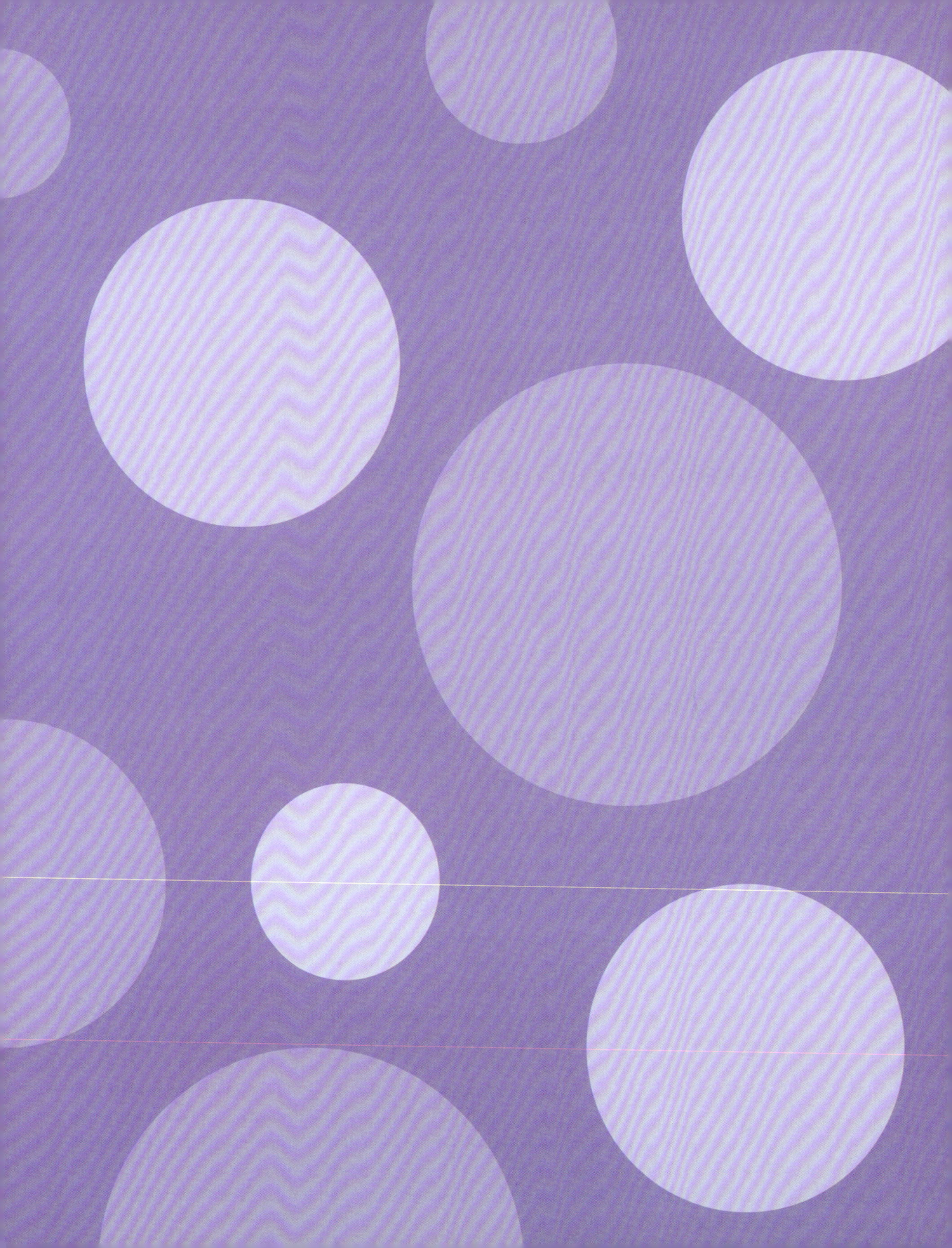

THE WHOLE BODY

🔴 **Contagious (depending on cause)**

Fevers

A fever is our body's response to infection. While a fever accompanied by other symptoms can be an indication of something more serious, in many cases a fever is simply a healthy immune system reacting to an infection in exactly the way it should and is usually nothing to worry about.

SYMPTOMS
+ **Higher than usual temperature (see below).**

Diagnosis

You'll need a good thermometer to measure temperature accurately – see First Aid Kit on page 7. An average temperature is around 36.5°C to 37°C (97.7°F to 98.6°F), although it varies from person to person and changes throughout the day. Body temperature is often naturally lower in older people. If you need to talk to a medical professional about a fever, it's useful to be able to tell them the person's temperature.

When to seek medical help will depend on the age of the person and any additional symptoms. See the tables on pages 25–6 for advice on when to seek help for babies and children under five, and children over five and adults.

Treatment

DO
- Drink more water than usual – the adult or child should be peeing every four to six hours and the urine should be light in colour.
- Make sure the room isn't too hot or cold.
- Rest.
- Take over-the-counter drugs that help to bring fevers down, such as paracetamol and ibuprofen, so long as there are no allergies (note that taking ibuprofen on an empty stomach might make the person vomit). **But *do not* give ibuprofen to children who have** CHICKENPOX.
- Wear loose-fitting, comfortable clothes.
- Try taking a tepid bath (with someone nearby in case of loss of consciousness).
- Eat, if possible.

DON'T
- Put lots of blankets on the bed to try to 'sweat it out', or cool the person down with cold water. Our bodies know what they are doing!
- Leave the adult or child at home alone if possible, in case they begin to get worse. Try to keep them to their own room (and ideally using their own bathroom) to avoid spreading infection.
- Mix with other people. Stay at home to avoid spreading infection.
- Drink alcohol or take illicit drugs.

Rashes: The glass test

If a baby, child or adult has any kind of rash then it's important to do the glass test. This simple test will tell you if you need to be worried. Take a colourless glass (not plastic!) tumbler and roll it firmly over the rash. If the spots do not fade under pressure, this is called a non-blanching rash. Seek urgent medical attention by calling 999.

Fevers in babies & children under five

Fevers are more serious in babies. If you are worried, trust your instincts and go to your nearest hospital (this also applies to children over five years old and adults).

Expected bodily response – if you observe these symptoms use at-home treatments	If you observe these symptoms, monitor closely and call 111 if they do not improve or if they worsen	Red flag situation – seek urgent medical attention; in the case of babies and small children, go to hospital or call an ambulance
A child or baby has a mild temperature of 37.8–39°C (100–102°F) within 48 hours of a vaccination.	A child or baby has a temperature of 39°C (102°F) or higher for more than five days.	A baby under three months has a temperature above 38°C (100°F) or below 36°C (97°F).
A child has a temperature of 38°C (100°F) or higher for less than four days and no other severe or long-lasting symptoms.	A feverish child is consistently off their food or a baby won't take the breast or a bottle.	A baby aged three to six months has a temperature of 39°C (102°F) or higher.
A child or baby over six months is feverish but able to eat and drink, and will settle.	A feverish child or baby is dehydrated – their nappies are hardly wet and their lips and tongue are dry.	A child or baby is breathing fast and noisily, is breathless and/or their stomach muscles are visibly working hard with every breath.
A child or baby's fever comes and goes, settling with children's paracetamol.	A feverish child or a baby over six months is consistently hard to settle and not interested in their toys and usual activities.	A child or baby is unusually cold to the touch and their skin is blue and mottled.
	A child or baby has had a viral infection such as CHICKENPOX in the last few days and the fever is getting worse or not reducing from 37.8°C (100°F).	A child or baby is sleepy, confused and difficult to wake.
	A child is complaining of pain that isn't responding to paracetamol. Severe crying and distress in a baby.	A child or baby has a fit or seizure (convulsions).
	A child or baby has a swollen limb and/or seems reluctant to put weight on any part of their body.	A child or baby has a rash that doesn't pass the 'glass test' (see opposite).

Fevers in children aged over five & adults

Expected bodily response – use at-home treatments	Monitor closely and call 111 if symptoms do not improve or if they worsen	Red flag situation – seek urgent medical attention; in the case young children, go to hospital or call an ambulance
A low-grade fever of 37.3°C to 38°C (99°F to 100°F), or a moderate fever of 38.1°C to 39°C (100.6°F to 102°F), with no 'red flag' symptoms.	A high-grade fever of 39°C to 41°C (102°F to 106°F).	A seizure, or loss of consciousness, confusion, not responding when spoken to.
The fever goes down in response to taking paracetamol/ibuprofen/a tepid bath.	Extreme sleepiness – feels or seems 'out of it'.	Has trouble breathing.
Accompanying symptoms such as irritability, achy muscles, lack of appetite, restlessness and not being able to sleep are common with fevers, but shouldn't last more than three days.	A fever that doesn't get better after three whole days, or the temperature rises further.	Fever and pain when urinating and the urine smells unusually bad.
	A moderate fever – 38.1°C to 39°C (100.6°F to 102°F) – that doesn't respond to any at-home treatments.	Fever and blood in stools.
	Vomiting that is causing dehydration – the person consistently can't hold anything down including water.	Fever and a stiff and rigid neck.
	Fever in someone who is immunodeficient, on immunosuppressants or taking any medication that might reduce the immune system's response.	Fever and discoloured, bad-smelling vaginal or penile discharge.
	Fever in someone who has an underlying health condition such as lung problems, HEART DISEASE, DIABETES, CHRONIC KIDNEY DISEASE, neurological dysfunction, SICKLE CELL DISEASE.	Fever accompanied by swelling in any part of the body.
		A rash that doesn't pass the 'glass test' (see page 24).

Septicaemia/sepsis

These terms are often used interchangeably for what is essentially the same thing: a very serious condition caused by an infection – bacterial, viral or fungal – and how the body responds to it. The infection overwhelms the immune system and the body isn't able to fight back.

Learning to recognise sepsis is very important as it's vital to get emergency medical attention as soon as possible. We can use the acronym 'TIME' to help us:

T = TEMPERATURE: Unusually high or low, often accompanied by shivering and muscle cramps.
I = INFECTION: Sepsis always starts with an infection of some sort, although it can be mild.
M = MENTAL DECLINE: The person may be very confused, slurring their speech or has become unresponsive.
E = EXTREMELY ILL: They may also be struggling to breathe properly.
If you suspect sepsis, call 999 immediately.

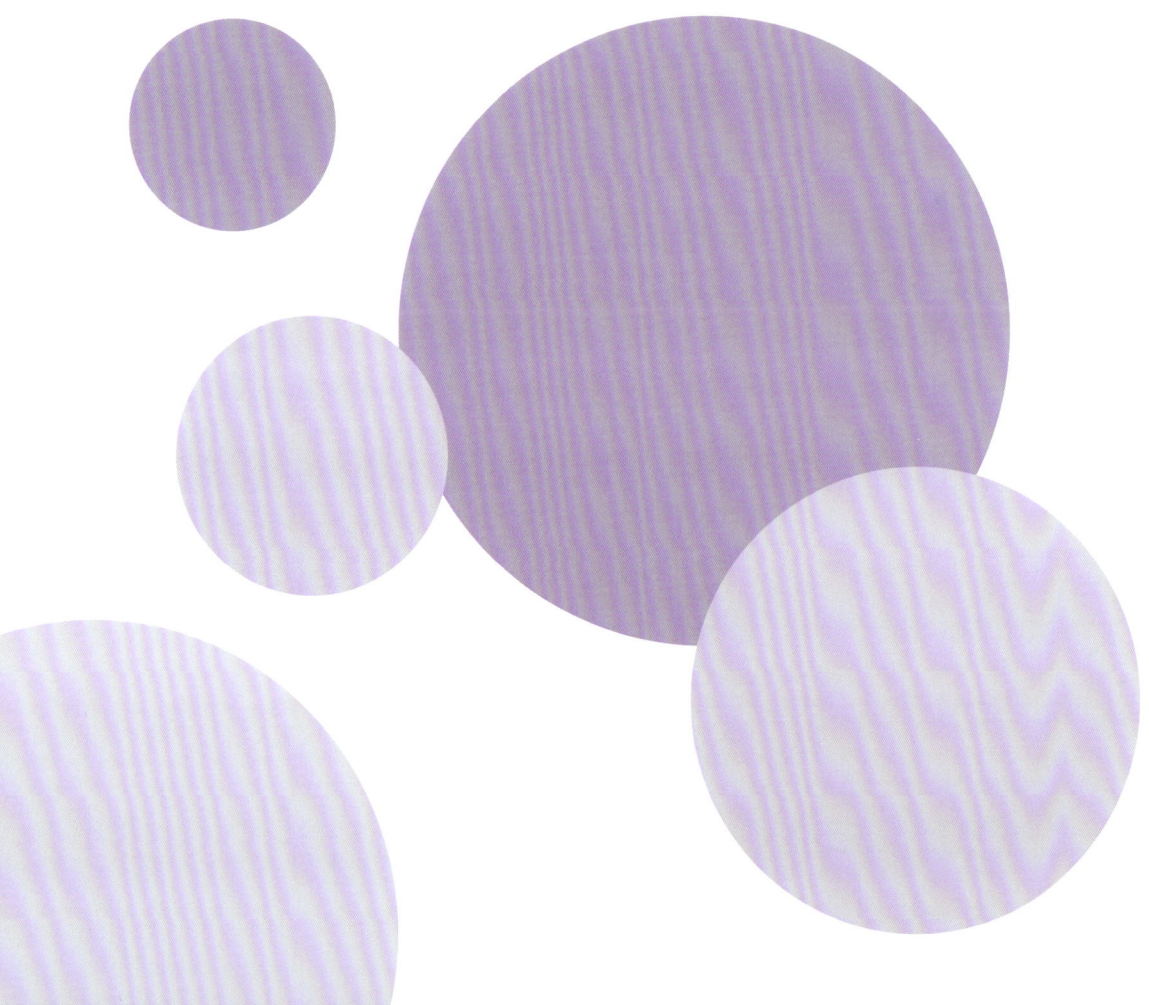

THE MUSCULO-SKELETAL SYSTEM

Our body is mechanically amazing. Your skeleton is made up of 206 individual bones, ranging in size from the largest, the femur (your thigh bone), to the tiny stapes (in your ear). Your joints work as hinges and your muscles make up a 'pulley system' so you can bend and move. As well as the muscles you consciously use to walk around, play sport, wave at someone, etc., you have 'involuntary' muscles that work away without you thinking about it – for example, your heart and those inside your digestive system.

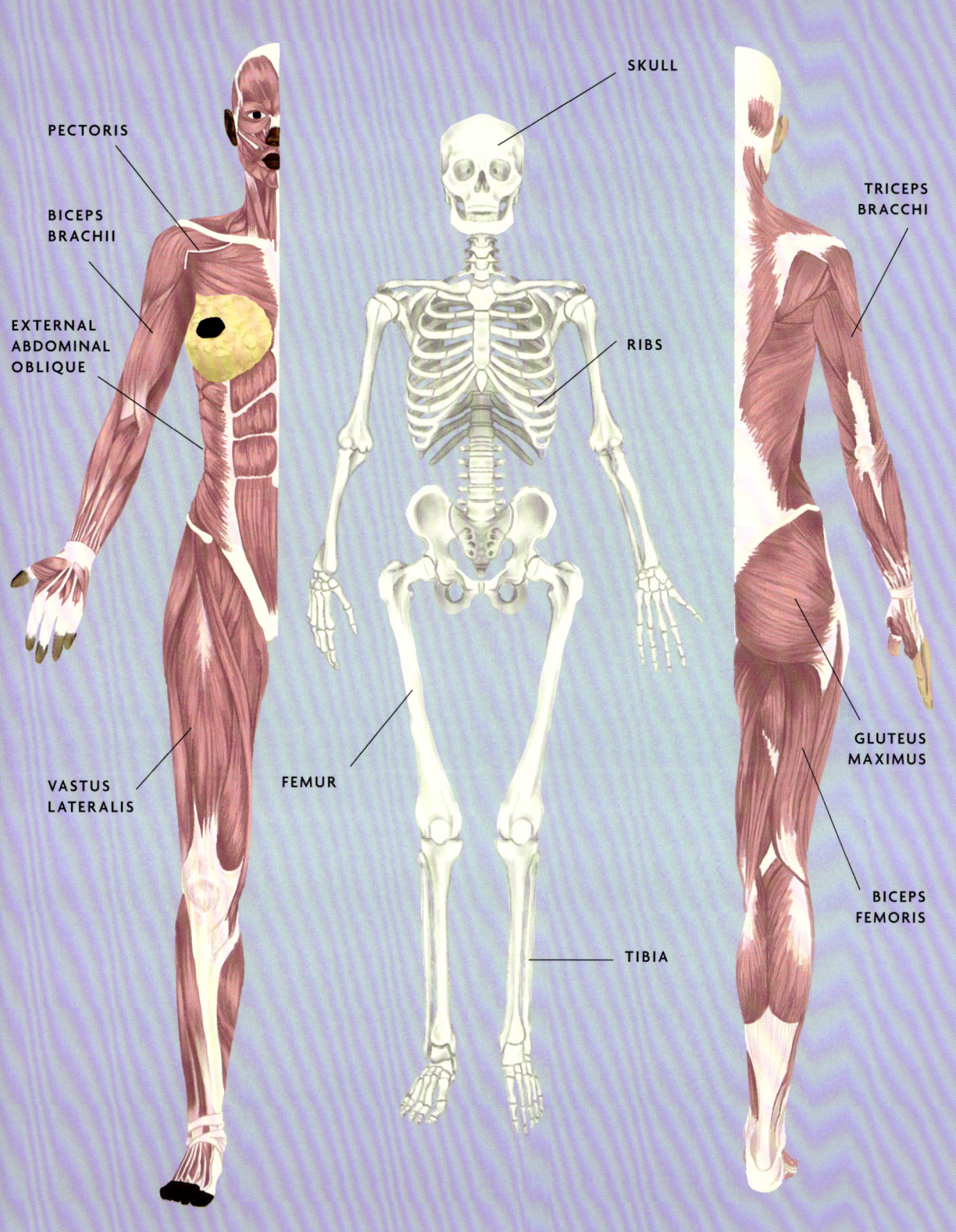

THE MUSCULOSKELETAL SYSTEM

Bones

Your skeleton literally holds you up; it protects important organs, and it's where red and white blood cells are made, in the bone marrow. Bone is a living tissue with its own blood supply and it's constantly being broken down and reformed again – this is also how the body repairs itself if a bone is broken or fractured.

Muscles

Muscles work by contracting and relaxing. Skeletal muscles – those we use to move – are attached to our bones. They tend to come in pairs, to give us a range of movement. So, in your knee, quadriceps at the front of your leg contract so you can straighten your leg. To bend your knee, the hamstrings at the back of the leg contract while your quads relax. This is basically how we walk. It's simple but at the same time very clever!

We also have cardiac muscles that make up the heart and 'smooth muscles', which are found in places like the stomach lining.

Eating for bone strength

Calcium: This mineral is essential for good bone health and for growing children. Too little calcium is one cause of OSTEOPOROSIS. Calcium is found in dairy products such as milk and cheese, green leafy vegetables like spinach and broccoli, and fish with soft, edible bones such as salmon and sardines. Some foods are 'calcium fortified' which means they have extra calcium added to them.

Vitamin D: We need vitamin D to help us absorb calcium. It's also important for our muscles. We can get some vitamin D from foods like fatty fish, and there are small amounts in egg yolks and red meat, plus it's added to some of our food. But the main source is sunlight. In the UK, the NHS recommends that everyone should consider taking a daily supplement containing 10 micrograms of vitamin D, or 400IU, during the autumn, winter and early spring months (if you see this in a multivitamin, then you are covered for the recommended baseline amount). Children, those with darker skin or those who spend very little time outdoors, should take this all year round.

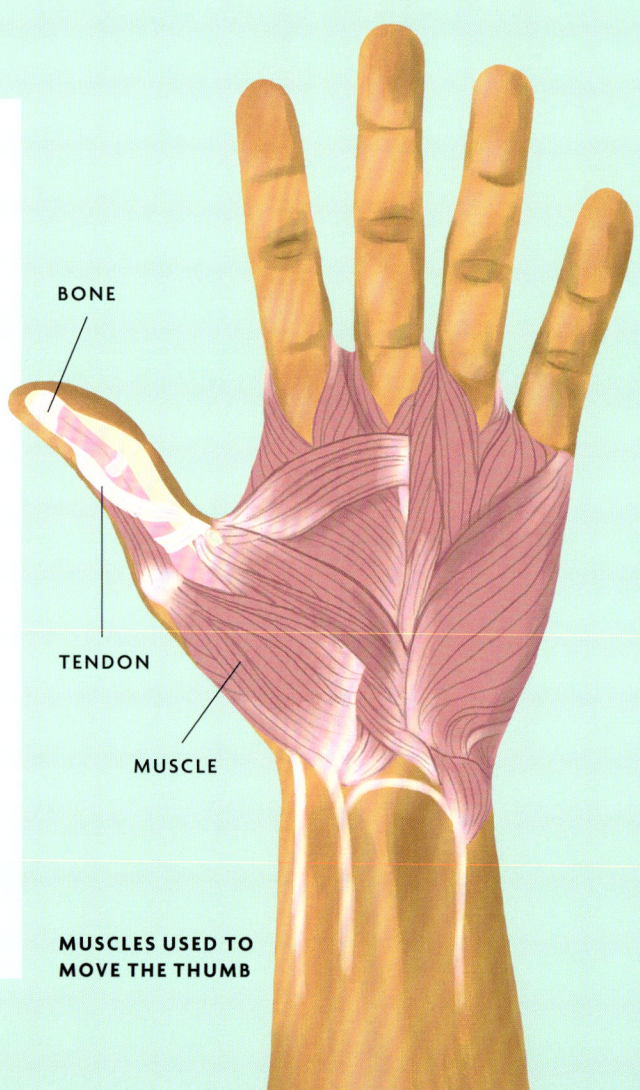

BONE

TENDON

MUSCLE

MUSCLES USED TO MOVE THE THUMB

Joints

We have different sorts of joints in our bodies. Some are essentially hinges, like the elbow or knee. Hips are ball-and-socket joints, which allow a range of movement in different directions.

- **Ligaments** keep bone joints together.
- **Tendons** hold the muscles to the bones they are responsible for moving around.
- **Cartilage** is a tough but smooth tissue found at the ends of bones, which reduces friction when they're rubbed together.
- **Synovial fluid** is what I like to call 'golden lubricant'. It helps with movement by stopping friction in joints, which damages them and causes us pain.

Fascia

This thin casing of connective tissue surrounds and holds every organ, blood vessel, bone, nerve and muscle in our bodies. It has its own nerve endings, which make it sensitive when it is stressed and tight. Sometimes patients tell me that they have some pain, but they don't feel like it's a muscle, a bone or ligament. This is likely their fascia tissue. It usually responds to massage, heat treatment and/or gentle exercise to loosen it up.

JOINTS USED TO MOVE THE KNEE

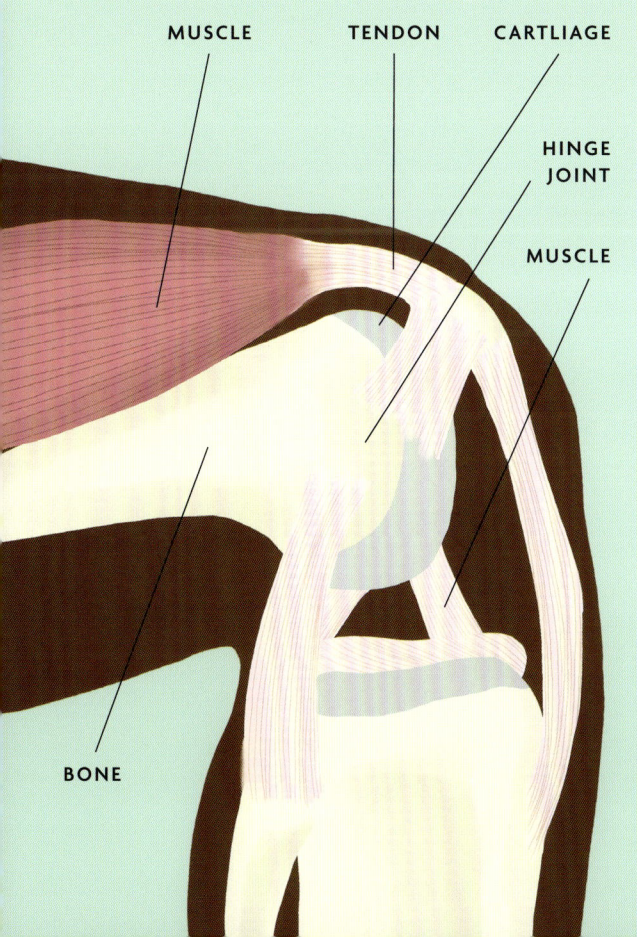

MUSCLE · TENDON · CARTLIAGE · HINGE JOINT · MUSCLE · BONE

Wear & tear

Our bones are really strong and regenerate themselves, but eventually they do wear down. Our joints and muscles are resilient but it's important to look after them if we want a healthy and happy life as we get older.

You can cause temporary damage to joints by twisting them beyond their normal range or putting repeated stress on them. This can cause the cartilage to wear away, meaning the bones rub together. We think if this as something that happens to older people, but I also see it in younger people as a result of putting stress on the joints through being very overweight or OBESE.

The best way to look after our bodies is with a good diet, so we're getting the right vitamins and nutrients to protect our bones and joints, and regular movement. These awesome machines we have been born with are capable of so much and they really want us to move!

Sprains & strains

A sprain is when you injure the ligament, the tissue that holds our joints together. A strain is an injury to a muscle or tendon – it's sometimes called a pulled muscle.

SYMPTOMS

+ Soreness around the injury, that can vary from moderate to intense pain if there is a serious tear.
+ Stiffness around the injury and difficulty moving it without pain.

Diagnosis
Self-diagnose from the symptoms shown.

Treatment
Most sprains and strains can be treated at home. A pharmacist can advise on over-the-counter pain relief and a physiotherapist can give you exercises to do as part of rehabilitation. See below for when to go to A&E.

The first 24 hours

The best approach has the acronym 'PRICE':
P= Protect: Support the injury, by wearing the right shoes, for example, and guarding against further strains.
R= Rest: Rest it as much as possible in the first day.
I = Ice: Apply an ice pack (or a bag of frozen veg wrapped in a tea towel) for 15–20 minutes every 3 hours.
C = Compression: Wrap a bandage or a long piece of fabric around the area if you can. Tie it firmly enough to add support but don't cut off the circulation. Take it off at night.
E = Elevate: Keep sprained knees, ankles and wrists raised on a cushion as much as you can during the first day.

Take over-the-counter painkillers (preferably oral paracetamol, or try low-dose codeine). Ibuprofen gel can also help but avoid heat treatments (see opposite).

Days two to three

When you can, gently and slowly move the injured area as much as possible every few hours. Gradually build up the range of movement over the coming days. Too much rest will cause the joint to stiffen up and it will take longer to heal.

Continue taking painkillers as you need them.

Up to two weeks

Most non-serious sprains and strains will heal within two weeks. Back injuries can take longer to get better (see BACK PAIN).

Avoid strenuous exercise (like running and weightlifting) for eight weeks following a painful injury to avoid further damage.

Listen to your body. It needs to move to get better, but if you try to do something and you feel it's screaming at you to stop, then do!

THE MUSCULOSKELETAL SYSTEM

Red flags

Look out for these warning signs that the injury could be more serious, such as a ruptured tendon or FRACTURE:

- You heard a cracking sound when the injury was sustained – in this instance don't try to move and call an ambulance.
- You can't move or put any weight on the joint without experiencing severe pain.
- The injured body part has changed shape beyond swelling.
- The injured body part is numb or tingling with pins and needles – this indicates the circulation has been cut off.

Go to a minor injuries unit or A&E straight away as you will likely need an X-ray. There's no need to go to the GP first. Note that in the UK, a physiotherapist can refer you for an X-ray.

Ice versus heat

It can be confusing whether to apply ice or heat to an injury as both have a role to play. Here's how to choose the most appropriate option.

Ice – restricts blood flow to an injured area. It brings down swelling and helps stop the body 'overreacting' to an injury. It's the best thing to do immediately after sustaining the injury.

Heat – encourages blood flow. We want this to happen as blood contains the nutrients that help us heal. Heat treatment is good for ongoing chronic injuries, tight muscles and 72 hours after an injury, once the swelling has gone down.

Healing times

Healing times can vary a lot depending on the extent of a sprain or strain. Muscle soreness from exercise should subside within three days but for injuries, healing times should be within the following parameters:

Muscle strain: From 0–2 weeks for a grade 1 strain, through to up to 6 months for a grade 3 strain.
Ligament sprain: From 0–3 days for a grade 1 sprain, through to 5 weeks, or up to 1 year for a grade 3 sprain.
Tendon injuries: From 3 weeks for tendonitis, through to up to 6 months for a laceration or tendinosis.

Knee pain

There are many causes of knee pain. It's important to know that sometimes knee pain can be caused by mild inflammation rather than an underlying condition.

SYMPTOMS

+ **Pain, swelling and/or stiffness in one or both knees.**

Causes

Some of the most common reasons for knee pain are:
- Kneeling for long periods.
- SPRAINS and STRAINS from exercise.
- Ligament damage from exercise or wear and tear.
- Wearing the wrong sort of shoes that don't support your knee joint.
- ARTHRITIS.
- GOUT.

Red flags

See a medical professional, who may recommend an X-ray, if the following applies:
- You are experiencing persistent and severe knee pain that is stopping you leading your normal life and doesn't respond to the at-home treatments below.
- The pain is keeping you awake at night.
- You have a weakness in the knee that is new and/or getting worse, particularly if you are losing muscle tone.
- Your swollen knee is hot, which can be a sign of infection.

Treatment

Most knee pain can be treated at home initially.
- If the knee is swollen, initially rest and keep it elevated as much as possible, until the swelling reduces.
- Apply ice if swollen (not heat, which can increase swelling).
- Think about your diet and avoid anything you know from experience will cause inflammation in your gut. Remember that everything in the body is interconnected.
- Take ibuprofen and paracetamol.
- Once any swelling has gone down, move your knee gently at regular intervals.
- A knee support may be helpful.
- Try sleeping on your side with a pillow between your knees.
- Walk and take gentle, though not high-impact, exercise if the pain is not too severe to promote better circulation, which is important for healing.
- When the pain subsides, consider strengthening exercises to support your knees in the future. Seek advice from a physiotherapist.

Knee pain in women

Knee pain is more common in women for a number of reasons:
- Women's wider hips can put extra stress on joints.
- A reduction in oestrogen and testosterone starting in PERIMENOPAUSE can mean more inflammation in the body, which can cause painful joints.
- Women are more susceptible to OSTEOPOROSIS, which causes knee pain.
- Research shows that being overweight or OBESE causes women's joints to wear more quickly than men's.

Back pain

Most of us will experience back pain from time to time. It can have many causes and most aren't usually serious. The main issue with ongoing back pain is when it affects our wellbeing, stopping us from doing things and even impacting our MENTAL HEALTH.

SYMPTOMS
+ **Stiffness and/or muscle aches.**
+ **Burning, shooting or stabbing pains.**
+ **Pins and needles, tingling or numbness.**

Causes
Some of the most common causes of back pain are:
- Stress.
- Poor sleeping position, such as not having the right neck support.
- Poor posture, particularly if you sit at a desk all day.
- Misalignment in your back, caused for example by carrying a heavy backpack on one shoulder.
- Repeatedly lifting heavy weights (see RSI).
- Lifting heavy items with a poor technique.
- Pregnancy.
- ARTHRITIS, ANKYLOSING SPONDYLITIS, PROLAPSED DISC and SCIATICA.

Treatment
Much of the same advice applies as for SPRAINS and STRAINS – rest in the first instance, then ice followed by alternating cold then hot treatments. Take ibuprofen and paracetamol if you are able. Topical pain relief, such as ibuprofen gels, might help, too.

Gentle exercise is often the best prevention and treatment for general back pain. Low-impact activities like swimming, Pilates and yoga are recommended. If you are overweight or OBESE, losing weight so your spine is under less pressure will almost always help.

Red flags
If you are experiencing any of the following, seek advice from a medical professional or go to A&E in an emergency.
- Extreme pain that doesn't improve with pain relief.
- If you have been experiencing ongoing pain for over four weeks.
- You have a history of cancer and you have recently lost weight for no apparent reason.
- You are struggling to walk or use your legs normally.
- Tingling or numbness that goes down into the buttocks and groin, and you have difficulty peeing or controlling peeing or pooing.
- Sudden pain in the upper back, especially if this spreads to the jaw, neck or chest and is accompanied by difficulty breathing (see HEART ATTACK).
- You have a FEVER or have recently had a bacterial infection.
- You have had a fall, which could indicate a FRACTURE.
- You have other serious health conditions, particularly if you are immunocompromised.

Frozen shoulder

Frozen shoulder, also known as adhesive capsulitus, is caused by the shoulder joint becoming thickened and stiff, therefore limiting movement. This can happen due to an injury, such as a rotator cuff tear, keeping the shoulder still for an extended period, underlying medical conditions (DIABETES, viral disorders, if you have had a STROKE), and we know that age is a common factor in frozen shoulder as it's more commonplace in people aged 40 and above. This is because as we get older the tissues in the shoulder naturally become more prone to inflammation and thickening.

SYMPTOMS

Stiffness and pain in the shoulder that goes on for a long time – sometimes for months – making it difficult, or even impossible, to move the arm. Patients often find that the symptoms have three phases:

- **Pain:** The shoulder is always sore, and feels worse at night when you are trying to sleep.
- **Stiffness:** While the pain may decrease, the amount of movement in the shoulder decreases too. If this phase lasts more than six weeks, your muscles may start reducing (known as 'muscle atrophy'), making recovery more difficult.
- **Recovery:** The range of motion comes back slowly. This may happen by itself, but the treatments below will help you to reach this phase sooner in many cases.

Diagnosis

Diagnosis by symptoms and examination by your GP. Sometimes you will be referred to an X-ray, ultrasound or MRI scan.

Treatment

It's important to start at-home treatment early.

- Treat the pain with over-the-counter pain medication, ibuprofen gel, and/or a heat rub such as Deep Heat.
- Try a cold pack – such as a packet of frozen vegetables wrapped in a tea towel – on a fresh injury to decrease inflammation.
- After a few days, use a heat pack or hot water bottle wrapped in a towel to encourage blood flow. Or try using a heat pack for 15 minutes then alternating with a cold pack. The heat will encourage blood flow, which decreases inflammation.
- A therapy called transcutaneous electrical nerve stimulation (TENS), which uses a low-voltage electrical current to block or change how the pain is perceived, is found by some to be helpful in managing the pain.
- Exercise is very important, when you can manage it. The finger walk exercise can help reduce stiffness. Face a wall and slowly walk your fingers up it until your arm is raised at shoulder level, and then gradually go higher if you can. Repeat regularly.
- A physiotherapist can advise on more exercises.

Red flags

See a medical professional if any of the following apply:

- The pain means you cannot live your life as normal and it's affecting your sleep.
- You have swelling, a FEVER and/or the joint feels hot to touch.
- If the frozen shoulder has been caused by an injury and isn't getting better, you may need an X-ray to check for a FRACTURE.
- If none of the above treatments help over a period of six months (if not severe), a GP may investigate the cause further and/or prescribe steroid injections.

Repetitive strain injury (RSI)

This is the general term for a STRAIN in the tendons, joints, ligaments or muscles, usually caused by repeating the same movement over and over again.

SYMPTOMS
+ Burning, throbbing or aching pain in the joints, forearms, shins or back that comes on gradually – it's rare for the symptoms to develop suddenly.
+ Weakness or stiffness in the area.
+ Tingling or pins and needles.
+ Cramps and/or swelling in the area.

Diagnosis
RSI is an injury, not an illness or condition, and can be self-diagnosed. You can consult a pharmacist or physiotherapist for further advice, and acupuncturists, chiropractors and osteopaths can be very helpful, too.

Who is more likely to develop RSI?
- People whose job means that they repeatedly move in the same way, such as hairdressers, carpenters, builders, etc.
- Those using vibrating power tools for long periods.
- Anyone whose job requires them to stand for long periods, particularly if they have poor posture.
- People who play a lot of sport, particularly tennis and golf. Runners can develop shin splints, which is a form of RSI.
- Those who have returned to a job or activity following a break.

Preventing RSI
- Be aware of your posture and how you stand when you carry out certain tasks.
- Mix up activities as much as possible, whether that's switching between work tasks, playing different sports or varying your training.
- Stretch regularly – you can find helpful NHS videos on YouTube.
- Maintain a healthy weight to avoid putting extra pressure on your joints.

Treatment
- Stay active. Don't rest the affected area for more than 72 hours (24 is often enough) as it will seize up and become more painful.
- Think about how you sleep. For example, if you have RSI in your hands and you sleep with them bunched up under you this will likely make the pain worse.
- Take painkillers such as ibuprofen and paracetamol and use pain-relieving gels on the area.
- Talk to your employer if your RSI is caused by or affecting your work to see what accommodations they can make, or to find out if different equipment is available.

Red flags
See you doctor if any of the following apply:
- You have been treating your injury at home for at least four weeks and following any advice from other health professionals and have seen no improvement.
- Your symptoms have been steadily getting worse.
- Painkillers aren't helping and the pain is stopping you living your life as normal.

Bunions

A bunion is a bony bump on the joint of the big toe where the edges of feet bones have protruded, causing joints to deform and toes overlap. It's the most common foot deformity.

SYMPTOMS
- A hard bump on the big toe joint.
- Red and sore skin where the bunion rubs against a shoe.
- Difficulty walking in more severe cases.

Other foot issues caused by badly fitting shoes

Bunionette: Very similar to a bunion but occurs on the joint of the little toe. The same advice applies as for bunions.

Hammer toe: An abnormal bend in the middle joint of usually the second toe, that can cause pain and rubbing. Devices like toe spacers and strapping can help, as can specific exercises – search for 'foot and toe exercercises' on Versus Arthritis (www.versusarthritis.org).

Plantar fasciitis: Pain in the heel and arch that comes on after resting. Stretch after exercising, make sure your footwear has good arch support and use an ice pack (such as a bag of frozen vegetables wrapped in a tea towel) for flare-ups.

Ingrown toenails: When the toenail – usually on the big toe – grows into the skin, causing pain and swelling. Soak the foot in warm salty water. Don't try to cut the toenail out, and see a doctor if it becomes infected.

Metatarsalgia: Pain and swelling in the ball of the foot. Try not to walk or stand for long periods if you can avoid it. Use soft insoles and try some foot and ankle stretches.

Causes
- Wearing shoes that don't fit properly and squash the feet and/or squeeze the toes.
- Wearing high heels, as they shift more weight onto the toe joint.
- Spending a lot of time on your feet wearing the wrong shoes.

Far more women develop bunions than men, due to wearing high-heels or other styles of shoe that squash the feet and/or put more pressure on the big toe joint. Bunions are more common in older women, but I have seen them on a 15-year-old as a result of wearing stilettos.

Treatment
- Ditch the high heels and make sure you are wearing shoes with a wide enough toe box, and space between the end of the big toe and the shoe.
- Take ibuprofen for the inflammation and soreness.
- Bunion pads (to protect from rubbing on the shoe) and toe splints are available from pharmacies.
- Losing weight if you are overweight or OBESE will relieve pressure on all the joints and lessen pain.
- Bunions can be removed surgically but this is not always effective and the recovery time is long. A bunion would have to be seriously affecting someone's life before surgery is considered.

> **Red flag**
> Foot problems are likely to be more serious if you have DIABETES – check with a pharmacist or your GP.

Fibromyalgia

Fibromyalgia is a long-term chronic inflammatory autoimmune condition. It's not well-understood and often goes unrecognised and undiagnosed. It's caused by inflammation and affects the whole body. It's more common in women and thought to sometimes be linked to ENDOMETRIOSIS.

SYMPTOMS

One of the difficulties with fibromyalgia is that it affects people differently. Not everyone will have all these symptoms, and they can get better and worse at different times.

+ Increased sensitivity to pain that usually comes on gradually.
+ Body pain and HEADACHES.
+ Muscles stiffness.
+ Difficulty sleeping or staying asleep.
+ 'Brain fog' including issues with memory, concentration and confusion.
+ Clumsiness.
+ Digestive issues, such as stomach pain, bloating and/or IRRITABLE BOWEL SYNDROME (IBS).
+ Low mood and/or loss of self-esteem.

Diagnosis

As we don't currently understand what causes fibromyalgia, there is no way to test for it, although two blood tests – called ESR and CRP – can check the levels of inflammation in the body.

Not all healthcare professionals are well-informed about fibromyalgia. The symptoms are often attributed to a MENTAL HEALTH CONDITION, CHRONIC FATIGUE SYNDROME or ARTHRITIS. Sometimes the severity of the brain fog makes people worried they have DEMENTIA. Doctors may carry out tests to rule these things out, however if you have fibromyalgia, blood tests may be painful and repeated trips to the surgery or hospital can be exhausting.

If you have the symptoms listed, keep a detailed diary so you can track how you feel day to day.

Treatment

There's currently no cure for fibromyalgia, but the symptoms, which will be different for everyone, can be managed. It can take trial and error to figure out what works for you, and different treatments can work at different times.

- **Lifestyle changes** such as exercise programmes and relaxation techniques like meditation.
- **Prioritising sleep** through establishing a good sleeping environment (no screens before bed, keep the bedroom cool, etc.).
- **Avoiding stimulants** like nicotine and caffeine and giving up alcohol.
- **Talking therapies** such as cognitive behavioural therapy and acceptance and commitment therapy. Some people find group therapy useful.
- **Low doses of antidepressants** such as amitriptyline/norotryptyline, can help relieve aches and pains related to nerve pain. This is because these two types of medications work on two chemicals – noradrenaline and serotonin – that lower the pain signals to the brain, helping to reduce the level of pain experienced.
- **HRT** can help some symptoms if you are MENOPAUSAL.
- **Acupuncture**, **physiotherapy**, **chiropractic massage** and **physical therapy** may also be beneficial for those who can tolerate them.

Fractures

A fracture is a medical term for a break in the bone.

SYMPTOMS

Fractures are usually caused by experiencing an injury. Someone may have a fracture if:
- A sudden, forceful trauma has been sustained, such as a fall from a height or being hit by something heavy.
- A person can't move after an injury or put any weight on a limb.
- A crack was heard at the time of the injury.
- There is a visible deformity, twist or change in shape to the area.

Different kinds of fractures

A partial fracture is an incomplete break of the bone.
A complete fracture is a break all the way through the bone, causing it to be separated into two or more pieces.
A stable fracture is when the two broken ends of the bone haven't moved out of place.
A displaced fracture is when there is a gap between the broken ends of the bone.
A compound or open fracture is when the broken bone pierces skin. This is serious as it can cause heavy bleeding.

Diagnosis
Fractures are usually diagnosed by X-ray. All suspected fractures should be treated by a medical professional.

Treatment
While you await medical attention:
- If there is bleeding from the wound, apply pressure with a bandage or clean cloth, but do *not* do this over a visible bone or where you think the fracture is.
- If the bleeding is heavy, tie a strip of cloth tightly around the damaged limb, above the wound, as a tourniquet, to reduce blood flow while you await help.
- Keep the person still and support the injured area with a cushion, rolled up clothing or a sling to stop it moving.
- If you suspect a broken back, or a break to a large bone like the thigh or hip, or the bone is visible, don't move the person and call 999 immediately. In these incidences the person should only be moved by paramedics.
- For smaller bones, go to A&E or an urgent treatment centre.
- The injury will swell, so in the case of a broken arm or hand, remove rings and watches as soon as possible.

A bag of frozen vegetables, ice pack or towel soaked in cold water will help relieve the pain and reduce swelling. Fractures will usually take from five weeks to three months to fully repair.

DO always seek medical help for a fracture, as left untreated, they can lead to a deformity in the bone.

DON'T ever try to push bones back together or 'pop' a dislocated joint back into place.

Shock
Sudden injuries like fractures can cause someone to go into shock, which can be life-threatening and cause the circulatory system to fail to provide sufficient oxygenated blood, depriving organs. Signs of shock are:
- Fast, shallow breathing.
- Fast or weak pulse.
- Skin feels cold to the touch, sweaty or clammy.
- Appearance is pale, especially lips and palms.
- Person may seem 'out of it'.

If you suspect someone is in shock:
- Lie them down with raised feet (if no leg injury).
- Use blankets or coats to keep them warm.
- Call 999 and tell the operator you think someone is in shock, and what has happened to them.

Osteomalacia

Osteomalacia means a softening of the bones. In children, this is commonly known as rickets. It means children don't grow properly and can have bone deformities, such as bowed legs. The most common cause is not getting enough vitamin D or calcium, although a rare genetic form of osteomalacia also exists.

SYMPTOMS
+ Slow growth.
+ Fragile bones that are more prone to fractures.
+ Dental problems such as delay in teeth growing or weak tooth enamel.
+ Skeletal deformities such as bowed legs, soft skull bones or thickened wrists, ankles and knees.
+ Pain in the bones.

Diagnosis
Visit your GP if you or a child in your care has these symptoms. They will diagnose by checking your symptoms and conducting an X-ray.

Treatment
Increase vitamin D and calcium levels through dietary choices or supplements – your GP will advise on how much. You should also increase the amount of time spent outside for safe exposure to sunlight.

Causes
In modern times, rickets had become rare in the West. However, in the UK there has been an increase in cases of the condition in those who have low levels of vitamin D. Those more at risk are:
- Children born prematurely.
- Children and adults with black or brown skin, as more sunlight is needed to get enough vitamin D.
- Those who have a diet lacking in calcium and vitamin D, especially as a consequence of living in poverty.

Who should take a vitamin D supplement?

The NHS recommends that the following groups should consider a vitamin D supplement:
- Everyone in the UK over four years old should take 10 micrograms of vitamin D daily from September to April.
- People with black or brown skin should take 10 micrograms of vitamin D daily throughout the year.
- If someone rarely goes outside (e.g. they are housebound) or they completely cover their skin when they do, 10 micrograms of vitamin D should be taken daily throughout the year.
- Babies from birth to one year should be given 8.5 to 10 micrograms of vitamin D daily if they are breastfed all or some of the time (the supplement can be given in a dropper), regardless of whether the breastfeeding parent is taking a vitamin D supplement.
- Children aged one to four (once they are no longer on formula, as this has vitamin D added) should be given 10 micrograms of vitamin D daily throughout the year.

Vitamin D supplements
Taking too much vitamin D – 100 micrograms a day or more – can lead to long-term damage to kidneys, bones and the heart.

The UK government offers free vitamin D supplements for people who need them – such as care home residents, people who are vulnerable due to other health conditions and families experiencing poverty. Speak to an allied health professional or social worker to find out more about this.

Osteoporosis

Osteoporosis is a disease that causes brittle, more-likely-to-break bones. It's more common in women, particularly POST-MENOPAUSE. Most people don't know they have it until they get a FRACTURE in a bone.

SYMPTOMS
+ **Bones fracturing.**
+ **Back pain.**
+ **Stooped posture, from bones gradually breaking or softening in the spine that make it a struggle to support the body.**

Causes
We all lose bone density as we age. This is called osteopenia, which doesn't always lead to osteoporosis, but can be a contributing factor. Other risk factors are:
- Smoking.
- Drinking a lot of alcohol.
- A family history of osteoporosis.
- A history of EATING DISORDERS.
- Long-term use of some medications, particularly steroids.
- CROHN'S DISEASE, HYPERPARATHYROIDISM (in which the body produces too much calcium) and other conditions which impair the digestive system's ability to absorb nutrients from food.
- Periods of inactivity, such as bed rest.

Diagnosis
The best way to diagnose osteoporosis is with a scan that measures the bone density, called a DEXA scan. However, they are not readily available on the NHS. Most people are diagnosed after they FRACTURE a bone unexpectedly, for example through a minor knock or slip, or even cracking a rib while coughing.

Prevention
It's much easier to treat osteopenia before it turns into osteoporosis.
- **Exercise:** As we age, everyone – but particularly women – should do some sort of strength and resistance training, alongside cardio exercise like brisk walking. This is by far the best way to guard against brittle bones as well as accidents like falls which can lead to FRACTURES.
- **Diet:** We all need enough calcium in our diets at every age, as well as vitamin D that helps our bodies to absorb it (see page 30). Adults need at least 700mg calcium per day, as part of a balanced diet.
- **Smoking and alcohol:** Quit smoking and limit alcohol intake, as both are associated with a loss of bone density.

Treatment
While there is no cure for osteoporosis, its symptoms can be managed via lifestyle changes such as exercise, and sometimes with drugs. Some medications that might be prescribed include:
- **Bisphosphonates:** These may be prescribed for six months or a year to build back bone density. They have to be taken on an empty stomach and can irritate the oesophagus.
- **Teriparatide:** Given to people who are at high risk of FRACTURES due to osteoporosis as a self-administered daily injection to stimulate the cells that build bones.

Osteoporosis & menopause

MENOPAUSAL and POST-MENOPAUSAL women are at the highest risk of osteoporosis due to a continual decrease in oestrogen. Hormone replacement therapy (HRT) can help to slow this down by supplementing oestrogen. There can be BREAST CANCER or THROMBOSIS or EMBOLISM risk factors associated with HRT for certain groups, although these are becoming better understood in medicine. But the benefits of HRT in terms of strengthening bones – even in those who already have osteoporosis, as well as those who are PERIMENOPAUSAL and want to future-proof their bones – are worth taking into consideration and discussing with your doctor when deciding whether to go down this route.

Muscle loss (sarcopenia) roughly starts in your 30s, and bone loss begins gradually in most people by their late-30s. Looking ahead to PERIMENOPAUSE, there is a lot you can do to slow the decline in bone density that comes with age; the best thing is weight-bearing and resistance exercise. You should do these at least twice a week, ensuring you work your full body (so the legs and lower muscles, hips, abdomen, chest, shoulders and arms). Your lower body should support all your own weight during weight-bearing exercise, so this can include aerobics or dancing and running. Swimming and cycling, while useful aerobic exercises, are not weight-bearing because the water or bicycle helps to support you. Resistance exercises, such as weightlifting or bodyweight exercises, improve muscle and bone strength. Ensure you are using correct form and consult with a fitness instructor or use reliable online videos for beginners to complete them correctly. As with any exercise plan, experiment to find something you enjoy as then you'll be more likely to stick to it. In addition, maintaining a healthy weight, good nutrition, not smoking and reducing alcohol intake will all reduce your chances of osteoporosis. See pages 8–10 for more details.

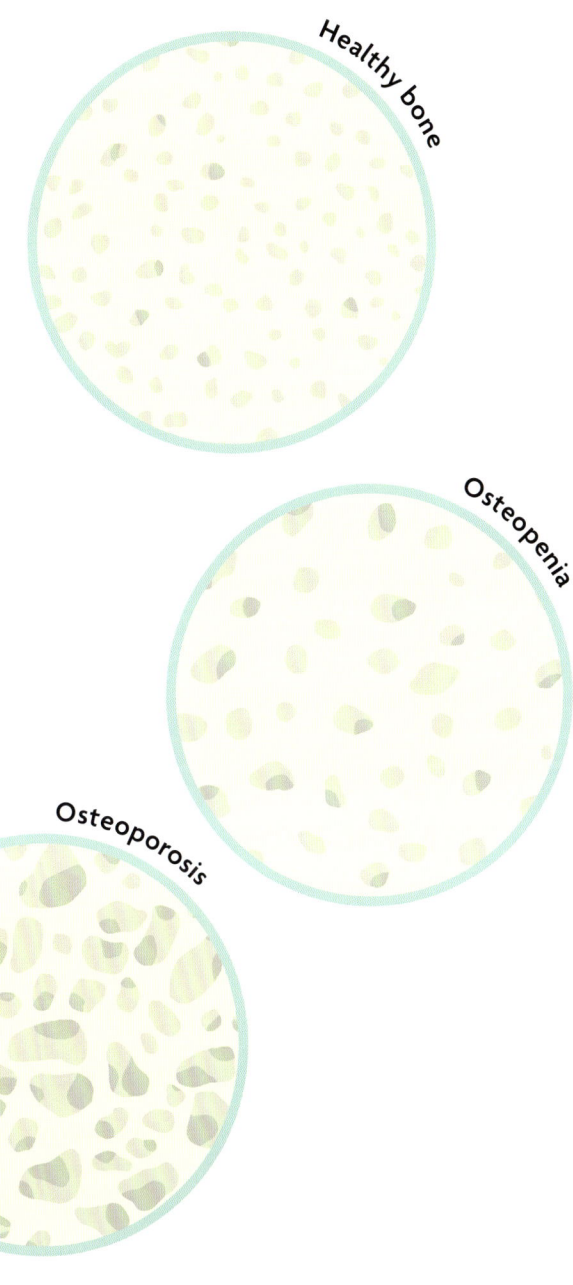

Arthritis

Arthritis is the inflammation of joints, causing pain and stiffness. It is more common in women and older people but can affect anyone at any age.

Two main types of arthritis

Osteoarthritis

Osteoarthritis occurs when the cartilage in the joint breaks down and two bones begin to grate together. This can cause changes in the bone and deterioration of the connective tissue that attaches muscle to bone and holds the joint together. This is the most common form of arthritis and the pain and stiffness it causes will usually worsen throughout the day. It may only affect one joint. Sometimes, an osteophyte – a bit of extra bone – is formed as bones try to renew themselves.

Rheumatoid arthritis

Unlike osteoarthritis, rheumatoid arthritis is an autoimmune condition and is characterised by joint pain and stiffness that is worse upon waking but improves with movement throughout the day. The immune system attacks a membrane inside the joint that helps it to move properly. The inflammation and swelling this causes can eventually destroy the cartilage and the bone within the joint. It often effects more than one joint and can run in families.

SYMPTOMS

+ Joint pain.
+ Inflammation (for rheumatoid arthritis only).
+ Stiffness.

Diagnosis

A physical examination to check the joints for swelling, redness, tenderness and warmth is usually carried out by your doctor alongside a conversation to establish medical history and understand symptoms. Sometimes an X-ray or a CT scan will be carried out to check the condition of the joint. A rheumatoid factor or HLA-B27 blood test will also be conducted if rheumatoid arthritis is suspected.

Living with arthritis can be exhausting, but finding positions for good sex is important for your overall health, so don't be embarrassed to seek advice.

Prevention & treatment

	Osteoarthritis	Rheumatoid arthritis
Prevention	**Maintain a healthy weight:** Being overweight or OBESE puts a lot of pressure on the joints. Building up the muscle around joints strengthens them and improves overall stability so they are less susceptible to damage.	**Eat a balanced diet:** Include plenty of fruit and vegetables to help to lower inflammation in the body and maintain good gut health. **Exercise regularly:** Exercise helps to maintain a healthy weight and strong, flexible joints.
At-home treatments	**Exercise:** A low-impact exercise that you can do regularly — such as swimming or yoga — will strength the muscles around the joint and improve blood flow. It's a myth that exercise 'damages' joints (although, of course, sports injuries can). **Paracetamol and over-the-counter anti-inflammatories (NSAIDs):** These are available as tablets or gels which can be rubbed into the joint and can often be used by people who can't take ibuprofen orally (check with your doctor or pharmacist if you are unsure). **Wearing a splint:** A splint on the affected joint(s) can support it by improving stability, particularly when resting. However, it's important to still move the joint as much as you are able. **Hot and cold packs**: Use cold packs if you are having a flare-up, to reduce swelling. Many people find alternating between hot and cold works for general pain management. **A capsaicin-based cream:** This can be massaged into the joint (some tiger balms contain this natural ingredient).	
Medical treatments	**Corticosteroid injections:** These will help with pain during a flare-up. However, they can cause weight gain, thinning of the bones and are linked to an increased risk of DIABETES, so they are very much a short-term treatment. **Sometimes removing fluid from around the joint with a syringe:** This can reduce swelling and pain.	**Removing fluid from around the joint with a syringe:** This can reduce swelling and pain, due to the more pronounced inflammatory response and fluid accumulation with the condition. **Disease-modifying anti-rheumatic drugs (DMARDs)**: For example, methotrexate — these will slow down damage to the joints caused by inflammation.

Gout

Gout is the sudden swelling of and severe pain in a joint. There's an old-fashioned myth that only older, wealthy people develop gout as it was believed to be associated with rich, meat-heavy diets, but this isn't true. It's caused by tiny urate crystals forming in the blood and becoming stuck in joints, causing inflammation and pain.

SYMPTOMS
- A very bad pain in the big toe joint, and/or ankles, feet, wrists, fingers or knees (some people can't even bear to have a duvet resting on the joint).
- Swollen joints.
- The skin over the joint is hot and shiny and may look red on those with paler skin.

Causes
There's no one cause for what we call 'primary gout', although secondary gout is often a result of KIDNEY DISEASE or taking certain medications, such as diuretics (also known as 'water pills') and BLOOD PRESSURE medication. Risk factors include:
- Genetics – having a family history of gout.
- Being overweight or OBESE.
- Gender, as men are four times more likely to develop gout than women.

Triggers
Triggers that can bring on an episode of gout are:
- Alcohol, as it can cause chemical compounds known as purines to accumulate in the body.
- A knock or injury to the joint.
- A FEVER.
- Eating an unusually large meal containing lots of red meat, which is high in purines that the body breaks down into uric acid. Elevated uric acid levels can lead to the formation of urate crystals in the joints. Note that diet is thought to be a trigger rather than a cause of gout.

Note that if you experience an episode of gout, you can expect another, usually within a year.

Diagnosis
See your GP if this is the first time you are experiencing symptoms of gout. Your doctor will usually diagnose gout by examining the joint. They may recommend a blood test to check kidney function and if they suspect that the symptoms may be caused by another condition, such as OSTEOARTHRITIS, you may be sent for an X-ray.

Treatment
- The first treatment is anti-inflammatories, although they may interact with other medications – check with your GP or pharmacist if you are unsure.
- A doctor can prescribe colchicine tablets, steroid tablets or steroid injections for severe cases.
- Keeping the joint cool with an ice pack can help with pain and swelling.
- If gout is left untreated, it can cause joint damage so treatment should be sought and applied.

Prevention
To prevent further attacks, it's important to maintain a healthy weight, keep CHOLESTEROL low, eat well, avoid too much red meat or strong cheese, stay hydrated and cut out alcohol. If you have more than two attacks per year, you could be placed on the long-term prophylactic medicine allopurinol.

> Genetic

Ankylosing spondylitis

Ankylosing spondylitis is a chronic autoimmune condition, thought to be genetic, that causes inflammation in the joints and ligaments of the spine and its neighbouring joints. It usually begins when people are in their teens or twenties and is a lifelong condition. Many people have a mild version, but in rare cases it can lead to the bones of the spine fusing together and causing disability.

SYMPTOMS

Most symptoms develop gradually and may come and go.

- Ongoing BACK PAIN, particularly in the early morning, that improves with movement.
- Stiffness in the back, and sometimes neck and ribcage, which restricts movement.
- Pain and swelling in other joints.
- Pain in the buttocks and back of the thighs.
- FATIGUE.
- Changes to the curvature of the spine.
- Inflammation in the eye.

Diagnosis

It's important to speak to your GP if you or your child are experiencing symptoms of ankylosing spondylitis, particularly as it's associated with other health conditions including IRRITABLE BOWEL SYNDROME (IBS) and ANAEMIA.

People with ankylosing spondylitis are more likely to suffer FRACTURES and go on to develop OSTEOPOROSIS. Diagnosis isn't straightforward and may include:

- An X-ray or MRI to pick-up inflammation and damage to the spine.
- A blood test to show inflammation (although there can be lots of reasons for inflammation).
- A genetic test to determine if someone has the gene variant – although not everyone who does will develop ankylosing spondylitis, and not everyone who has the condition has the gene variant.

Treatment

While there is no cure for ankylosing spondylitis, treatments to manage the symptoms include:

- Exercises and physiotherapy.
- Ensuring you get enough good-quality sleep, e.g. avoiding caffeine and screens before bed.
- Wearing the right footwear, paying attention to posture and generally making sure the back and other joints are supported.
- Taking or applying anti-inflammatories.
- Anti-TNF drugs, which work by targeting the substance in your body that causes inflammation.
- Steroids can treat the pain caused by flare-up in the short term.
- In extreme cases, surgery may be required.

THE SKIN

Your skin is your largest organ. It's made up of three layers: the epidermis on the outside, the dermis in the middle, then the subcutis underneath. Our skin is one of the main lines of defence that stops bugs getting into our bodies.

Lots of bacteria and fungi live harmlessly on our skin all the time and some are even helpful – so while it's important to keep ourselves clean and particularly to wash our hands regularly to avoid microbes and viruses making us ill, it's not usually necessary to use harsh cleansers or to scrub the skin.

As our largest organ, when we are not in the best of health – tired and run down, with poor gut health, or with an underlying condition – it often shows on our skin. If we are dehydrated our skin will become dry. It is also susceptible to the elements. Many people find that central heating dries out their skin in the winter and some of us get heat rash in the summer.

The majority of conditions that affect the outside layers of our skin are harmless, although they can be unpleasant and not feel great if they are visible. If you have a condition like DIABETES or EHLERS-DANLOS SYNDROMES, for example, you might find that scrapes and cuts take longer to heal. But for the most part, skin has an impressive ability to mend itself.

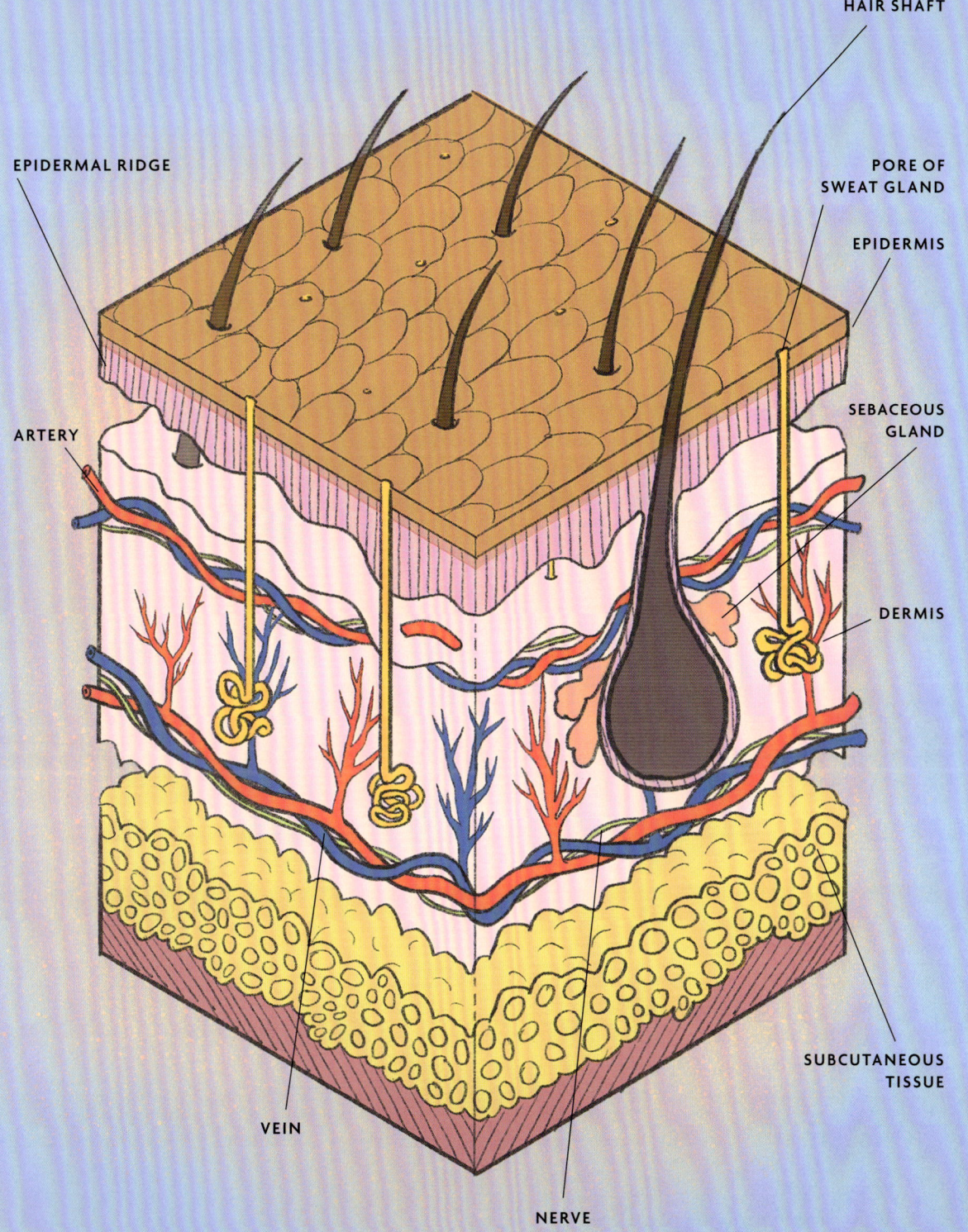

🟢 Non-contagious

Eczema

Eczema, causing itchy skin, is a lifelong condition which varies in severity over time. Some may experience improvement or outgrow it, but for many it remains a chronic condition with periods of flare-up and remission. There is no cure for eczema and it can be hereditary.

SYMPTOMS
- Dry, itchy patches of skin that may appear darker or lighter than your skin tone.
- May occur behind the knees, on the inside of the arms or anywhere there are creases or folds in the skin.
- It's so tempting to scratch, but this releases histamines, which makes you want to scratch even more, creating that horrible itch-scratch cycle. It then dries out and damages the skin further.
- Deep scratching can cause bleeding, inflammation, hardness of the skin, scarring and infection.

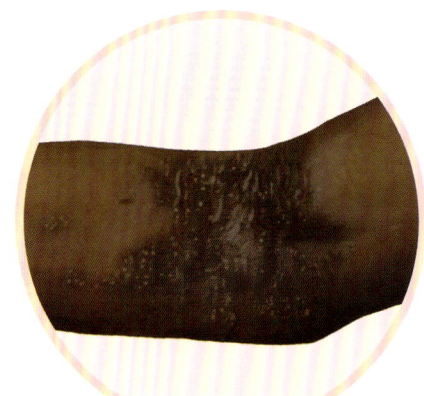

Diagnosis

Consult a GP if you think you or your child has eczema. A pharmacist can be your first port of call for mild cases. Also see a GP if over-the-counter treatments are not helping. Eczema can run in families and can be confused with PSORIASIS.

Treatment

Eczema cannot be cured but it's important to manage it before it causes scarring or infection. Treat early, rather than waiting until it increases in severity.

- Potential triggers should be investigated first. These can be allergies, for example to pollen, cigarette smoke or something in the diet. Stress can be a factor. Keep notes on what you are eating and doing to identify the triggers.
- Gut inflammation can trigger eczema: see page 76 for more on inflammation.

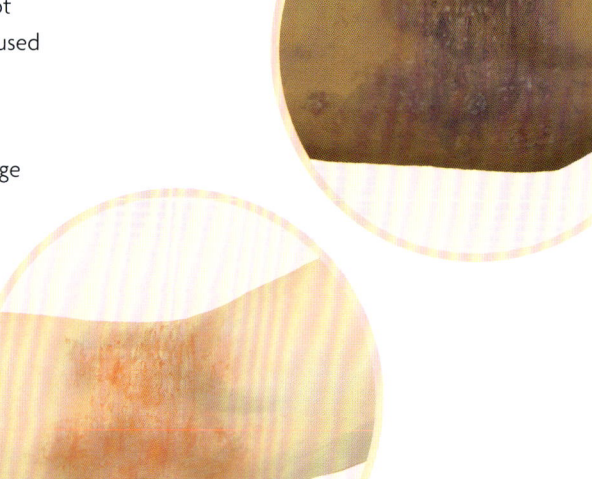

- Emollients are the mainstay of any treatment. Moisturise the affected area a few times a day and use emollient bath products, too.
- Over-the-counter antihistamines work well if the eczema is related to allergies – speak to a pharmacist for advice. Just bear in mind that they can make you sleepy, so these medications should be taken at night.
- Antibiotics can be prescribed if the eczema becomes infected – if it is constantly opening-up, oozing, weeping or forming crusts.
- Steroid treatments may be prescribed by a GP for more serious flare-ups, and it's better to start steroids as early as possible. There's a myth that steroids stop you building up immunity, but that's not the case with eczema treatments. They are a good way of giving you relief and stopping that itch-scratch cycle.
- A dermatologist referral may be necessary for severe, chronic eczema.

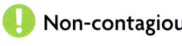 Non-contagious

Acne

This skin condition occurs in different places on the body when the hair follicles become plugged with oil and dead skin, causing whiteheads, blackheads and pimples. It's very common, but the fact that a lot of people come to me with it shows how upsetting it can be to suffer with acne. Acne is associated with the teenage years, but it affects many people of different ages. There's a myth that people who suffer with acne don't wash often enough or look after their skin properly, but this is completely untrue. Blackheads are black because the sebum on the skin's surface oxidises, producing pigmentation. Spots are not filled with dirt. There's no evidence that diet or sexual activity plays a role in acne, either.

SYMPTOMS

Acne can take many different forms:
+ Blackheads are small black or yellow spots.
+ Whiteheads are exactly the same as blackheads, but they may be firmer and won't empty when squeezed.
+ Pustules are small red bumps which may feel tender or sore.
+ Papules are like pustules but have a white tip in the centre caused by a build-up of pus.
+ Nodules are small hard lumps that build up beneath the surface of the skin and can be painful.
+ Cysts are pus-filled spots and lumps that look similar to boils. They carry the greater risk of permanent scarring.

Causes
The main causes are genetic factors, stress and hormones (particularly in girls and women).

Treatment
Although acne can't be cured, there are lots of different treatments to try that may improve the situation.

At-home treatments
- Try not to wash the affected area more than twice a day as this can irritate the skin and make the acne worse. Use products designed for acne-prone skin, as these will contain non-comedogenic (non-pore blocking) ingredients.
- Don't squeeze or pop blackheads or spots, and especially don't use a needle as this can cause infection and permanent scarring.
- Avoid applying excess makeup, as this can worsen the breakout by trapping bacteria and oils under the makeup, therefore further clogging pores and irritating inflamed skin. Always make sure you take off all makeup before bed.
- If the skin is also dry, use fragrance-free or water-based emollient.
- Steaming the skin over a bowl of hot water or in a hot bath or shower can help, particularly for those with oily or acne-prone skin. It helps to loosen and release trapped sebum, dirt and dead skin cells that clog pores and contribute to acne breakouts. Use steam cautiously however, as overheating or steaming for too long can dry out the skin, causing irritation. Other skin conditions, such as rosacea, can be aggravated by steaming.
- Exercise can help, although be aware that sweat can irritate acne, so wear loose-fitting clothing made of natural fibres if you have acne on the body.
- Wash your hair regularly, especially if you have acne around the hairline, so that dirt or excess oil doesn't transfer from your hair to your face.
- Try to notice if anything triggers your acne so you can avoid them – keeping a diary of flare-ups will help with this.
- Do a little research to figure out what sort of skin you have (dry, oily, normal, combination or sensitive). This will help you choose from the wide range of over-the-counter creams, lotions and gels.
- Salicylic and azelaic acids can help dissolve build-ups of oil and dead skin in the hair follicle.

Medical treatments
- If the cause of acne is thought to be bacteria on the skin, a GP might prescribe an antibiotic cream such as Clindamycin or another cream with a mixture of a steroid and antibiotics.
- The combined contraceptive pill or hormonal coil (such as the Mirena coil) will regulate periods and is an option for women whose acne is affected by their hormones.
- Hormonal, cystic acne in women from their 20s onwards can be treated with Spironolactone.
- Topical retinoids reduce inflammation and help deal with bacteria. They make your skin more sensitive to sunlight so should only be used at night, and you should wear SPF 50 during the day if you are using them.
- Isotretinoin (known as the brand name Roaccutane in the UK) is a strong drug that can be prescribed by a dermatologist when acne is severe and causing scarring. It has potential side effects, such as dry skin and HEADACHES and, less commonly, mood changes and frequent infections, so its use should be considered carefully. It is important not to use this if you are PREGNANT or could get pregnant because it can affect the foetus, so you must use CONTRACEPTION alongside it. This should also be avoided if you have LIVER DISEASE.

Acne or rosacea?
Rosacea is sometimes confused with acne as it can look like a rash and involve small pimples. The skin will look red and might feel hot. Rosacea is generally concentrated in the centre of the face, in a butterfly shape, and has triggers including alcohol, spicy food, sunlight and caffeine. It's rare in young people and more common in those over 30.

🟢 Non-contagious

Psoriasis

Psoriasis is a common autoimmune condition, which means the immune system attacks its own cells, and flare-ups may be triggered by stress or illness. People who have other autoimmune conditions, such as IRRITABLE BOWEL SYNDROME or RHEUMATOID ARTHRITIS, are more likely to suffer from psoriasis.

SYMPTOMS

- Itchy, inflamed and sore patches, commonly on elbows, knees, the scalp or the back of the neck. Unlike eczema, these do not usually appear in the skin's creases.
- Patches may appear silvery and raised, and are known as plaques.
- Psoriasis on the scalp can easily be mistaken for dandruff and in extreme cases can cause hair loss.
- Nails and toenails can become pitted and crumbly.
- Sunlight exposure in the summer may cause flare-ups, meaning it can be mistaken for sunburn on some skintones.

Diagnosis

Psoriasis is usually diagnosed by a doctor examining the skin. If they are uncertain, a skin biopsy may be performed. A medical professional may use a questionnaire to determine how serious the psoriasis is, taking into consideration how much the symptoms are affecting the person, as well as other health conditions, such as HIGH BLOOD PRESSURE or DIABETES.

Treatment

Psoriasis can't be prevented or cured but there are various treatments that will help to manage it.

- Non-greasy emollient creams are the first line of treatment.
- Coal tar-based ointments and over-the-counter shampoos can be used if the scalp is affected.
- For more serious flare-ups, steroids may be prescribed or a GP may refer you to a dermatologist.

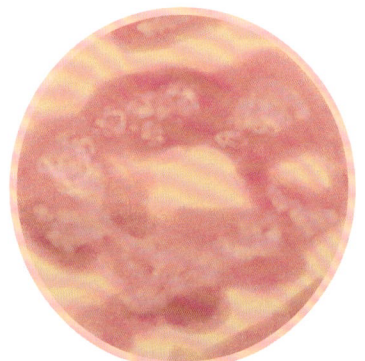
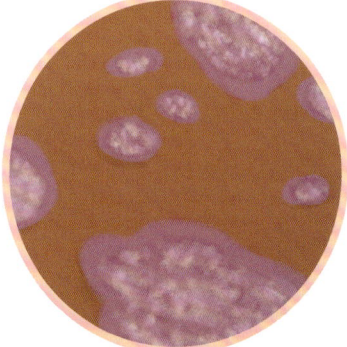
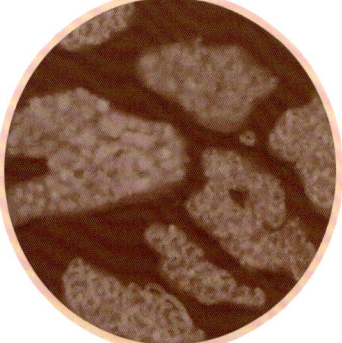

🟢 **Non-contagious**

Hives (urticaria)

Hives (urticaria) are raised bumps with a smooth surface. Hives can look dramatic, but they are not usually dangerous, unless they occur in the throat and restrict breathing. They can get worse during PERIMENOPAUSE.

SYMPTOMS

+ Hives can be different shapes and sizes, sometimes merging together.
+ They may be red on someone with white skin but harder to see on black or brown skin.
+ They happen as a result of your immune system responding to something it thinks is a threat. This might be:
  - An allergy to food, detergents or medicine.
  - Insect bites.
  - Exposure to heat or cold weather.
  - Pressure on the skin, rubbing or scratching.
+ They may last a few hours or be a longer-term issue.

Diagnosis

If you roll a glass over a patch of hives they should disappear, and they shouldn't be accompanied by a FEVER. If this is not the case, it could indicate another condition. A pharmacist can recommend a treatment for hives, and they are usually very short-lived – the majority will disappear within 24 hours. Hives that stay for more than six weeks are considered chronic hives, which can last months or even years.

Treatment

- Antihistamines to relax the immune system.
- A topical cream to stop the itching.
- Sometimes steroid creams might be prescribed if the hives persist.

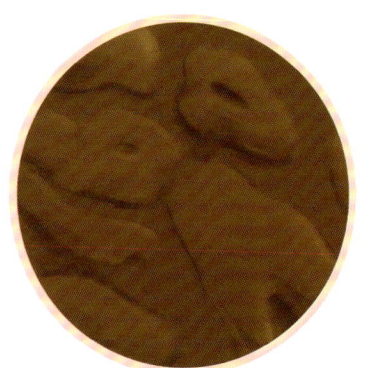
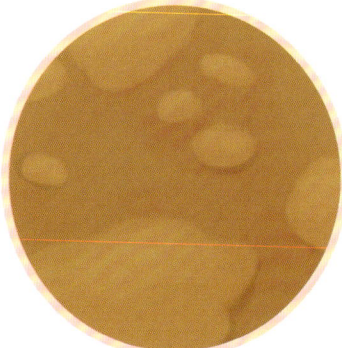
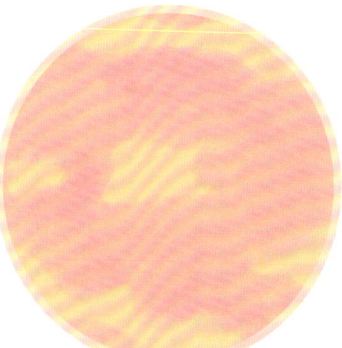

⚠️ Contagious

Viral skin infections

Viral skin infections are caused by various viruses that manifest on the skin, often as rashes. These can be localised or systemic and may be contagious depending on the causing virus.

Chickenpox

Chickenpox is a highly contagious viral skin infection. It's spread by coughing and sneezing, by direct contact and through the fluid from the poxes, or spots. If someone has been in contact with someone who has had chickenpox, they should avoid immunocompromised people and PREGNANT women. Chickenpox is very common in children under 10; adults who did not have it in childhood are susceptible, too. Vaccination is now available as part of the NHS childhood vaccination programme.

SYMPTOMS

+ Short-term FEVER.
+ Aches and pains.
+ Itchy spots all over the body that become a blistering rash.
+ Note that it takes about 10 to 21 days for the chickenpox infection to become obvious. It is infectious during this time and until all of the spots have formed scabs.

Diagnosis

If you're unsure whether it's chickenpox, speak to a doctor. If you are taking your child to a surgery, let the receptionist know they have (suspected) chickenpox before you arrive.

Treatment

- Calamine lotion applied regularly, and antihistamines, can ease the itching.
- Try to minimise scratching to avoid infection and scarring.
- Paracetamol can help with any aches and pains.
- Avoid ibuprofen or NSAIDs (non-steroidal anti-inflammatory drugs) as they increase the risk of complications. Don't use aspirin, as taking it to treat chickenpox is associated with a rare but serious brain condition called Reye's syndrome.

Shingles

Shingles is a viral infection caused by a reactivated chickenpox virus. It manifests as a blotchy rash on one side of the face. Seek help from a pharmacist if you suspect shingles, or from your GP or 111 for those under 18, pregnant or immunocompromised.

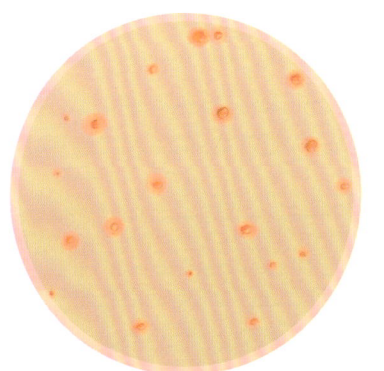
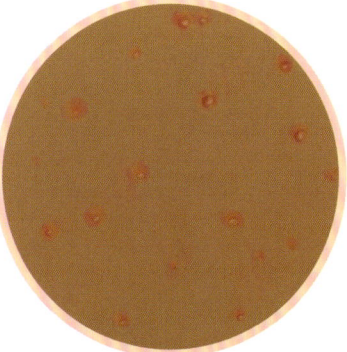
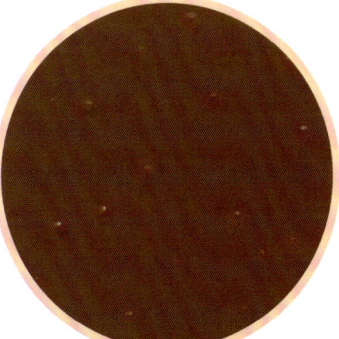

⚠️ Contagious

Bacterial skin infections

Anything that compromises the skin barrier can cause an infection – a wound, persistent scratching, an insect bite. Staphylococcus and streptococcal bacteria are the two main culprits. Skin infections can also be caused by an infection in another part of the body spreading to the skin. Children under five and adults over 65 are particularly vulnerable to skin infections, as well as anyone who is immunocompromised, such as those having treatment for cancer, who have HIV, or who have had an organ transplant. Visit a GP if any skin infection lasts more than two weeks without improving.

Common bacterial skin infections

Condition	Symptoms	Treatment
Boils	A hard, raised bump that fills with pus.	Most boils will go away on their own. Ensure you wash towels and bedding regularly at a high temperature, avoid the swimming pool or gym and don't share towels. A warm, damp cloth can ease symptoms and, if pus leaks out, clean the area with antibacterial soap.
Cellulitis	Darker and swollen patches of skin appear, often on the feet and legs. The patches feel hot and sore, and may blister. Cellulitis can spread quickly and needs fast medical attention to avoid more severe symptoms such as FEVER and dizziness.	Visit your GP on first symptoms as you will need antibiotics, then contact them again if symptoms do not improve after two to three days of antibiotics. Regularly moving the area, raising it on a pillow, and taking paracetamol or ibuprofen can help to ease symptoms.
Impetigo	Superficial reddish sores with a yellow crust. Impetigo is common in children and very infectious, although very rarely serious.	Impetigo often goes away on its own. To avoid infecting others, it's very important to keep skin, nails, clothes and bedding clean.

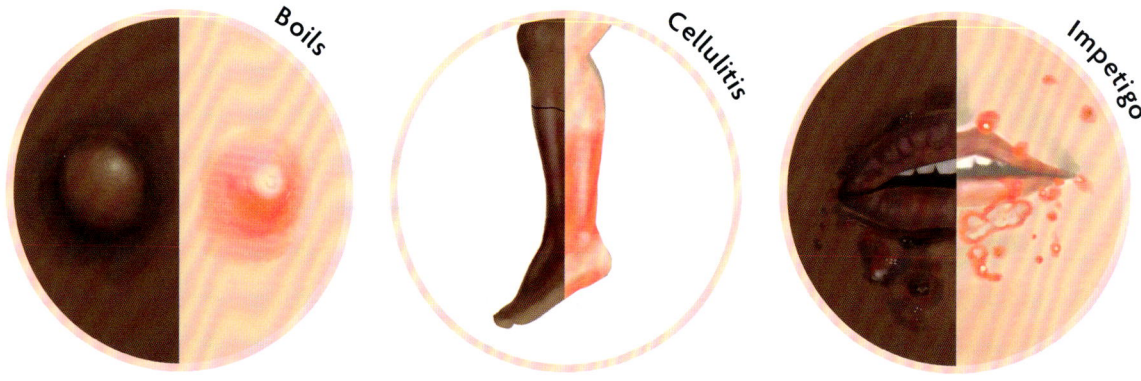

Boils · Cellulitis · Impetigo

Condition	Symptoms	Treatment
Folliculitis	Small, raised, sometimes itchy bumps on the skin that can occur anywhere there is hair – often on thighs, arms and buttocks – as they are caused by bacteria getting into the hair follicles and causing inflammation.	Folliculitis usually resolves within 10 days but visit your GP if the area becomes very painful, hot or swollen. A warm compress can ease symptoms and it's important to regularly clean the area with soap and water.
Paronychia	An inflamed red bump that may have pus, below or next to the fingernail or toenail. It's common if you're a nail biter and in children who suck their thumbs, and also in people who have their hands in water a lot for work.	Mild cases will go away on their own, or try soaking in warm salty water four times a day for several days. If symptoms persist, seek pharmacist advice.
Infected bites	If you have an allergic reaction to a bite (see HIVES), scratching the area can introduce bacteria and cause a further infection. The skin around the bite may feel hot, be swollen or leak pus or fluid. Take precautions to avoid bites by using repellent and keeping your skin covered. If you do get bitten, an antihistamine cream can reduce itching.	Pharmacists can advise on treatments for infected bites. These may include antihistamine and steroid creams or antibiotics.

Red flag

Always seek medical advice if you have a skin infection accompanied by a FEVER. This can be a sign of SEPSIS, which is very serious.

Avoiding infection

It's so important to keep all cuts and grazes clean and covered as this really helps prevent infections. 'Letting the air get to it' is a myth – wounds heal better when kept slightly moist.

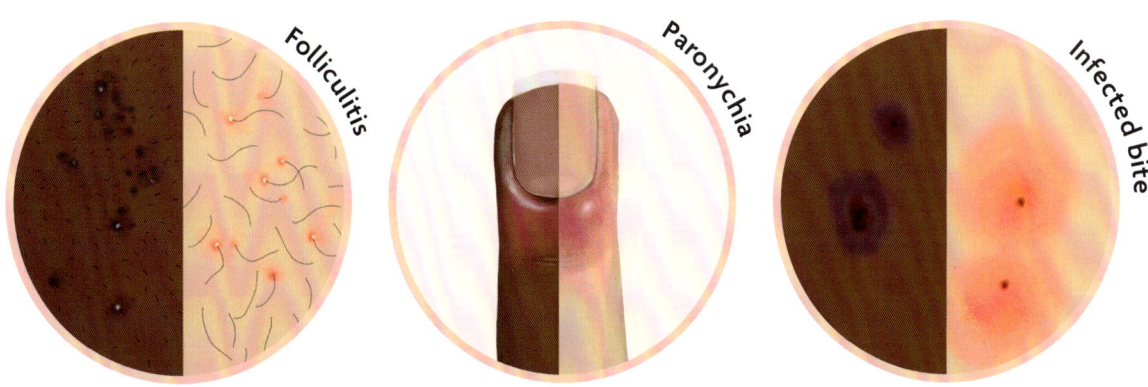

Folliculitis

Paronychia

Infected bite

⚠️ **Contagious**

Fungal skin conditions

This could sound a little off-putting, but fungi are very much a part of our body's make-up – we were born with fungi and we will die with fungi. Fungal infections might look unpleasant but, unless you are suffering from other health problems, they aren't usually serious and most only affect the outer layer of skin, although they are infectious and can spread to other parts of the body and to other people.

The most common type is caused by the yeast Candida. It feeds on the sugars on our skin and likes moist, damp conditions. When our natural balance of bacteria is out of sync, Candida can flourish and become a problem (for example, if you have been taking antibiotics). Candida can be found:

- In armpits and groins.
- Around the genitals.
- Between fingers and on nails.
- In the crease underneath breasts.
- In the mouth.

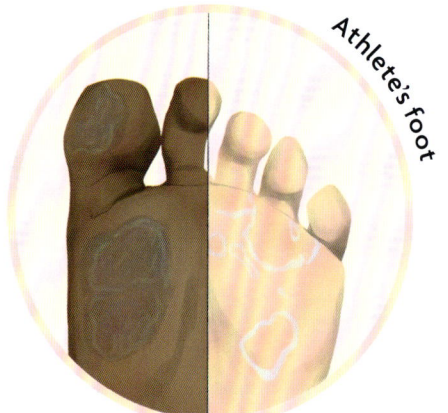

Athlete's foot

Treatment & prevention

Depending on the type of infection, here's how to keep it in check and stop it spreading to others:

- Keep the affected skin clean and dry. Wash between the creases and the toes, dry well, using a hairdryer if necessary.
- Don't share towels or bathing suits.
- Wash bathmats, towels and bedsheets at 60°C (140°F).
- Don't wear clothing that is not breathable for long periods.
- If someone you live with has a fungal infection, particularly athlete's foot, carefully clean the shower and bathroom and wash floors where they walk barefoot.
- Avoid transferring fungi from public spaces like swimming baths and saunas. Aqua socks are good to use.
- Wear open-toed sandals where possible in hot weather.
- Use a cream containing the antifungal ingredient Clotrimazole.

There are lots of over-the-counter powders and creams available to treat fungal/yeast infections, but prevention and early intervention is best. Ideally, we don't want to use antifungals too often as the fungi develop resistance.

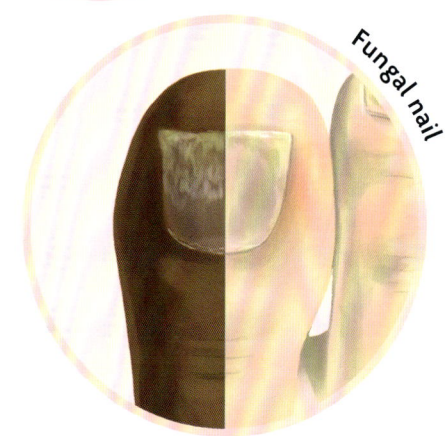

Fungal nail

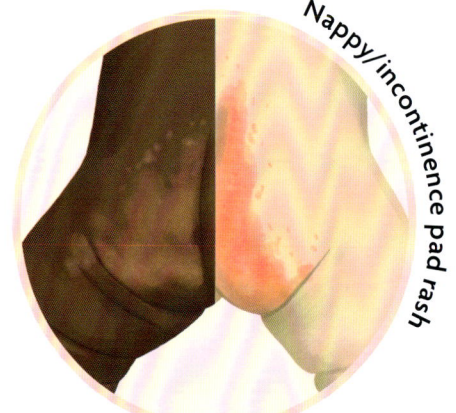

Nappy/incontinence pad rash

Common fungal infections

Condition	Symptoms	Treatment
Athlete's foot	Itchy patches and sometimes small blisters between toes and/or scaly patches on the sides or sole of the foot. Can be confused with ECZEMA.	Keep the feet clean and dry and avoid sweaty footwear. Use over-the-counter antifungal creams and powders if that doesn't help.
Fungal nail	Yellow, white or brownish patches on the nail, which might become brittle and flaky or pitted. Common in older people and diabetics.	Keep the feet clean and dry or try over-the-counter treatments like nail paints (which will take effect when the new nail grows through). For serious or persistent cases, a GP may prescribe antifungal tablets. In rare cases, nail changes can indicate SKIN CANCER.
Nappy/ incontinence pad rash	Angry, sore rash, sometimes scaly, around the bottom and genitals, where the skin has been in contact with a wet nappy/incontinence pad.	Keep the area clean and dry, as the yeast feeds on the poo and pee on the skin. Use a barrier cream to soothe and protect the area.
Oral thrush	Reddened, sore skin inside the mouth with white patches that peel. Can be sore and cause an unpleasant taste. (See page 230 for vaginal THRUSH.)	Practise good oral hygiene. Over-14s can use warm salty water as a mouthwash. Always remove dentures at night and clean them well. Sterilise baby bottles, breast pumps and dummies. See a GP if it doesn't clear up.
Ringworm	A round-shaped, often itchy rash with a paler area and maybe bumps in the middle. It can affect any part of the body, including the scalp and nails, and is more common in hot, humid weather. (Don't worry, it's not actually a worm!)	A pharmacist will recommend an antifungal cream or gel. Keep the area clean and dry and wear loose-fitting clothing. It's important to keep applying the treatment for at least a week after it has gone to avoid it coming back. Occasionally, for very persistent cases, you might need to take antifungal medication.

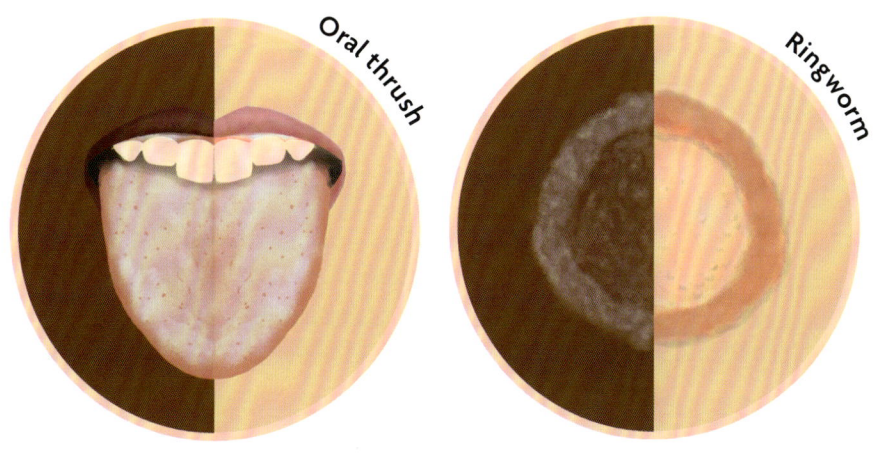

Oral thrush

Ringworm

🟢 Non-contagious

Skin cancer

Skin cancer is an out-of-control growth of abnormal cells in the dermis – the outer layer of the skin. A lesion or a growth can sometimes grow quite slowly over time, making it more difficult to notice, but it can also grow very rapidly. Not all unusual growths are cancerous. Some are benign – harmless, in other words – although they should always be checked by a doctor. Skin cancer can be relatively easy to treat and completely curable if caught early, so it's important to stay vigilant.

Basal cell carcinoma

This is the most common type of skin cancer. It spreads slowly and is rarely fatal when caught early.

Appearance
A pinkish or transparent patch on white skin and a darker, glossy patch on black skin, with pearly edges and a dip in the middle. Often appears on areas that see the sun the most, such as the head or neck.

Treatment
Cryotherapy (freezing), photodynamic therapy (using light), surgery and sometimes radiotherapy.

Squamous cell carcinoma

The second most common type of skin cancer is usually caused by too much UV light. It can be treated relatively easily and completely cured if caught early, though if left too long it can spread and become disfiguring.

Appearance
Can appear as a wound that won't heal, or as a thick, rough, scaly patch that's crusty and may bleed. Can also resemble warts.

Treatment
Depending on how far it has progressed and where it is, the cancer can be removed by cryotherapy (freezing), photodynamic therapy (using light), laser surgery or radiation.

How to check your skin

A lesion will look very different from any other part of your skin. I recommend that you do a head-to-toe check once a month on yourself and your children. Use this simple guide, known as the 'ABCDE' criteria, to help you know what to look for. Consult your GP if the answer is yes to any of the following:

A = asymmetry: Do any of the moles look different on one side to another?
B = border: Are the edges of a mole or pigmentation spot blurred, uneven or red?
C = colour: Most moles will be the same colour all over. Do any contain different colours?
D = diameter: Are any moles larger than 6mm (¼in)?
E = evolving: This is very important. Have any moles changed shape, colour or texture? Have they started to itch or bleed?

Photograph moles and pigmentation spots; it's often hard to notice changes from month to month otherwise. You can then zoom in to get a better look. Photos will be useful for the GP if anything changes in the future and you need to get it checked. You can also use your phone to video your body, to help you see bits of you that are difficult to photograph.

When doing a self-exam, ensure you:
- Remove nail varnish and check nail beds as cancer can form there, too.
- Remove all makeup.
- Check your scalp, feeling all over with your hair loose. Get someone else to look at the bits you can't see.

Melanoma

A more serious form of skin cancer that can spread to other areas of the body. It can be fatal if diagnosed late.

Appearance
A mole that has become a melanoma looks asymmetrical with an uneven border. It can have different colours on any skin type – brown, tan, black, red, pink, blue or white. It will often grow quite quickly and can bleed easily.

Treatment
Depending on location and how advanced the cancer is, the cancer will be cut out and sometimes followed by radiotherapy and/or chemotherapy.

Merkel cell carcinoma

This rare but very aggressive skin cancer often but not always appears on sun-exposed areas of the body and is less distinctive than other skin cancers.

Appearance
Tumours appear as a pearly pimple-like bump, sometimes skin-coloured or red, purplish or blue. The bumps are not usually sore so may go unnoticed at first, but they grow and change appearance quickly.

Treatment
Serious but treatable, usually with radiotherapy, immunotherapy or chemotherapy. This cancer has a high risk of returning so needs to be monitored.

Actinic keratosis

This is a pre-cancerous condition that I see frequently. It is caused by abnormal cells that are linked to an increased risk of developing cancer but that are not themselves cancerous.

Appearance
Small, dry, scaly or crusty patches of the skin. May be skin-coloured or light or dark tan, or a combination of colours. Because of their rough texture, actinic keratosis patches can be easier to feel than see, particularly in places such as on the scalp. They are caused by exposure to UV light and often occur on the shoulders, face, neck and ears.

Treatment
Usually easily treatable with a diclofenac topical gel.

Skin cancer risks
Everyone, regardless of skin colour, can get skin cancer, although those with pale skin, freckles and numerous moles are at a higher risk. Exposure to UV light is one of the leading causes so high factor sunscreen is essential. Avoid using tanning beds.

Sunlight is formed from UVA rays (responsible for burning and tanning the skin, as well as contributing to skin aging) and UVB rays (which cause sunburn). Most sunscreens will have a UVA (up to 5 stars) and UVB (SPF number) rating so you can see how well they protect you. Both UVA and UVB can cause skin cancer so it's important to choose a high rating for both categories.

The Sun Protection Factor (SPF) refers to how many times longer the sunscreen provides protection from burning versus exposure without it, so if you are in the sun for longer than this time you will need to reapply the sunscreen. Always reapply sunscreen after getting wet or towelling the skin dry to ensure adequate protection. You can also protect yourself and your children by avoiding the sun at the hottest part of the day and wearing wide-brimmed sunhats or loose, long layers. Young children and babies should avoid strong, direct sunlight.

THE BLOOD

Blood is the most amazing transportation system for all the things that our body needs to work and stay healthy. Just some of its key jobs are:

- Carrying oxygen from the lungs and delivering it to every cell in our bodies.
- Removing waste products such as carbon dioxide and urea from cells so they don't poison us.
- Transmitting messages in the form of hormones – for example, adrenaline is transmitted to tells our lungs, muscles, etc. that there may be a threat we need to be ready for.
- Supplying our immune response and fighting infections from bacteria and viruses.

What is blood?

Blood is made up of four main components that each do different jobs:

Plasma

Plasma carries antibodies and proteins and helps maintain blood pressure, among other things. People who have suffered major physical trauma or have cancer, LIVER DISEASE or severe infections may need a plasma transfusion.

Red blood cells

Made in the bone marrow and super flexible so they can get around the tiniest capillaries. They only last for 120 days before being replaced. Their main job is transporting oxygen and carbon dioxide, and they use the protein haemoglobin to do this.

White blood cells

Also made in the bone marrow and make up a key part of our immune response.

Platelets

Help our blood to clot so we can heal. Too many can lead to STROKES and HEART ATTACKS, while too few can cause excessive bleeding.

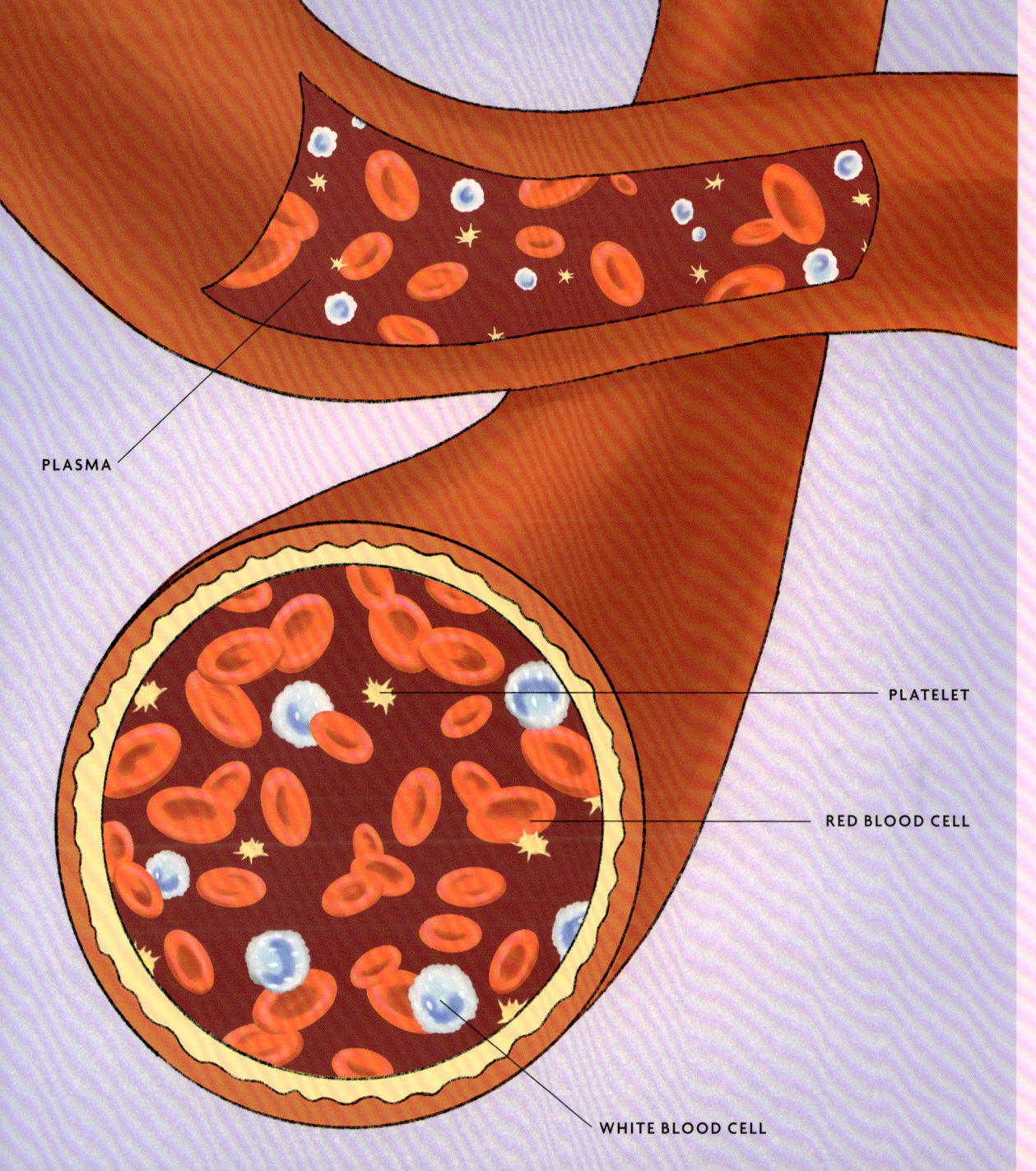

Anaemia

Anaemia is the general term for having fewer red blood cells than normal, or red blood cells having abnormally low haemoglobin levels. This means that your blood can't carry enough oxygen around your body. It's often linked to, or a result of, other health conditions.

SYMPTOMS

Mild anaemia:
+ Feeling TIRED and/or weak.
+ HEADACHES.
+ Difficulty concentrating.
+ Irritability.
+ Loss of appetite.
+ Numbness, coldness or tingling in the hands and feet.

More severe anaemia:
+ Shortness of breath.
+ Chest pains.
+ Light-headedness when standing from a seated position.
+ Rapid or irregular heart rate.
+ Sores in the mouth, ulcers, inflamed tongue.
+ Desire to eat ice or non-food items.
+ Paler skin than usual.
+ Brittle nails.
+ Low sex drive.
+ Blue tone to the whites of the eyes.

Diagnosis

If you have some symptoms of mild anaemia and no other health concerns, the best treatment is to up your iron intake through foods such as red meat, kidney beans, spinach or fortified foods, and consider an over-the-counter iron supplement. See if this improves your symptoms over the course of a few weeks.

We use a blood test to check for anaemia. A full blood count will look at all the deficiencies that can cause anaemia, and because anaemia can be a sign of other health issues, the underlying cause may need further investigation.

Note that women who have HEAVY BLEEDING during their periods sometimes have anaemia that goes undetected because the iron loss during menstruation isn't addressed. So when checking iron levels ensure your doctor conducts a haematinic blood test, which comprises ferratin, folate, iron and B_{12}.

Women and girls who are menstruating lose 1mg of iron with each 'normal' monthly period.

Causes

The body needs the correct amounts of iron, ferritin, vitamin B$_{12}$ and folate to make healthy red blood cells with enough haemoglobin. If not, we can become anaemic. There are many reasons why levels of these micronutrients could be low:

- Diet, for example vegans may not get enough vitamin B$_{12}$ from food alone.
- Chronic inflammation in the body caused by a range of conditions, including cancer, ENDOMETRIOSIS, ULCERATIVE COLITIS and RHEUMATOID ARTHRITIS.
- Any condition that means your body struggles to absorb nutrients, such as COELIAC DISEASE or CYSTIC FIBROSIS.
- Surgery that has removed part of your gut, a gastric bypass or gastric sleeve.
- Some medications, like steroids, can remove iron from your system.
- Sudden or ongoing slow blood loss, e.g. from STOMACH ULCERS, BOWEL CANCER or HEAVY BLEEDING during a period.

Treatment

- Supplements, to top up low vitamin and iron levels. If you are taking iron tablets, it's usually recommended to take them three times a day so the iron can be more easily absorbed. Taking too much iron in one go can result in black poo and constipation, so people stop taking them and the anaemia comes back.
- If you menstruate, consider a regular iron supplement, particularly if you have a chronic inflammatory condition such as ADENOMYOSIS, ENDOMETRIOSIS, FIBROMYALGIA or an autoimmune condition.

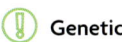 Genetic

Haemolytic anaemia

Haemolytic anaemia occurs when the red blood cell count becomes too low because the red blood cells are destroyed faster than the body can make them. It can be caused by an infection like MALARIA, an inherited condition (such as hereditary spherocytosis or hereditary elliptocytosis), a reaction to certain drugs or by someone receiving a transfusion of blood that doesn't match their own blood type.

SYMPTOMS

The symptoms of haemolytic anaemia are similar to anaemia and can also include:
+ Jaundice and pain in upper right abdomen, where the liver is positioned.
+ Fast heartbeat.
+ Low blood pressure.
+ Blood in your pee.

Diagnosis

- Physical examination looking for signs of jaundice, pallor and an enlarged spleen.
- A single blood test that will be checked in the lab for the following investigations: to check reticulocyte count (measures the number of young red cells which will show as elevated); a direct Coombs test (identifies antibodies attached to red blood cells which can occur in autoimmune haematinic anaemia), and an indirect bilirubin, because elevated levels would suggest increased red blood cell breakdown.
- Other tests can include a urine test or bone marrow biopsy if the above tests are inconclusive.

Treatment

Treatment is to identify and treat the underlying issue causing the haemolytic anaemia.

Genetic

Thalassaemia

This inherited blood disorder is due to a gene variant that causes abnormal haemoglobin – the substance that allows red blood cells to carry oxygen. There are different types of the condition, and it varies in seriousness from no symptoms to severe symptoms. The severity depends on how many defective genes are inherited.

SYMPTOMS

- ANAEMIA.
- OSTEOPOROSIS.
- Enlarged spleen.
- Jaundice.
- Dark urine.
- Slow growth in childhood and delayed puberty.
- Irregular facial bone structure.

Diagnosis
Thalassaemia is diagnosed via blood test. This may be genetic testing, prenatal testing (if there's a family history) or a newborn blood spot/heel prick test (for all newborn babies).

Treatment
The treatment will be defined by the form of the disease and whether there is too little iron in the blood. In more serious cases, blood transfusions are often necessary.

The only cure is a bone marrow/stem cell transplant, which is only attempted in very serious cases and when a compatible donor – usually a sibling – is available.

Only people who inherit the gene from both parents can be born with thalassaemia. Those with the mildest form may not know they have it. If there is any family history, or you suspect there is, and you want to have a child, speak to a doctor to find out about genetic testing.

Genetic

Haemophilia

Haemophilia is a rare inherited blood disorder where the blood doesn't clot properly, leading to sometimes life-threatening complications, such as haemorrhaging (bleeding inside the body). Most people who have haemophilia are male, although women can also have it, or be carriers, and symptoms are likely to be more severe in biological males.

SYMPTOMS

- **Excessive bleeding from small wounds, nosebleeds, etc.**
- **Bruising easily.**
- **Pain around the joints.**

Diagnosis
In the UK, all newborn babies are screened for haemophilia, so most people will know if they have it.

You can only get haemophilia if one or both of your parents has it or carries the gene – although this doesn't mean they will definitely pass it on to you. You can be a carrier and have no symptoms of haemophilia (although some carriers who menstruate have HEAVY BLEEDING during their periods). People who are or may be carriers who want to have children can be tested and receive advice from genetic counsellors.

Treatment
There is no cure for haemophilia, but it can be managed with regular injections of a medicine that helps the blood to clot. People with haemophilia will sometimes need to be treated for bleeding from wounds that won't stop.

Genetic

Sickle cell disease

Sickle cell is an inherited condition that varies in severity. It's so-called because the red blood cells are an unusual shape, meaning they can become stuck in blood vessels, leading to pain and serious complications. There is a myth that only Black people have sickle cell disease; this is not true, but it is more common in people of African or Caribbean descent.

SYMPTOMS
- **Frequent infections.**
- **Slow growth in children.**
- **ANAEMIA.**
- **Leg ulcers.**
- **Bone and joint pain.**
- **Experiencing sickle cell crises (see below).**

Diagnosis
Babies born in the UK are given a newborn blood spot test (formerly known as the heel prick test) soon after birth, where a blood sample from the foot is tested for rare diseases, including sickle cell. If you were born outside the UK and you have any family history of sickle cell speak to your GP about being tested.

Treatment
Sickle cell disease is a lifelong condition that will require ongoing support from a specialist.

Symptoms of a sickle cell crisis
A sickle cell crisis occurs when the unusually shaped red blood cells form a blockage, causing extreme pain and restricting blood flow to organs. It can lead to STROKES and HEART ATTACKS, so it's important to know the signs if you have or think you may have sickle cell disease:
- Severe pain in one area.
- Swelling of hands and feet, or stomach.
- Chest pain and shortness of breath.
- FEVER.
- Painful, long-lasting erections in men (see PRIAPISM).

Leukaemia

Leukaemia is an umbrella term for cancers that affect the blood and bone marrow. It usually starts in the bone marrow – where blood is made – or in the lymph system, and then spreads to other parts of the body. It's caused by a problem with the way the body makes white blood cells, a key part of the immune system, which makes those with leukaemia more susceptible to infection. There are different types of leukaemia that vary in how quickly the disease progresses, and in treatments and prognosis. Some factors seem to increase the risk – such as previous chemotherapy, exposure to radiation, other blood disorders, chemicals found in cigarettes and some manufacturing processes – but we don't yet know what causes leukaemia.

SYMPTOMS

- **FATIGUE**, feeling weak.
- Being ill often.
- Looking 'washed out'.
- Unusual bruising and bleeding, such as nosebleeds, bleeding from the gums or small cuts bleeding more than you would expect.
- Losing weight without trying to.

Symptoms cross over with other conditions and in some cases come on slowly, so they can go unnoticed. But equally, there are other explanations for these symptoms aside from leukaemia, so if you experience these symptoms, it's important not to panic.

Diagnosis

If a doctor suspects leukaemia, they will do a blood test to check, which may be followed by a biopsy of the bone marrow.

Acute myeloid leukaemia (AML)

The 'acute' part of the name means it comes on quickly and needs immediate treatment. This rare type of leukaemia is most common in people aged over 75.

ADDITIONAL SYMPTOMS

- Faster onset of leukaemia symptoms.

Treatment

Chemotherapy is usually the main treatment. In some cases, radiotherapy is needed or a bone marrow or stem cell transplant. As with most cancers, if someone is young and healthy, and the disease is caught early so treatment can begin quickly, then they have a much better chance of recovery. It can be harder to treat leukaemia that has changed from 'chronic' (see below) to acute.

Chronic myeloid leukaemia

This type of leukaemia develops more slowly, over years. It's most common in people aged over 65 but is still rare.

ADDITIONAL SYMPTOMS

- Swollen glands around the armpits, neck and/or groin.
- Swollen stomach, which may be painful or uncomfortable.
- Night sweats.
- HEADACHES.
- Aching joints or bones.

Treatment
Treatment depends on factors such as age and how advanced the disease is, but the most likely treatment is targeted cancer medicines called tyrosine kinase inhibitors (TKIs). Chemotherapy or a stem cell transplant may follow if the leukaemia doesn't respond to medication. The outcomes for this type of leukaemia are generally very good, although people sometimes have to take medication for the rest of their lives.

Chronic lymphocytic leukaemia

This kind of leukaemia is managed with treatment and develops slowly, so it doesn't always need to be treated straight away. It's a rare disease that is even more uncommon in those under 40, and it mostly affects men.

ADDITIONAL SYMPTOMS
- Swollen glands around the armpits, neck and/or groin.
- Swollen stomach, which may be painful or uncomfortable.
- Night sweats.
- HEADACHES.
- Ongoing aches and pains.
- FEVER.
- A rash that looks like bleeding or bruises under the skin and doesn't fade with the glass test (see page 24).

Treatment
May be treated with targeted cancer medicines called tyrosine kinase inhibitors (TKIs). Some people will have chemotherapy and radiotherapy if other treatments aren't working well. In rare cases, the spleen – the organ that filters the blood and controls blood cells – may be removed.

Multiple myeloma

Multiple myeloma is a cancer of the bone marrow that affects the plasma cells, meaning the body struggles to make the correct antibodies. It also prompts bones to break down faster, which leads to a lot of calcium in the blood, which can cause kidney damage. The disease may not cause any symptoms in its early stages, and it's most common in men aged over 60.

SYMPTOMS
- Feeling TIRED and weak.
- Being thirsty all the time and needing to pee more often.
- Feeling confused/less alert.
- Painful bones that may fracture more easily.
- Frequent infections.
- Constipation.
- Numbness and tingling in hands and feet.
- Lower back pain, caused by kidney problems.

Diagnosis
The doctor will order a blood test and probably a Bence Jones urine test, to check for proteins that can indicate this type of cancer. This may be followed by a bone marrow biopsy.

Treatment
Even though multiple myeloma is a cancer, not everyone who has it will need treatment straight away. It can be very slow growing and not cause symptoms, in which case someone will be monitored by a specialist. Anti-cancer drugs and steroids are usually the first step, sometimes followed by or alongside chemotherapy and radiotherapy; it depends on the health of the patient and how advanced the myeloma is. Some people may need a bone marrow transplant.

THE IMMUNE SYSTEM

Our immune system is a complicated but ingenious network of organs, cells and proteins that protects us from harmful substances such as bacteria, viruses, fungi and cancer cells. Any organisms that can get inside us and make us sick are called pathogens. Our white blood cells are always actively seeking them out and using proteins called antibodies to neutralise them, so they are no longer harmful. Through exposure to different pathogens, our bodies figure out how to fight them. This is how vaccines work; by training the immune system to make the right antibodies to react to a disease.

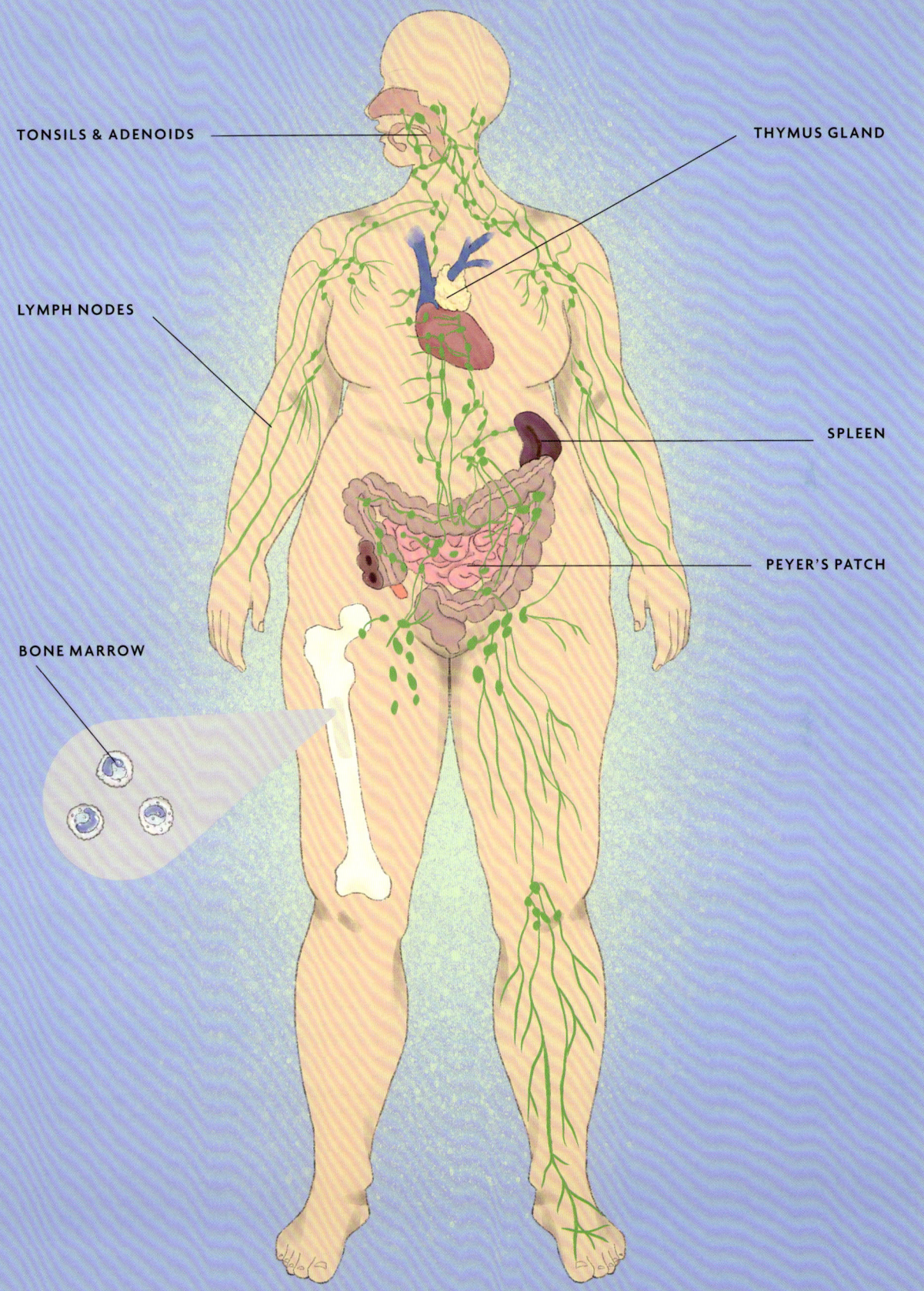

How can we support the immune system?

Avoid stress: Easier said than done of course, but it's important to know that the hormones that are produced when we experience some sort of stress to our bodies – cortisol, adrenaline and noradrenaline – can damage our natural, healthy immune response. When our body is stressed, such as when we are under more physical, emotional or mental pressure than usual, it can lead to or exacerbate chronic inflammation (see below).

Have a healthy lifestyle: Our bodies – and therefore our immune systems – work best when they have all the nutrients they need to fuel the work they do for us. Being deficient in vitamins and minerals through poor diet, or due to alcohol consumption or recreational drug use, inhibits our immune response. Exercise increases blood flow and reduces stress, while the right amount of sleep helps us deal with inflammation.

Look after the gut: Two thirds of our immune system is located in our gut. The microbiome is the name for all the bacteria and fungi that live happily and healthily in our gut and interact with our immune system. When this is disrupted, it can cause inflammation in the body.

Inflammation

Inflammation is the process by which our white blood cells deal with toxins. It's the body's natural and important response to a threat to its wellbeing. Increased blood flow to the area brings more white blood cells and substances that trap invaders and repair cells.

Inflammation is a good thing when it promotes healing. For example, a SORE THROAT or a swollen sprained ankle might be painful and not much fun, but it's a sign that the immune system is working well.

Inflammation is a problem when the body overreacts to a threat, making us more sick in the process; when the immune reaction lasts too long, resulting in 'chronic inflammation'; or if the immune system starts attacking healthy tissue, such as with AUTOIMMUNE DISEASES, CARDIOVASCULAR DISEASE, DIABETES, neurodegenerative diseases such as ALZHEIMER'S DISEASE or PARKINSON'S DISEASE and certain types of cancers.

Antibiotics

Antibiotics will treat bacterial infections only (so not COLD or FLU viruses, or fungal infections) and penicillin is the most widely used. They can be taken orally, injected, put on the skin in a cream or given via IV. They should only be prescribed if an infection:

- Carries a serious risk to health.
- Is unlikely to go away otherwise or will take a long time to clear up by itself.
- Is highly contagious and likely to spread to others.

Finishing the course

You **MUST** finish the course because, even when symptoms have gone, there may still be some bacteria left in your system which can reproduce, making you sick again. In addition, bacteria that reproduces this way may develop a resistance to the antibiotics so they won't work any more – creating a so-called 'Superbug'. Superbugs, such as MRSA and C. diff, are a growing problem globally. In the West in particular, we have over-prescribed antibiotics which, combined with their use in animal farming, has given bacteria increased chances to adapt. These superbugs put a big strain on the health system and threaten lives.

Infectious diseases

These are the foreign bodies, or 'pathogens', that can get into the body and cause us to be ill.

Types of pathogens

Pathogen	Description	Examples of conditions it can cause
Bacteria	Single-cell organisms that can cause infection (but not all do).	Strep throat, URINARY TRACT INFECTIONS, tuberculosis.
Viruses	Tiny bundles of DNA that can reproduce only when they get inside a living cell of an organism (plant, animal or human).	The common COLD, FLU, HIV.
Fungi	Plant-like organisms that often live on us harmlessly but cause problems when they grow out of control.	ATHLETE'S FOOT, RINGWORM, THRUSH, lung and nervous system infections.
Parasites	An organism that lives on or in its host and depends on it for survival, but may cause infections.	MALARIA, HEADLICE, pinworms.
Prions	A rare, abnormal version of a protein that affects the normal proteins it encounters when it enters the body.	Creutzfeldt-Jakob disease (CJD).

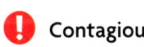 Contagious

Food-borne bacterial infections

What we generally refer to as 'food poisoning' is often caused by bacteria being in something we have eaten, usually introduced during food preparation or through not washing hands properly after handling infected raw meat or coming into contact with infected animals. You can also ingest the bugs via contaminated water – drinking it or swimming in it. These bugs are very common and our bodies can usually deal with low levels without us becoming unwell.

SYMPTOMS

+ **Gastroenteritis (inflammation of the gut).**
+ **Nausea and vomiting.**
+ **Diarrhoea.**
+ **Stomach cramps and general muscle aches.**
+ **Sometimes a FEVER.**

Causes

There are numerous bacteria that cause upset stomachs. The most common are:

- **Salmonella**, a bacteria commonly found in raw meat.
- **E. coli** has strains that live harmlessly in the gut, but some cause illness which can be serious.
- **Campylobacter** is a very common cause of diarrhoea.
- **Listeria** is sometimes found in unpasteurised dairy products, which is why PREGNANT people are advised to avoid them.

These bacteria can enter our systems via:
- Raw or undercooked meat, fish, seafood and eggs.
- Unwashed, contaminated fruits and vegetables.
- Contaminated water or unpasteurized milk.
- Infected animals.
- Being in contact with an infected person.
- Listeria can also be present in unpasteurised dairy products, chilled foods like processed deli meat and smoked/cured fish.

Prevention
Food-borne bacterial infections can largely be prevented by good hygiene, e.g. hand washing, and making sure you handle and cook food correctly.

Treatment
For most of us, if we are in good health, unpleasant though the symptoms are, they will resolve within seven days. To help manage symptoms at home and aid your recovery, follow these tips:
- When you have sickness and diarrhoea, dehydration is the main issue. Sip water, as well as diluted fruit juices and sports drinks. Ice lollies can also help.
- Avoid food until your stomach feels more settled and don't eat if you don't feel hungry.
- It's usually best not to take medication to stop diarrhoea, so your body can get on with getting rid of what it needs to.
- Wash your hands thoroughly after going to the toilet to avoid infecting others – these bugs are very contagious.
- Stay away from anyone vulnerable to infections.
- Don't go back to school or work until the diarrhoea has stopped.
- If you take an oral contraceptive then remember this may stop working when you have sickness and diarrhoea.

Red flags
Food-borne bacterial infections are more serious for those who are:
- Under five.
- Over 65.
- PREGNANT.
- Immunocompromised or have another health condition.
- Experiencing IRRITABLE BOWEL SYNDROME (IBS).
- Taking antibiotics.

Seek urgent medical attention if the person suffering from the infection:
- Is very confused and/or delirious.
- Is dehydrated to the point where they aren't peeing at all, or not able to take on fluid due to vomiting.
- Has blood in their diarrhoea.
- Has had diarrhoea for seven days.

See also advice on FEVERS.

Other common causes

Viruses, parasites and fungi can also cause gastroenteritis symptoms, when the stomach and intestines become inflamed.

Norovirus
Very common, particularly in the winter. This virus is highly contagious and spreads person-to-person through close contact or eating or drinking something handled by an infected person. The treatments (and the red flags) are the same as for food-borne bacterial infections, listed above.

Giardiasis
Caused by a parasite picked up from contaminated water (or more rarely from food handled by someone with the parasite or food washed in contaminated water). Symptoms include terrible-smelling diarrhoea, burps like rotten eggs, bloating and gas. You may need to give a stool sample to be diagnosed and take antibiotics.

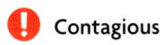 Contagious

Viral diseases

Viral diseases are infections caused by viruses. They range from mild to servere, and include the common COLD, FLU or coronavirus. They are contagious and spread in various ways, usually infected droplets (e.g. coughing, sneezing) or on surfaces (via hands or worktops, etc).

Measles

Measles is a highly contagious disease that can be fatal. Symptoms start 10–14 days after exposure to the airborne virus, which is spread by droplets from an infected person. Measles is particularly dangerous for children under 5, anyone who is immunocompromised, PREGNANT women or adults over 30. In some cases it can cause complications such as blindness, ENCEPHALITIS, severe dehydration, hearing issues, or severe breathing problems including PNEUMONIA. Being vaccinated is the best way to avoid getting and spreading measles. Two doses of the MMR (Measles, Mumps and Rubella) vaccine gives lifelong protection and is offered to all children, but you can also request it at any time for free on the NHS.

SYMPTOMS

+ **FEVER.**
+ Cough.
+ Red, watery eyes and/or runny nose.
+ Rash (harder to see on darker skin) that usually starts on the face and neck and spreads over the whole body after three days.
+ Small white spots inside cheeks (may help diagnosis in people with darker skin).

Diagnosis & treatment

Measles is diagnosed by symptoms but it is highly contagious so your GP might ask for a video or telephone consultation. The rash lasts five to six days and you can feel really rotten. There is no specific treatment but ensure you stay hydrated, use soaked cotton wool to gently remove any crusts from the eyes and take paracetamol to reduce your temperature. Beware that ibuprofen can sometimes make the rash worse in children. You are infectious from four days before the rash appears and for four days after. You must stay off nursery, school or work for this time and avoid contact with babies, anyone PREGNANT or with a weakened immune system.

Red flags

If you are PREGNANT or have a child under one who has come into contact with measles, call 111. If your child has a FEVER that is not coming down with paracetamol, difficulty breathing, is taking on less fluids, not producing wet nappies, or seems seriously unwell, call 111 or visit A&E. MENINGITIS can be mistaken for measles so be aware of symptoms and seek immediate help if required.

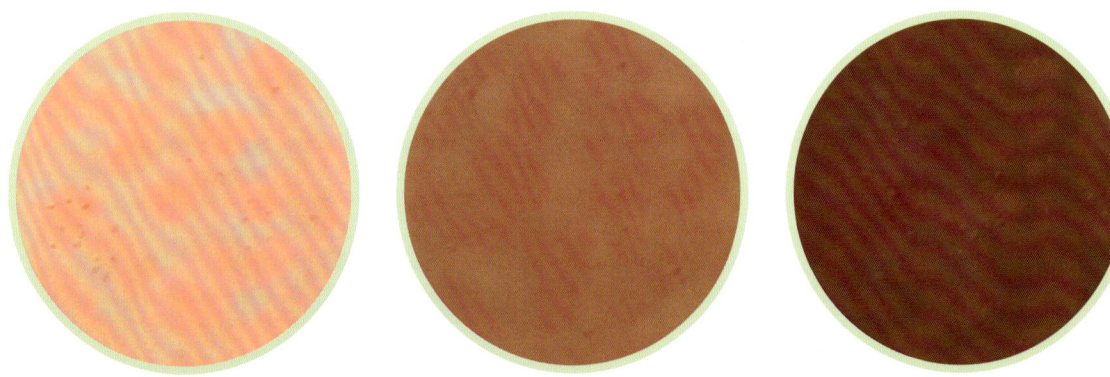

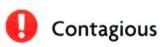 **Contagious**

Mumps

Mumps is a highly contagious viral infection. It tends to incubate for 12–25 days before symptoms show and is infectious during this time. For most people, it will resolve in a couple of weeks. It can cause TONSILLITIS and QUINSY, and, rarely, serious complications, such as VIRAL MENINGITIS or a permanent reduction in fertility for males. The MMR vaccine prevents mumps.

SYMPTOMS

+ Swollen, painful parotid glands on either side of the neck, making you look a bit like a hamster.
+ HEADACHE.
+ FEVER.
+ Feeling achy and exhausted.
+ Dry mouth.
+ Loss of appetite, nausea or abdominal pain.

Diagnosis

Call your GP surgery if you suspect mumps as they may want you to come in so they can confirm the diagnosis. Always tell the surgery before you visit as mumps is very contagious. Seek advice from your midwife if you are PREGNANT and suspect mumps.

Treatment

Like lots of viruses, mumps can usually be treated effectively at home with lots of fluids, painkillers and a warm compress to the swollen glands. If you can't control a FEVER, are vomiting or have diarrhoea that goes on for more than two days, are showing signs of severe dehydration or the pain is acute and not responding to painkillers, seek urgent medical attention.

Don't go back to work or school until at least five days after your symptoms started showing (it may take longer than this to start to feel better anyway).

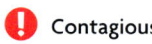 **Contagious**

Rubella

Sometimes called German measles, rubella is a highly contagious, airborne virus. Symptoms start two to three weeks after exposure. It can pose a serious risk to those who are immunocompromised or PREGNANT. Being vaccinated with the MMR vaccine is the best way to avoid getting and spreading rubella.

SYMPTOMS

+ FEVER.
+ Cough and SORE THROAT.
+ Sneezing and runny nose.
+ HEADACHE.
+ Sore eyes.
+ Aching fingers, wrists or knees.
+ Spotty rash (harder to see on brown or black skin) that starts on the face or behind the ears and spreads all over the body.

Diagnosis & treatment

Rubella is diagnosed by your GP but it is highly contagious so they might ask for a video or telephone consultation. There is no treatment and it usually gets better after one week. To manage your symptoms, stay hydrated, take paracetamol and get plenty of rest. You are infectious for one week before symptoms start until five days after the rash first appears, so stay away from nursery, school or work throughout this time and avoid contact with babies, anyone PREGNANT or with a weakened immune system. To limit the spread of infection, wash hands with soap; do not share eating or drinking utensils, clothes, towels or bedding; and use tissues to catch sneezes, disposing of them into the bin immediately.

> ### Rubella in pregnancy
> Exposure in the first 20 weeks of PREGNANCY can cause MISCARRIAGE or serious problems for the baby after birth. Always contact a midwife if you get a new rash while PREGNANT.

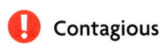 Contagious

Glandular fever (mono)

Glandular fever, also called infectious mononucleosis, or 'mono', is sometimes referred to as the 'kissing disease' as it's spread by saliva. It's caused by the Epstein-Barr virus and mainly affects young adults. It can linger and make you feel terrible, but you are unlikely to get it more than once.

SYMPTOMS

- FEVER.
- Feeling hot and shivery.
- Very SORE THROAT.
- Swollen glands in the neck, armpits or groin.
- FATIGUE.
- HEADACHE.
- TONSILLITIS.

Diagnosis

Glandular fever is diagnosed by physical examination and sometimes an antibody test, but this may not detect the infection during the first week of the illness.

Treatment

There is no specific treatment; it's just about trying to relieve the symptoms. If you develop a strep A infection or TONSILLITIS, you may need antibiotics for that. Unless the symptoms become severe the main advice is to:

- Stay hydrated.
- Take paracetamol, aspirin or ibuprofen.
- Gargle with warm salty water to treat a SORE THROAT.
- Rest.

Note that ibuprofen should only be given to children under 16 who have a rash after consulting a doctor.

There is no need to isolate but the official guidance is to not kiss anyone for three to six months after having the infection! You can remain contagious for up to a year after your symptoms go away.

FATIGUE can last for some weeks after the illness has passed. If this happens, there is a small risk of developing CHRONIC FATIGUE SYNDROME.

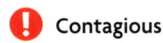 Contagious

Scarlet fever

This highly contagious infection, caused by the group A strep bacteria, is especially common in young children. It can occur at the same time as CHICKENPOX, which makes it more serious.

SYMPTOMS

- FEVER and FATIGUE.
- SORE THROAT.
- Swollen neck glands.
- A rash of small, raised bumps on the chest and stomach that looks pink/red on white skin but can be easier to feel for on darker skin – usually comes on after the other symptoms.
- 'Strawberry mouth' – a white coating on the tongue that peels, leaving it swollen, bumpy and sore.

Diagnosis & treatment

Scarlet fever can make you feel really horrible, but it is easily treated with antibiotics, so see a doctor as soon as possible. Treat the symptoms at home as with any FEVER. If you fall ill again a few weeks after you have recovered from scarlet fever, see a doctor as this could be rheumatic fever – a rare complication of scarlet fever caused by the immune system attacking healthy tissue.

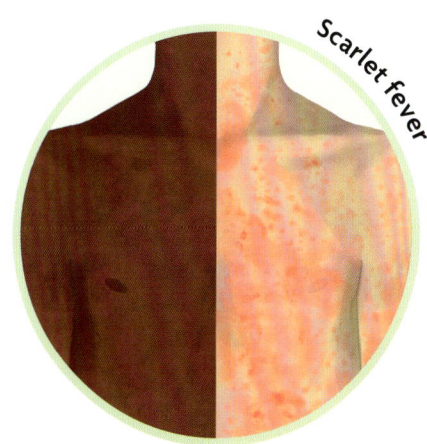

Scarlet fever

🟢 Non-contagious

ME/Chronic fatigue syndrome (CFS)

Myalgic encephalomyelitis (ME) is also known as chronic fatigue syndrome (CFS). It's a neurological condition with symptoms that can affect different parts of the body – the most common of which is feeling extremely TIRED all the time, to the point where it gets in the way of living your 'normal' life. We don't know what causes it but some people start experiencing symptoms following a virus or bacterial infection.

SYMPTOMS
- Feelings of extreme exhaustion.
- Brain fog.
- Trouble sleeping.
- Feeling much worse after physical activity.
- General pain or aches.
- Unusual sensitivity to light or noise.

Symptoms may come and go in terms of severity but are chronic (i.e. they persist for a long period of time).

Diagnosis
As ME/CFS shares symptoms with other conditions and not enough is known about it, it is underdiagnosed. The first step is to rule out other causes of the symptoms (such as ANAEMIA) and possibly run blood and urine tests. Then, if the symptoms and medical history meet the guidelines, ME/CFS will be diagnosed.

Treatment
While there is no cure for ME/CFS, it is possible to manage the symptoms, and the best way to do this varies by individual. Medication may be prescribed, such as painkillers or sleeping tablets. Some people find it helpful to seek support from a therapist to discuss ways to deal with the challenges that living with the condition presents.

 Non-contagious

Long Covid

Since the Covid-19 epidemic, we've seen increased reports of long-term symptoms and debilitation, but there's lots more work to be done to better understand post-viral infection and its consequences.

SYMPTOMS
- Debilitating FATIGUE and/or insomnia.
- Muscle weakness, pain and joint pain.
- Feeling out of breath.
- Fast heart rate.
- Menstrual cycle or erectile dysfunction.
- Changes to smell and/or taste.

Diagnosis & treatment
Diagnosis is based on patient history but you may have blood and other tests to rule out other conditions. The NHS now offers post-Covid-19 rehab, including breathing physio and MENTAL HEALTH support, if needed. As there is no cure, managing the symptoms is key. Avoid over-exertion or too much alcohol, and keep sleeping hours consistent. Keep a diary of triggers that worsen symptoms and stay well hydrated.

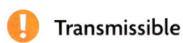 Transmissible

HIV & AIDS

The human immunodeficiency virus (HIV) attacks cells that help the body fight infection. AIDS stands for acquired immunodeficiency syndrome and occurs when the effects of HIV on the immune system means it can no longer fight infection. HIV can't survive outside the body for long – it can't be spread by saliva, urine, touching or anything similar. It can only be spread by semen, vaginal fluids, breast milk or blood (such as through sharing needles). It can also passed from mother to unborn baby in instances where the mother is not receiving HIV treatment. It is possible to get it through oral sex, but the risk is low. There is still no cure for HIV but people who have it can be treated with drugs that allow them to lead long, normal lives well into parenthood and old age. Anti-placental transference drugs also allow HIV-positive mothers to safely have children without transferring the virus, and other medications allow couples to have unprotected sex in order to get PREGNANT without transferring the virus.

SYMPTOMS OF HIV

- FLU-like symptoms two to six weeks after infection (although not everyone has this after being infected).
- Swollen lymph glands in the neck, armpits or groin.
- Mouth sores.

These symptoms will go away but can recur. The virus will continue to gradually damage the immune system over time, eventually leading to AIDS if left untreated. Over time, symptoms become more serious, and can include PNEUMONIA, skin infections or death, if there is no treatment.

Prevention

The best way to prevent HIV is to practise safe sex. A drug, known as pre-exposure prophylaxis (PEP), can be prescribed to people who are at risk of contracting HIV – such as having a sexual partner who is HIV positive – although it isn't suitable for everyone. It also must be taken soon after having sex, and a maximum of 72 hours after (see right).

Diagnosis

It is very easy to get tested at GP surgeries, sexual health centres and clinics run by charities, where a sample of blood or saliva is taken. You can even do it by post. You may need to repeat the test a few times over a period of months if there is a chance you could have become infected.

Treatment

If there is a chance you could have been exposed to HIV, speak to a medical professional as soon as possible as the emergency drug post-exposure prophylaxis (PEP) can stop you becoming infected if taken within 72 hours after exposure. Even if you cannot take the drug in that time, early diagnosis hugely improves the outcome so get tested as soon as possible.

The treatment for HIV is antiretroviral medications. They stop the virus from replicating in the body, allowing the immune system to repair itself. With the right combination, the level of virus in the body can become so low that it is not damaging the immune system any more and can't even be detected by a test. After six months of clear results, while the virus may still be in your system, you are no longer able to give it to other people, but you must continue taking the medication for life to maintain the lower virus levels.

⚠️ Transmissible

Malaria

Malaria is a potentially life-threatening parasitic infection of the blood cells, spread by bites from the Anopheles mosquito (not from person to person). Malaria-carrying mosquitos are not found in the UK, but they are common in many tropical and subtropical regions around the world.

SYMPTOMS

Symptoms can be mild to very serious. They tend to appear seven days to several months after being bitten by a mosquito carrying the disease. The most common are:
- FEVER and sweating.
- Feeling sleepy and 'out of it'.
- Chills.
- HEADACHE and confusion.
- Muscle aches.
- Loss of appetite.
- Yellowing to the whites of the eyes or skin.
- SORE THROAT and/or cough.
- Trouble breathing.

Where swelling occurs on the brain symtomps can include:
- SEIZURES.
- Life-threatening coma.

Diagnosis & treatment

If you think you have malaria, it's important to seek medical help quickly. Diagnosis is usually via a blood test by a tropical diseases specialist. Treatment is by antimalarial drugs.

Prevention

- Ensure you know in advance if the region of the country you are travelling to carries a malaria risk – go to www.fitfortravel.nhs.uk for more information.
- If you need to take antimalarials, leave enough time to get a prescription (only one type is currently available over the counter). You will need to start taking them before you travel and continue after you return.
- Prevent mosquito bites by using a repellent containing permethrin. Treat clothing and camping gear with it too. Cover up with long-sleeved and full-length clothing, especially near undisturbed water sources or places with a lot of animals (which mosquitos will be using as hosts).
- Take a sleeping net to your destination if recommended.
- Previous time spent in a malarial region does not make you immune, as any resistance is believed to decrease quickly.

Dengue

Similar to MALARIA, this is a virus spread by infected mosquitos, usually only found in tropical places, although it has been reported in some parts of southern Europe. Dengue doesn't always cause symptoms, although in rare cases it can lead to complications like ENCEPHALITIS. Some people will have painful joints and muscles, high FEVER, a rash, nausea and vomiting, skin itching and a HEADACHE.

There is currently no vaccine so it's very important to use repellent and mosquito nets when travelling in areas with dengue.

See a doctor if you have symptoms of dengue after travelling to an affected area. Do not take NSAIDs (non-steroidal anti-inflammatory drugs) such as aspirin or ibuprofen. There is no cure but in severe cases your symptoms may need treating in hospital.

⚠️ Transmissable

Lyme disease

Lyme disease is a bacterial infection that is spread by the bites of infected ticks.

SYMPTOMS
Early (1 day–12 weeks after bite):
+ Bull's-eye rash in the area local to the bite.
+ Local area warm to touch.
+ Rash can be itchy and painful.

Dissemination (3 days–12 weeks after bite):
+ FEVER and/or chills.
+ HEADACHE.
+ Large lymph nodes.
+ Muscle or joint pain.
+ SORE THROAT.
+ FATIGUE.

Late dissemination (months or years after):
+ ARTHRITIS-like symptoms, facial palsy and neck stiffness.
+ Tendon pain.
+ Abnormal heart rhythm.
+ Behavioural or psychological changes, such as depression or uncharacteristic anger.

Diagnosis
The earlier Lyme disease is diagnosed the better (ideally within three days of early symptoms). Be alert to symptoms if you have been bitten by a tick or found ticks on your skin or clothes. Diagnosis is by patient history and blood test.

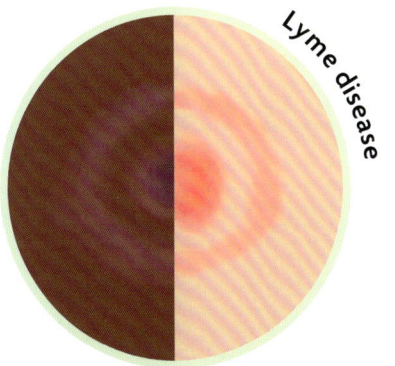

Lyme disease

Treatment & prevention
If identified early, Lyme disease is treated with antibiotics that quickly reduce its effects. Most cases go away with early treatment, but left untreated it can cause long-term damage such as ARTHRITIS.

Although not all ticks carry the disease it's best to avoid bites in the first place and exercise particular caution in grassy and wooded areas. Wear long trousers, treat clothes and skin with insect repellent in high-risk areas, stick to clear paths where possible and check clothing, skin and pets regularly for ticks. If you find a tick on your skin, use tweezers to get as close to the skin as possible, then slowly pull upwards to remove and avoid squeezing it. Then treat the area with soap and water or antiseptic.

Scabies
Scabies is a highly transmissible mite infection, resulting from direct skin-to-skin contact with an infected person. It's most common in moist parts of the body (such as between fingers and toes, in armpits, buttocks or at folds in the waist, wrists, elbows or penis). Symptoms appear one to four days after exposure but the mites can incubate for up to eight weeks. Symptoms include intense itching that is worse at night, tiny bites, hives and bumps on the skin and you may also see burrow marks where the mites leave eggs. Diagnosis is by physical examination and it is treated with a topical cream that should be used for at least two weeks, even if symptoms desist. The whole household should be treated. Wash clothes, towels, curtains and bedding at 60°C and deep-clean mattresses and furniture. While animals can catch scabies they do not incubate the type that usually infects people. A more severe form is crusted scabies, presenting as a thick skin crust. This can be life-threatening so seek immediate help.

Autoimmune diseases

An autoimmune disease is a condition that results from the immune system mistakenly targeting and attacking a healthy, functioning part of the body. There are around 80 different autoimmune diseases, ranging in severity from mild to disabling.

    Common autoimmune diseases include RHEUMATOID ARTHRITIS, FIBROMYALGIA and CROHN'S DISEASE. Living with an autoimmune disease can be challenging, but medicine is making advances in understanding our immune system and inflammation. While autoimmune diseases can cause serious complications, I have many patients who have learnt to manage their symptoms with little impact on their day-to-day lives. A frustration is that diagnosis is difficult and autoimmune conditions are still not well understood, so it can take a long time for people to get an answer as to what is behind their symptoms.

The wider impact

Any condition that causes chronic pain and discomfort will, of course, have a wider impact on different areas of the person's life. In addition to getting the right medication, it's important to seek help and support so that life can be lived as fully as possible. For example:

- **At work:** You should be able to ask your employer for accommodations so you can carry on doing your job.
- **Sex:** It's not talked about enough, but those with conditions such as ARTHRITIS and ANKYLOSING SPONDYLITIS often find that their symptoms affect their sex life. They may need to experiment with different positions, for example, and information and support is available.
- **PREGNANCY:** If you have an autoimmune condition and are thinking of becoming PREGNANT, you'll need some information regarding the medications you take. Make sure the midwives and other medical professionals understand your condition and how this needs to be taken into consideration in your birth plan.
- **Mental health:** Being in constant pain takes an emotional toll. Therapy can help you deal with this and contribute to pain management.

Giant cell myocarditis

This rare autoimmune disorder causes inflammation of the heart. It progresses very quickly – within five months the symptoms can become severe without treatment – and can lead to life-threatening complications. It usually affects people between the ages of 20 and 40, and often those who are otherwise very fit and healthy. This is because these individuals tend to have a more robust immune system, that can lead to an overzealous response against the heart muscle tissue.

SYMPTOMS

+ Shortness of breath.
+ Chest pain.
+ Heart palpitations.
+ FATIGUE.
+ Swollen ankles.

Diagnosis

Giant cell myocarditis can only be diagnosed through a biopsy, so you will be referred to a specialist and may undertake less invasive tests first to rule out other causes.

Treatment

Immunosuppression drugs will be used to try to stop the immune system from attacking the heart. Some people will require a heart transplant.

Vasculitis

This is the name for a group of conditions caused by the immune system attacking the blood vessels in the body, making them inflamed and narrow. It can be a minor issue if it affects just one small part of the body, but very serious if it affects vital organs.

SYMPTOMS

A range of different symptoms can be experienced by people suffering from a vasculitis condition. It will depend on which blood vessels or organs are being affected the most. It can occur alongside other autoimmune conditions. Common symptoms include:
+ Loss of appetite.
+ Feeling very TIRED.
+ Unintended weight loss.
+ General aches and pains throughout the body.

Diagnosis

Vasculitis is often hard to diagnose. A doctor will usually order blood and urine tests and talk to you about your symptoms. You may need to have dye injected into your bloodstream to see how narrow your blood vessels are. A biopsy of the affected organs might also be necessary.

Treatment

The main treatment is steroid medicines or other drugs that suppress the immune system, so it stops attacking the blood cells. Of course, this can mean that you are more susceptible to infections.

Lupus

Lupus is a chronic condition that causes inflammation and pain all over the body. The cause is not known, and it's most commonly diagnosed in women aged 15 to 45. Many people who have lupus experience flare-ups, where their symptoms get worse, though the reason for this is generally unclear. Lupus was once seen as a deadly condition, but now lots of people live with it.

SYMPTOMS

There are many different symptoms – the more common ones include:
+ Rashes and sensitivity to sunlight.
+ Painful joints and muscles.
+ Feeling very TIRED all the time.
+ FEVER.
+ HEADACHE.
+ Hair loss.
+ Unintentional weight loss.
+ Mouth ulcers.
+ Swollen glands in the neck, armpits and/or groin.

Diagnosis

Lupus is hard to diagnose, not least because it affects people in different ways. A doctor will do a blood test to look for high levels of anti-double stranded DNA, anti-Smith, anti-U1RNP, anti-Ro/SSA and anti-la/SSB antibodies that attack the body. They may also recommend X-rays of potentially affected organs.

Treatment

Treatment is focused on managing the symptoms and preventing organ damage, as this is the most serious consequence of lupus. The earlier treatment is started, the more effective it will be. Anti-inflammatory medication, like hydroxychloroquine and steroid medications, are often prescribed.

Anti-NMDA receptor encephalitis

This occurs when the immune system attacks the NMDA receptors located in the brain, which are key for memory. About 40 per cent of cases are in people under the age of 18, and it's more common in women than men. Sometimes a non-cancerous tumour may be connected to the overproduction of the antibodies responsible.

SYMPTOMS

Often, the symptoms progress quickly, requiring hospitalisation. Sometimes, someone will appear to have flu, with a FEVER and HEADACHE, before other symptoms come on later.

+ Trouble speaking.
+ Difficulty understanding and remembering things.
+ Changes in behaviour and/or agitation.
+ Abnormal movement in the arms, mouth and legs.
+ Loss of consciousness.

Diagnosis

Anti-NMDA receptor encephalitis can be difficult to diagnose. Diagnosis will usually involve bloods tests and a lumbar puncture, to check for markers of inflammation and specific antibodies. Other tests such as an MRI and ECG may be used to rule out other causes.

Treatment

Treatments include replacement plasma exchange, immunoglobulin therapy to try to make the immune system behave normally and steroids, alongside the removal of any tumours. While anti-NMDA receptor encephalitis can be life-threatening, most people make a full recovery within two years.

Guillain-Barré syndrome

This is a rare neurological condition that causes the immune system to attack the peripheral nervous system. We don't know why this happens, but it seems to be linked to a viral or bacterial infection. Anyone experiencing symptoms needs treatment in hospital as it can cause paralysis and breathing problems.

EARLY SYMPTOMS

+ Difficulty breathing.
+ Difficulty swallowing.
+ Double vision.
+ Tingling in the back and/or legs that becomes sharp pain.
+ Facial drooping.

Note that these symptoms are similar to those caused by a STROKE; **ALWAYS** go to A&E if you have any sign of these symptoms.

Diagnosis

In hospital, blood and breathing tests will be carried out as well as an electrical test on the muscles and a lumbar puncture.

Treatment

Those with the syndrome will often need to be helped to breathe and supported while the body recovers. Most people do fully recover, but it can take time and some will be left with nerve damage, residual muscle weakness and CHRONIC FATIGUE SYNDROME. Reoccurrence has been reported in up to 3 per cent of previously affected patients.

Connective tissue disorders

The inside of our bodies is covered by a network of connective tissues: literally tissues that support and form a separation between different organs. These connective tissues are where much of the body's fat is stored, too. Connective tissue disorders can either be inherited, such as Ehlers-Danlos syndrome or, more rarely, Marfan syndrome and osteogenesis imperfecta. Alternatively they can be acquired at some point in life, such as RHEUMATOID ARTHRITIS, LUPUS, scleroderma, Sjögren's syndrome or relapsing polychondritis.

Ehlers-Danlos syndromes (EDS)

EDS is a group of 13 genetic conditions with a range of symptoms that can be experienced differently by different people, varying in severity. It's described as a 'connective tissue disorder' as it affects tissues that support, protect and give shape to organs and other parts of the body, impacting the joints and skin in particular, but not exclusively. It's rare, but is possibly underdiagnosed.

Lots of people with EDS have hypermobility. This can cause thin/stretchy skin and joints that are super-flexible, making them prone to injury. Some people also suffer from digestive and bladder issues.

Diagnosis

See your GP if you have painful joints, FATIGUE, you bruise/cut easily and don't heal well, or if you have problems with digestion or URINARY INCONTINENCE. There is no test to diagnose EDS, so your GP will take your medical history and refer you to a specialist rheumatologist. You may also be referred for genetic testing, as we know some of the genes that cause EDS.

Treatment

There is currently no cure for EDS but treatment for symptoms is available (such as pain management and physiotherapy) as well as support to help you live your life the way you want to. It's a lifelong condition that needs to be carefully managed.

Types of EDS

Type	Symptoms
hEDS (hypermobile EDS)	Joint hypermobility, chronic pain (around 90 per cent of people diagnosed have this type).
cEDS (classical EDS)	Fragile, stretchy skin, scarring caused by loss of collagen.
vEDS (vascular EDS)	Fragile skin, blood vessels and organs. Higher risk of lung collapse and aneurysm.
pEDS (periodontal EDS)	Severe GUM DISEASE, tooth loss and darker patches of skin on shins.
kEDS (kyphoscoliotic EDS)	Spinal curve and decreased muscle tone.

THE ENDOCRINE SYSTEM

While we all know what the digestive system and the nervous system are, we tend to be less familiar with the endocrine system. A 'system' just means a group of organs and tissues that work together to do the complicated tasks needed to keep us alive and healthy. The job of the endocrine system is to make and release the hormones that send messages around the body to tell it what to do – a bit like the nervous system but using chemical transmitters. It is involved in everything that goes on inside you, from your metabolism (how you convert food to energy) to sexual function, to heart rate, blood pressure and how your body responds to stress.

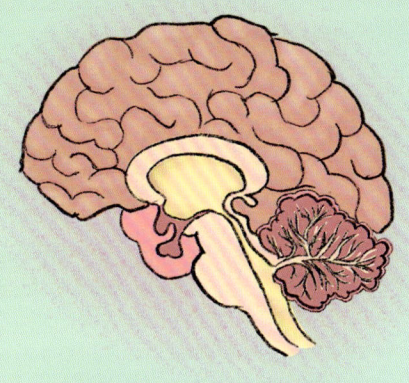

HYPOTHALAMUS, PINEAL BODY & PITUITARY GLAND

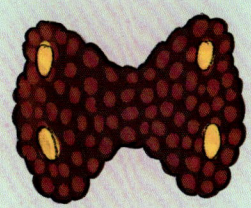

THYROID

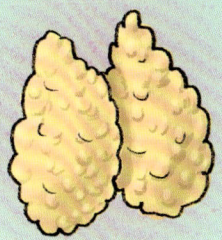

THYMUS

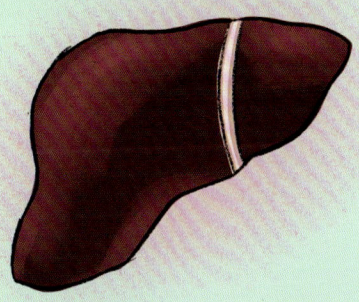

LIVER

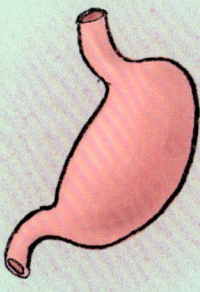

DIGESTIVE TRACT

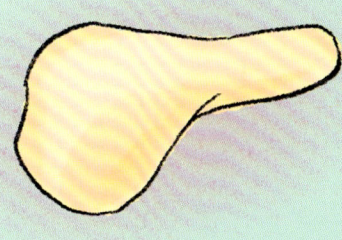

PANCREAS

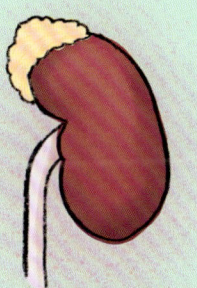

ADRENAL GLAND

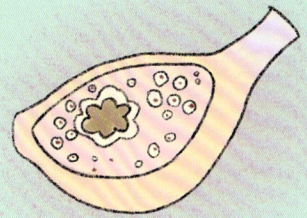

OVARY

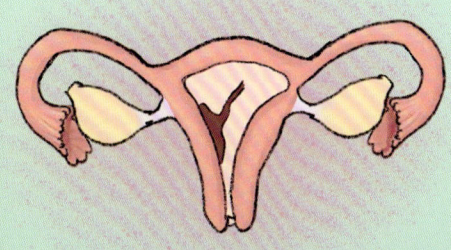

UTERUS

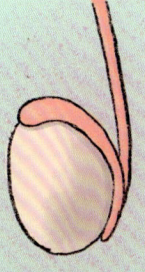

TESTES

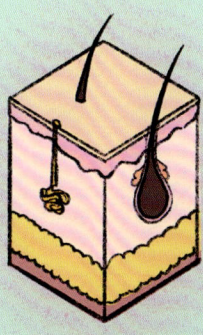

SKIN

THE ENDOCRINE SYSTEM

What is a gland?

A gland is a group of cells that makes and secretes substances that the body needs to function. Endocrine glands make and secrete hormones.

The main glands of the endocrine system are:

- Pituitary
- Adrenal
- Pineal
- Pancreas
- Thyroid
- Parathyroid
- Thymus
- Ovaries in women
- Testes in men

What can go wrong with the endocrine system?

Hormones are amazingly clever and complicated chemicals that have a massive bearing on how we function and feel. If you have too much or not enough of one hormone, or the receptors that are supposed to pass on the message aren't sensitive enough or are too sensitive, it will affect how well your body is able to do something. For example, if you have TYPE 1 DIABETES, it's because there is not enough insulin in your body. Women who have too much androgen in their bodies can have polycystic ovaries.

Problems occur because everything is interconnected. We don't always know why hormone levels become out of balance, but when they do, it can have a big knock-on effect throughout the body.

A doctor who specialises in the endocrine system, who looks at hormone disorders, is called an endocrinologist.

Diabetes

Diabetes is a chronic disease that results in high levels of blood sugar due to low levels of the hormone insulin. Left untreated, or not managed correctly, this causes symptoms in the short term; in the long term, it results in serious lifelong complications and damage. It is completely possible to live a normal life with diabetes and many people do. It's important that it's diagnosed and monitored to make sure you are getting the right treatment. The two main types are type 1 and type 2 diabetes.

Type 1 diabetes

This is an AUTOIMMUNE DISEASE where the body's immune system mistakenly destroys the insulin-producing cells in the pancreas so the body can't control blood-sugar levels. It can develop at any age but most people are diagnosed before the age of 40. Only 10 per cent of people with diabetes have type 1.

SYMPTOMS
+ **Feeling very thirsty.**
+ **Peeing more than usual.**
+ **A fruity smell on the breath, like pear drops or nail varnish remover.**
+ **Cuts and scrapes taking a long time to heal.**
+ **Weight loss.**

Left untreated or not managed properly, type 1 diabetes can cause:
- Diabetic ketoacidosis (DKA), a life-threatening condition (see page 91).
- Chronic KIDNEY DISEASE.
- Nerve damage, causing pain, tingling, itching and numbness.
- Poor circulation which, combined with nerve damage, means that the body struggles to heal itself, and sores and infections can develop in feet and legs in particular, even leading to amputation.

Diagnosis
A doctor will take samples of your blood and sometimes urine. If this suggests you have diabetes, you'll be referred to hospital for further tests to confirm the diagnosis.

Treatment
There is no cure for diabetes but it's possible to live a normal life with the correct treatment. You will have regular monitoring to make sure that you are getting the right dose of insulin and to keep an eye out for complications like cardiovascular issues. A specialist nurse or endocrinologist will tell you what you need to do on a day-to-day basis to manage the condition. Diet is an important part of this.

Many type 1 diabetics now have a wearable glucose monitor so they can constantly check their levels with an app. Some inject insulin or have a pump inserted underneath the skin that injects it automatically, and some have both. Different people will prefer different approaches, which may change over time. The injections are with a tiny needle and most people don't find them particularly painful. There is help available if you have a needle PHOBIA.

Research is being conducted into the possibility of implanting healthy insulin-producing cells from a donor or a pancreas transplant into diabetes patients – although this is currently only in experimental stages.

Type 2 diabetes

This occurs when the body doesn't produce enough insulin to deal with sugars in the blood, or the body's cells don't react to the insulin in the way they should (insulin resistance). This type of diabetes usually occurs as people get older and is linked to being overweight or OBESE and eating a high-sugar diet. Research has linked type 2 diabetes with having more fat around the pancreas and liver.

SYMPTOMS

+ Feeling very thirsty.
+ Peeing more than usual.
+ Having blurry vision.
+ Feeling very TIRED.
+ Itching around the genitals.
+ Losing weight without meaning to.
+ Sometimes there are no symptoms at all.

Left untreated, type 2 diabetes can lead to:
- Nerve damage/loss of feeling.
- HEART DISEASE and STROKE.
- Sores and infections in feet and legs.
- Vision problems.
- Kidney damage.
- ERECTILE DYSFUNCTION.

Diagnosis

A HbA1c blood test is used to check your blood-sugar levels. You might need more than one to check your levels at different times and to see how you respond to eating something sugary.

Treatment

Diet and lifestyle are big parts of effective treatment, as well as understanding your condition and what you need to do to manage it. There is lots of information at www.diabetes.org.uk.

You will usually be prescribed metformin if diet and exercise are not enough to get your blood sugar to within the right range, and some people do experience side effects. There are other medicines that can be tried.

Some people with type 2 diabetes will need to take insulin – for a short period or longer term – if other medications don't work.

Pre-diabetes

This means that you have blood-sugar levels above the usual range, but not yet high enough to be diagnosed with type 2 diabetes, although you are at a greater risk of developing it. You will be offered regular (usually yearly) blood tests and information on how to change your diet and lifestyle to reduce the risk of developing diabetes and all the health complications that come with it.

Gestational diabetes

This can occur in PREGNANCY with women who have never had issues with their blood sugar before. It can happen to anyone, although the main cause is lifestyle and having a higher baseline weight when you get PREGNANT.

Risks for the mother
- Pre-eclampsia.
- Developing type 2 diabetes later in life.
- Delivering a large baby.
- Needing a C-section.

Risks for the baby
- Respiratory distress syndrome.
- Low blood sugar/sugar withdrawal after birth.
- Developing OBESITY and/or diabetes in later life.

You will be screened for diabetes as part of your antenatal care if you are thought to be at risk. Talk to your midwife if you develop any symptoms of diabetes while PREGNANT.

Diabetes insipidus

This is a rare form of diabetes. Usually, a hormone called arginine vasopressin (AVP) or sometimes called antidiuretic hormone (ADH) tells the kidneys how much to dilute the urine – your pee is more yellow when you are dehydrated as this hormone tells your kidneys to hold onto as much water as they can. In diabetes insipidus, the message doesn't get through, so you pass more water than you should and feel thirsty and dehydrated.

SYMPTOMS

+ Peeing a lot, even at night – a healthy adult will pee four to seven times a day, children more often.
+ Peeing small amounts and often feeling like you need to go again (although this shouldn't be uncomfortable – as with a UTI).
+ Feeling very thirsty a lot of the time.
+ Experiencing symptoms of dehydration, such as HEADACHES, FATIGUE, or even collapse and SEIZURES.

Diagnosis & treatment

As the symptoms are similar to type 1 and 2 diabetes, which are more common, the doctor will want to rule these out. You will have blood tests and urine tests, and sometimes a 'water deprivation test' to see how your body responds to not drinking water.

There is medication that can replicate the job of AVP and stop the symptoms.

Diabetic emergencies

If you suffer from type 1 or type 2 diabetes, there are two types of emergencies that can occur – hypoglycaemia or hyperglycaemia. These are potentially life-threatening if not caught in time and treated.

Hypoglycaemia (low blood sugar)

This is when someone's blood-sugar level is at 3.9mmol/L or below.

SYMPTOMS

+ FATIGUE.
+ Sweating and/or shivering and shaking.
+ Restlessness or confusion.
+ Dizziness, feeling light-headed.
+ In extreme cases, having a fit or seizure, losing consciousness.

If someone is conscious & responsive

Give them something sugary to eat or drink. Fruit juice, sweets or dextrose tablets if they can chew are all good. Assess their blood sugar every 15 minutes using their own monitor or app so you know when it is stable again. If they do not have a monitor then call an ambulance as the paramedics will have one. Don't leave them alone.

If someone is unconscious

Call an ambulance. Put them in the recovery position to prevent their tongue from blocking their airway.

Hyperglycaemia (high blood sugar) leading to diabetic ketoacidosis

A short-lived blood-sugar spike is not serious if someone is able to take their medication and get their levels down. The danger is when a lack of insulin causes the liver to break down fat in your body, creating high levels of ketones in your blood. This affects type 1 diabetics and type 2 diabetics when their body doesn't use insulin properly, leading to a build-up of sugar in the bloodstream.

SYMPTOMS

+ FATIGUE or trouble staying awake.
+ Increased thirst.
+ Needing to pee a lot.
+ Confusion.
+ Nausea.
+ Laboured breathing.
+ A fruity smell to the breath.
+ Blurred vision.
+ Loss of consciousness.

Diabetics may be able to test ketone levels. A high risk reading of 1.6 to 3mmol/L indicates they should speak to their doctor. Over 3mmol/L is a medical emergency and you should call an ambulance or get them to A&E. If someone is unconscious always call an ambulance. If you can't find out their ketone levels but they have a number of the symptoms above, get help as soon as possible.

Thyroid conditions

Your thyroid is a gland in your neck. Its main job is controlling your metabolism – how your body uses energy from the food you eat. However, it has an impact on many things, such as heart rate, mood, bone health, BLOOD PRESSURE, body temperature and PREGNANCY. To do this, it produces hormones that work as messengers to tell other parts of the body what to do. Too much or too little of these hormones will lead to you experiencing symptoms. There are a number of conditions that can cause this and they are split into two main categories – hypothyroidism or hyperthyroidism – depending on whether your thyroid is producing too much or not enough hormones. Thyroid conditions can affect anyone but are more common in women.

Hypothyroidism

This occurs when your thyroid isn't producing enough hormones (also known as an underactive thyroid).

SYMPTOMS

- Feeling TIRED and low.
- Your heart beating slower than usual.
- Putting on weight for no apparent reason.
- Feeling the cold.
- Dry skin and hair.
- Abnormal bone development.
- Stunted growth.
- Heavy periods.

Diagnosis

See a doctor if you think you have an issue with your thyroid and always get lumps checked out. Thyroid issues can lead to further complications – such as problems with the eyes – if left untreated. If the doctor suspects a thyroid issue they will arrange for a blood test to check your hormone levels.

Hyperthyroidism

When your thyroid is over-producing hormones (also known as an overactive thyroid).

SYMPTOMS

- Feeling anxious, irritable or restless.
- Faster heartbeat than usual.
- Difficulty sleeping.
- Losing weight without trying to.
- Feeling sensitive to heat.
- Clammy or sweaty skin.
- Irregular menstrual cycle or a lack of periods.

Treatment

Thyroid conditions are usually treatable but not curable.

For an underactive thyroid, hormone replacement therapy in the form of a regular pill is the most common treatment.

For an overactive thyroid, you will be prescribed medication to control this or in some cases, radiotherapy will be used to reduce its size. Sometimes a section of the thyroid is removed in surgery.

Conditions that can cause hypothyroidism or hyperthyroidism

	Hypo- or hyper-thyroidism?	What is it?	Symptoms & treatment
Hashimoto's thyroiditis	Hypo	An autoimmune disease that causes the immune system to attack the thyroid.	It can cause low levels of thyroid hormones and associated symptoms. People with other autoimmune conditions seem to be more susceptible.
Prenatal hypo-thyroidism	Hypo	Thyroid hormones pass from mother to foetus and sometimes the body struggles to make enough.	FATIGUE, coldness, joint or muscle pains, constipation, low mood/DEPRESSION, hair loss in a PREGNANT woman. Treatment is with medications.
Postpartum thyroiditis	Short period of hyper followed by hypo	Inflammation in the thyroid after giving birth causing either an underactive or overactive thyroid.	Can be treated with medication and will resolve in 12–18 months of giving birth in 4 out of 5 cases.
Graves' disease	Hyper	An autoimmune disease that causes an overactive thyroid.	In addition to the typical symptoms, sufferers also often have bulging eyes and thick, discoloured skin on shins and feet. A common cause of hyperthyroidism, particularly in women.
Benign thyroid tumours	Either	Small, non-cancerous growths that start in the cell layer on the inner surface of the thyroid and cause it to produce too many hormones.	This can occur in people who have had radiotherapy to the head/neck/chest area. Treatment often includes surgery to remove the growth.
Goitre	Either	A swollen thyroid, making a lump in the neck. It can cause an overactive or underactive thyroid.	Some people experience no symptoms. Others can have a cough, a wheeze, feel like something is pressing on their windpipe or have a scratchy/husky voice. It's usually not serious but always get it checked. Not all goitres require treatment.
Thyroid cancer	Either	A cancerous tumour in the thyroid.	A hard, painless lump in the neck that gets bigger, often accompanied by a SORE THROAT, changes to the voice, weight loss and a cough. Most thyroid cancers can be treated successfully.

Adrenal gland conditions

You have two tiny adrenal glands, one on top of each kidney. The hormones they produce are involved in many processes, including controlling your salt levels, which affects BLOOD PRESSURE, cortisol levels, metabolism, sexual characteristics and how your body responds to illness.

Common adrenal gland conditions

	What is it?	Symptoms	Treatment
ADDISON'S DISEASE	Adrenal glands don't produce enough cortisol.	FATIGUE, low mood, thirst, losing weight without trying to, muscle weakness.	Lifelong medication. Sufferers can be susceptible to an ADRENAL CRISIS.
Cushing's syndrome	Adrenal glands produce too much cortisol, often in long-term steroid users or caused by a non-cancerous tumour.	Weight gain in the upper body, particularly in a 'hump' on the rear neck, a puffy face, low sex drive, skin that bruises easily and purple stretch marks.	Stop or reduce steroids or surgically remove or treat the tumour with radiotherapy. Medication can reduce the impact of cortisol.
Hyperaldosteronism	Over-production of aldosterone, causing HIGH BLOOD PRESSURE and low potassium.	HEADACHES, dizziness, vision issues, muscle weakness/spasms, HIGH BLOOD PRESSURE, TIREDNESS and excessive thirst.	If caused by a benign tumour, it can be removed or treated with radiotherapy. The main issue is to control BLOOD PRESSURE.
Congenital adrenal hyperplasia	An inherited condition where the body lacks enzymes needed to make certain hormones.	Dependent on which hormones are affected, it can impact on how the body deals with stress and affect growth or sexual development.	Usually hormone replacement medications. It is often diagnosed in newborns but milder cases may not be clear until later in childhood.
Virilisation	Over-production of male sex hormones. It can affect people who take anabolic steroids.	Increased body hair, male pattern baldness, ACNE, a deeper voice and tumours. Symptoms show before puberty and are more apparent in girls.	Surgery to remove tumours, corticosteroid or anti-androgen medication, dependent on the cause.

Causes

Adrenal gland conditions can have many different causes, and treatment will depend on what each individual cause is. The main causes are:

- Infection.
- Tumour (benign or cancerous, though cancer here is rare).
- Genetic variant.
- Certain medications.
- Issues with the PITUITARY GLAND.

Addison's disease

Addison's occurs when the adrenal glands don't produce enough cortisol. It can usually be easily treated with medication, though it is a lifelong condition. Sufferers can be susceptible to an adrenal crisis (see below).

SYMPTOMS

- FATIGUE.
- Low mood.
- Feeling thirsty but not hungry.
- Unintentional weight loss.
- Muscle weakness.

Diagnosis

Your GP will examine your skin and test for low BLOOD PRESSURE if Addison's disease is suspected. You will then be referred for a blood test and, if that shows signs of Addison's, you'll need a synacthen stimulation test to confirm the diagnosis – this involves three blood samples taken over a period of an hour before and after an injection of synacthen (a synthetic copy of the adrenocorticotrophic hormone) to see how your adrenal glands respond. Your thyroid gland may also be tested or you may have a CT or MRI scan.

Treatment

A corticosteroid medicine, such as hydrocortisone and fludrocortisone, to replace cortisol and aldosterone, usually taken as a tablet two to three times a day.

Adrenal crisis

People with Addison's disease may experience sudden worsening of symptoms, caused by a fall in cortisol levels. It's easily treatable so long as it's recognised early, however it is possible to die from an adrenal crisis if it is not treated, or to suffer long-term complications.

SYMPTOMS

- Muscle weakness and cramps.
- Loss of appetite, but craving salty foods.
- Increased thirst.
- Difficulty concentrating, dizziness and fainting.
- Darkening lips or gums.
- Abdominal pain, vomiting and diarrhoea.
- Sleepiness or drowsiness.
- HEADACHES.
- FEVER.

Treatment

Someone in an adrenal crisis needs a hydrocortisone injection immediately. If they do not have access to this call 999 and tell the operator that the person you are with has the condition.

Pituitary gland disorders

This pea-sized gland on the underside of the brain is actually the kingpin of the whole endocrine organisation. It issues instructions to almost every part of the body, including the other glands, telling them how to function. Some of the major things it has a hand in are sexual development, childbirth, growth, metabolism, how your body responds to stress and how much water and salt is in your body. So if anything goes wrong with the hormone production here, it can have a big (and complicated) knock-on effect on your body's systems and processes.

Causes

A major cause of pituitary gland disorders are benign (non-cancerous) tumours that can grow here and stop the gland working as it should. Large tumours can press on the optic nerve causing vision problems. A disruption of blood flow to the organ, such as from an EMBOLISM or THROMBOSIS, can also cause a pituitary gland disorder.

Diagnosis

Pituitary gland disorders can be diagnosed with an MRI or CT scan. The levels of hormones can also be measured by blood tests and urine tests, which may be repeated a number of times to get a fuller picture.

In the case of overproduction or underproduction of growth hormones in particular, it's important to get a diagnosis quickly, as although treatment is usually effective, not all physical changes can be reversed. Plus this comes with an increased risk of other health complications.

Treatment

Pituitary gland disorders that stem from a tumour can be managed with surgery and/or radiotherapy. Sometimes medication will help to shrink a tumour. Those that are not caused by a tumour are treated with hormone replacement therapy (cortisol, thyroid hormones and growth hormones can all be used).

The pituitary gland is referred to as the 'master gland' even though it's the size of a pea. It's a small package with a big role.

Examples of pituitary gland disorders

	What is it?	Symptoms
Acromegaly	A rare condition in which the pituitary gland produces too much growth hormone, causing a range of symptoms that come on over time.	Swelling of hands and feet; growth of nose and tongue; larger, protruding jaw. Thicker body hair; patches of skin that look thicker, velvety, oilier and darker (on all skin tones); skin tags. Increased sweating and body odour. Deeper voice; larger chest. Degenerative ARTHRITIS; a lack of energy and weakness; HEADACHES; loss of sight or double vision. Menstrual cycles may be disrupted and breasts get bigger. Men can have ERECTILE DYSFUNCTION and the thyroid gland gets larger. Children grow unusually tall.
Hypopituitarism	When the pituitary gland does not make enough hormones.	Vary from person to person and can come on quickly or over time. Adults who have gone through puberty can have problems with fertility and sexual function. Children may not go through puberty. Children can have stunted growth and adults may lose bone or muscle mass. It can also lead to HYPOTHYROIDISM.
Growth hormone deficiency	A condition where the pituitary gland produces too little growth hormone.	Slow growth, short stature, and various metabolic and physiological issues.
CUSHING'S SYNDROME	Caused by problems in the pituitary gland as well as the ADRENAL GLAND.	See page 94.
ADDISON'S DISEASE	Caused by problems in the pituitary gland as well as the ADRENAL GLAND.	See page 95.

THE HEAD & NECK

THE BRAIN & NERVE NETWORK

The nervous system is made up of the brain, the spinal cord and the nerves. It works as the body's high-tech, complex communications system. As well as being responsible for all the thinking, feeling, processing and understanding that we do to make sense of the world around us, the brain fires messages at superspeed around the body in the form of electrical impulses interplaying with hormones to let different parts know what they should be doing.

The central & peripheral nervous systems

The central nervous system is the name for the brain and the spinal cord, while everything else is the peripheral nervous system. Any issue relating to the nervous system is known as 'neurological'. There are hundreds of neurological disorders that disrupt this communication system in different ways. This means that there are many different symptoms associated with neurological conditions – for example, the fits associated with EPILEPSY or the facial muscle weakness caused by Bell's palsy.

Neurological conditions

We use the term 'cognitive function' to refer to any complex brain activities, such as understanding language, speaking, reasoning or spatial awareness. The main things that affect our cognitive function are age, lack of sleep (this is a big one), stress, poor diet, drugs and alcohol, brain injuries, tumours and neurological diseases like PARKINSON'S DISEASE and MENINGITIS.

Some neurological conditions (particularly if caused by infection) can clear on their own. Some require a lot of treatment, and those that we expect to get progressively worse, are known as degenerative neurological conditions.

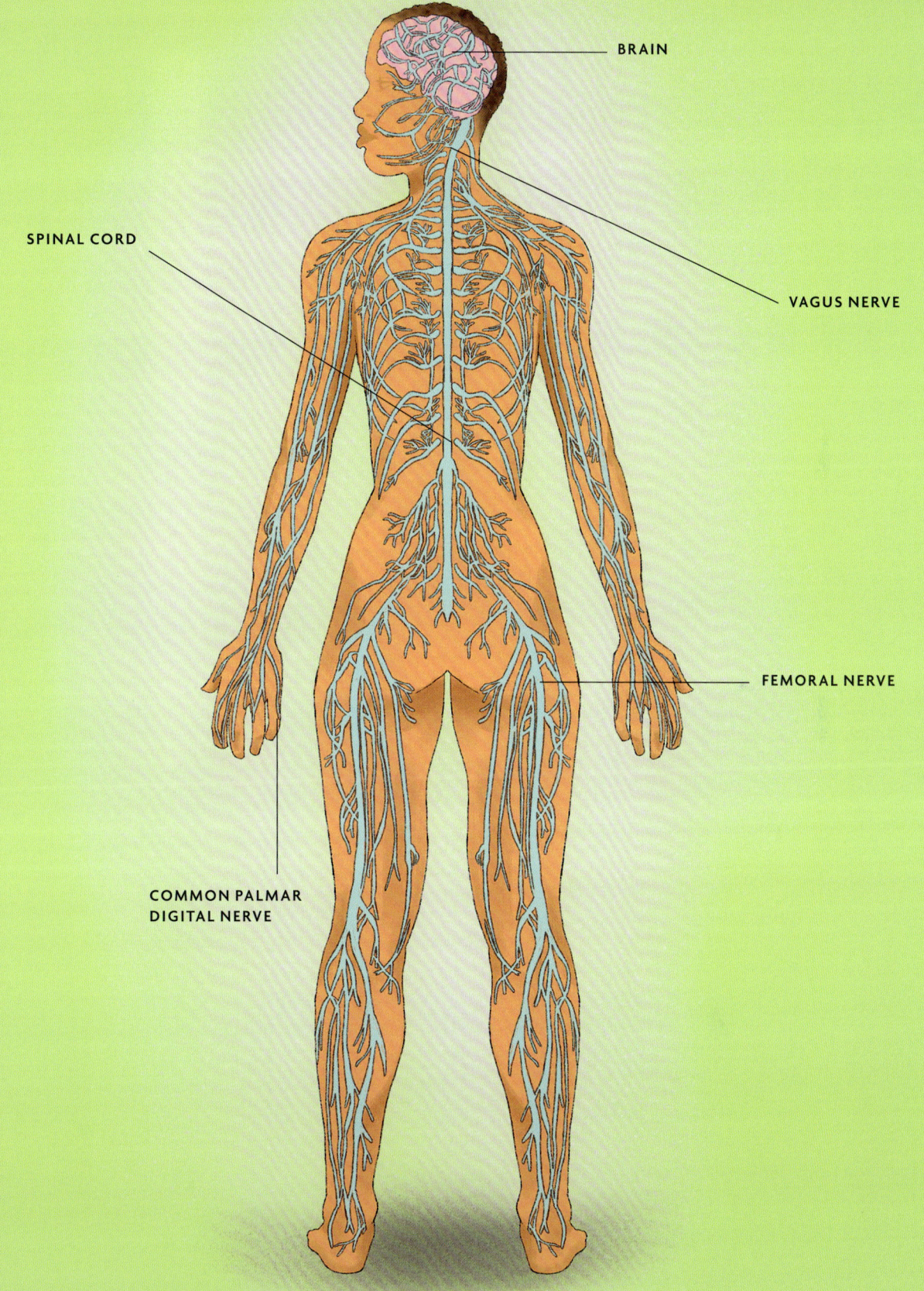

Mental health

The World Health Organization defines good mental health as 'a state of mental wellbeing that enables people to cope with the stresses of life, realise their abilities, learn well and work well, and contribute to their community. It has intrinsic and instrumental value and is integral to our wellbeing'.

When we are not in good health we struggle to do things we want and live up to our potential. If we are physically unwell, we often need professional medical advice or care from family and friends. This is also true when we are going through a period of mental ill health.

The joy and the challenge of being a human is that we have these amazing, complex brains that medicine is still trying to understand. When we go through a traumatic experience, a sudden life change or a chemical change happens in our bodies or brains, that can affect how well we are able to cope. Anyone can suffer from a period of poor mental health, and statistically, most of us will at some point. Sometimes there is no reason we can put our finger on. Mental illness is certainly NOT caused by being 'weak' or 'not good enough'.

When to seek help

Although at certain points we will all feel sad, if such bad feelings are stopping you living life, it's time to take action.

Firstly, look after your overall health with good sleep, nutrition and exercise (see pages 8–9). Human contact is also vital as we are wired to be social animals. If these things make little difference, speak to your GP, or self-refer to your local mental health team through the Every Mind Matters website (www.nhs.uk/every-mind-matters). For children, you can self-refer through Child and Adolescent Mental Health Services (CAMHS) by searching for your local service. In the NHS, you now have the legal right to choose your mental health-care provider, and your mental health team, through the 'right to choose'.

Alternatively, if you are able, you could pay privately for therapy. As there are many different approaches to therapy, it can take time to find the right one for you. Don't give up.

Where to find support
- **Samaritans**: www.samaritans.org
- **MIND**: www.mind.org.uk

Neurological red flag symptoms

People often come to me with neurological symptoms that they are worried might be a sign of something serious. While they can usually be explained by something straightforward, these are the neurological symptoms you should *never* ignore:
- An unrelenting HEADACHE that doesn't go away, particularly if it makes you vomit.
- A strange numbness or tingling on *one side* of the body only.
- Feeling unbalanced.
- Sudden changes to vision or loss of vision.
- Memory or cognitive changes, particularly forgetting words, difficulty speaking or slurred speech.
- Personality changes.

Anxiety & generalised anxiety disorder (GAD)

Anxiety is how our bodies and brains respond to something we perceive as a threat. We all encounter things that make us anxious, but generalised anxiety disorder is when we frequently feel uncontrollably anxious – not about one particular event, like a job interview, but in a way that affects our daily lives.

SYMPTOMS

- **Feelings of fear, dread and uneasiness.**
- **Trouble concentrating or making decisions.**
- **Feeling irritable, angry, tense or restless.**
- **Nausea and/or digestive problems.**
- **Heart palpitations, light-headedness.**
- **Sweating, trembling or shaking.**
- **Trouble sleeping.**
- **Feeling TIRED and 'wound up' frequently.**
- **Tingling or numbness in the hands or feet.**

Diagnosis

It's a good idea to write a list of your symptoms, triggers and underlying concerns before you talk to a doctor or therapist, to help them understand your particular experience. You may experience these symptoms sometimes, often or all the time. There is not always an identifiable trigger for anxiety – someone may not be able to explain what they are 'worried about'.

There is a seven-question survey you can find online called the GAD-7, which I use in my surgery. This survey gives a good indication of how mild or severe your anxiety is and allows you to carefully consider your symptoms. There is no physical or medical test for anxiety. It exists on a spectrum so it's not a case of you either have it or you don't.

See a GP or self-refer to your local mental health team if your anxiety:

- Is not helped by any of the management techniques discussed opposite.
- Is stopping you living a life that is 'normal' for you, for example, going to work or to your place of study.

Treatment

The first thing to do is to try to develop your own personal coping strategies to address your anxiety and its causes – everyone's experiences of anxiety, and therefore the best way to address it, will be different. Treatments can range from lifestyle changes to management techniques, talking therapies or medication, or could be a combination of them.

Lifestyle changes

- Limit alcohol intake. Alcohol may feel like a short-term reprieve, but it will only compound the problem in the long term.
- Make a list of the things you find calming, such as spending time with pets, friends, family or in nature, and certain smells or places that make you feel calm, and incorporate these into your day as much as possible.
- Exercise is great for the nervous system. Find exercises that work for you.
- Look after your gut health. In particular, complex carbohydrates are linked to serotonin production which alleviates the symptoms of anxiety, while low potassium is connected to anxiety and DEPRESSION.

Anxiety management techniques

- These techniques are all essentially aimed at calming your nervous system.
- Breathing techniques are central and useful for anyone in a stressful situation.
- Writing down your worries and dedicating a specific time to do this can help to contain them.
- The anxiety self-care section of the MIND website also has lots of management techniques to try.

Talking therapies

- Cognitive behavioural therapy (CBT) is often used as it takes a practical approach to managing symptoms.
- Applied therapy helps you to practice relaxing your muscles in anxious situations.

Medication

- If the above has little or no effect then a GP may prescribe medication, such as selective serotonin reuptake inhibitors (SSRIs) or sleeping tablets. These can have side effects such as drowsiness, HEADACHES, difficulty concentrating and gut-related symptoms including nausea, constipation or diarrhoea. Some people can also develop a dependency.
- If there is an underlying cause for the anxiety, then drugs will not help with this.
- In the short term, beta blockers can be prescribed off-licence to help in managing the physical symptoms of anxiety by preventing adrenaline from making contact with the heart's beta receptors.

What is a panic attack?

- Unlike ANXIETY, which is ongoing and chronic, panic attacks are severe and intense.
- They usually last for five to twenty minutes.
- They often appear suddenly without warning.
- Physical symptoms include a racing heart and chest pain (it can feel like you are having a HEART ATTACK), shaking, stomach knots or cramps, diarrhoea, nausea and/or vomiting.
- You may feel disconnected from your body or surroundings.

What to do if you have a panic attack

- Focus on breathing slowly and deeply (a prior knowledge of breathing exercises will be useful).
- Try to stay where you are if you can.
- Focus on what's immediately in front of you: what can you see, hear, smell and taste?
- Remind yourself that it will pass; you just need to get through the next few minutes.

See a GP or mental health professional if you are regularly experiencing panic attacks.

Be conscious of the way you speak to yourself. It can either heighten your anxiety or bring your anxiety down. Focus on your strength, your resilience and your ability to overcome challenges, rather than be consumed by fear.

Obsessive compulsive disorder (OCD)

This is a disorder which causes people to have unpleasant, obsessive thoughts and compulsive repetitive behaviours that they can't control. It's very different to just 'preferring it when things are tidy' or 'being fussy' and can make life incredibly difficult for sufferers.

The OCD spiral

Obsessive thoughts
Thoughts that take over your brain and you can't get rid of them.
'What if I left the iron on…'

Anxiety
The thought makes you feel anxious, fearful or disgusted.
'I'm terrified the house will burn down.'

Compulsion
You take a particular action to get rid of the all-consuming anxiety.
'I will drive all the way home to check.'

Temporary relief
The hit of feel-good brain chemical dopamine when the all-consuming thought and resulting anxiety is stopped strengthens a sense that giving in to a compulsive behaviour is actually a good thing. Invariably the loop will start again.
'I feel better now I know the iron wasn't on. But did I check it properly and unplug it from the wall?'

Diagnosis

OCD behaviours are a problem when they are impacting your quality of life and/or relationships. People are sometimes reluctant to seek help because of a perceived stigma. Some OCD involves intrusive thoughts that are sexual or violent, even though the person would not act on them, and this can make people feel ashamed. However, OCD is unlikely to get better by itself – you will need support. There is no shame in OCD or any other MENTAL HEALTH CONDITION. Visit your GP, who will take a note of your conditions to diagnose you.

Treatment

- Treatment is usually a talking therapy, like cognitive behavioural therapy (CBT).
- Sometimes antidepressants such as selective serotonin reuptake inhibitors (SSRIs), which can alter the balance of the chemicals in the brain, will be prescribed.
- The right treatment plan will depend on the type of OCD and any other issues the person is experiencing. For example, DEPRESSION and EATING DISORDERS are common in people with OCD.
- Important lifestyle factors include getting enough sleep, trying to stick to a regular routine and eating well. Some people report that meditation is beneficial.
- Many people feel tempted to use drugs and alcohol to quiet the intrusive thoughts. This is understandable when someone is in distress but will inevitably make symptoms worse in the medium and long term.

Addiction

Addiction is a medical condition and a lifelong disease. It is not down to a lack of willpower or some sort of personality defect. And it's not just obvious addictions, such as to alcohol and drugs, that can damage your health – addiction can affect many areas of life and can be detrimental to your wellbeing in a number of ways.

How addiction works

A vicious cycle
Like OCD, addiction often involves a loop: feeling a compulsion to seek out whatever you are addicted to; gratification followed by remorse and regret; then returning to the addiction to numb the negative feelings.

Brain chemistry
We know that addiction can change the way the brain is wired, which is known as neuroplasticity. Our brains are designed to seek rewards. But the 'buzz' you get from the thing you are addicted to overwhelms the brain's reward centres. As it adapts to this, it becomes more used to it, coming to crave it, and you need more of the substance or behaviour to get the same buzz.

SYMPTOMS
- Inability to stop, even if you want to.
- Increased tolerance, so needing to have or do more over time.
- Physical symptoms when you cannot access the thing you are addicted to, such as shaking, feeling nauseous or difficulty thinking clearly.
- Covering up or downplaying how much of the substance you use or how often you do the activity, particularly to those close to you.
- Feelings of helplessness and/or guilt.
- DEPRESSION.
- Being withdrawn.
- Putting the object of the addiction first, at the expense of relationships, work and socialising.

Types of addiction

Substance addiction
When your brain craves a particular substance, such as alcohol, nicotine (from cigarettes or vapes), illegal drugs, prescription drugs (like codeine, opioids, Adderall, sleeping pills), caffeine or sugar.

Behavioural addiction
When your brain craves a dopamine hit from particular activities, such as gambling, excessive exercise or dieting, or risky behaviours like shoplifting, sex, pornography, social media, gaming or doomscrolling.

Where to find support
The following organisations offer addiction support and advice:
- **Oasis Project** (support for women and children): www.oasisproject.org.uk
- **Alcoholics Anonymous**: www.alcoholics-anonymous.org.uk
- **Frank**: www.talktofrank.com
- **Samaritans**: www.samaritans.org
- **MIND**: www.mind.org.uk

Treatment

It is crucial to seek help for an addiction. Remember, it can happen to anyone. The long-term effects of addiction can be severe, and the longer it goes on the harder it is to treat.

- Support groups, therapy and group therapy are known to be beneficial. Often it takes trial and error to find the most supportive approach for you.
- Some addictions – such as heroin, and sometimes alcohol and cocaine – come with serious physical withdrawal symptoms that may need to be treated in a rehab facility.
- Understand your triggers so you can avoid situations that will likely activate the compulsive behaviour.
- Find ways to manage stress. Addictions often come from a coping mechanism. You can't meditate your way out of an addiction, but anything that makes you feel healthier and calmer will be supportive.
- Be prepared for relapse. Statistically, this is likely to happen to you at least once; there is no shame in it. Do not to let a slip send you back into the vicious addictive cycle. Get support as soon as possible.

Eating disorders

People develop a difficult relationship with food for many reasons. Eating disorders take different forms and exist on a spectrum of severity. There can be an assumption that an eating disorder is simply someone wanting to be thin, but the reality is often more complicated and links to conditions such as OCD and ANXIETY. Young women are the most at-risk group, but anyone can develop an eating disorder. The body wants and needs to be well-nourished, so it's always worrying when someone's psychological distress gets in the way of that.

Common eating disorders

Not everyone's issues around food will be easy to neatly categorise. Weight is not always an indication of whether someone is living with an eating disorder either, as it can be well hidden.

Anorexia
Defined by an intensely restricted diet, meaning the body is not getting adequate nutrition, resulting in low body weight. Often manifests as a PHOBIA of weight gain and distorted body image. Excessive exercise and using laxatives are also common.

Bulimia
Usually uncontrollable binge eating – often a type of 'bad' food someone has been trying to avoid – followed by a 'purge', where they make themselves sick and/or use laxatives to relieve the feeling of being uncomfortably full and to compensate for calories consumed. This is sometimes followed by fasting, until the cycle starts again.

Binge eating disorder
This involves compulsively eating large amounts of food rapidly and in secret until uncomfortably full, despite often feeling disgust, shame or guilt about doing so. This can cause someone to put on weight as they are not compelled to purge in the same way as someone with bulimia.

Pica syndrome
Eating non-food items, for example ice, soil, chalk, hair, cloth, wool, pebbles, toilet paper, laundry detergent or cornstarch. People who have learning disabilities, neurodevelopmental conditions such as AUTISM SPECTRUM DISORDER or MENTAL HEALTH CONDITIONS such as SCHIZOPHRENIA are more susceptible to developing this syndrome. It can also occur during PREGNANCY or be a sign of being ANAEMIC.

Rumination disorder

A person routinely regurgitates food that they have previously swallowed, re-chews it and then either swallows it or spits it out. In infants, rumination disorders tend to develop between three and twelve months old and often disappear on their own, but it's more complicated when adults and children are affected.

Avoidant restrictive food intake disorder (ARFID)

A lack of interest in eating or a distaste for certain smells, taste, colours or textures, sometimes triggered by trauma or stress. Lots of kids (and adults) are fussy eaters, but this is extreme and means someone is not getting enough calories or nutrients.

Orthorexia

Not a clinically recognised diagnosis but rather a term that refers to a fixation with 'clean' eating, so avoiding any foods perceived to be 'bad' or 'unhealthy'. There is a lot of confusing information about nutrition on social media, which can fuel people's anxieties around food to the point that it leads to disordered eating.

Night eating syndrome

Frequent excessive eating at night, either before going to bed or after waking up, as an attempt to get back to sleep.

Diagnosis

An eating disorder is a medical condition; the diagnosis is based on a discussion of eating habits as well as factors like weight and blood tests. However, you can get treatment for an eating problem without being diagnosed with an eating disorder.

It's so important to seek help if you're struggling with issues around food that are affecting your wellbeing. Left untreated, an eating disorder can seriously impact your health in many ways, including tooth decay, OSTEOPOROSIS, gut irritation, severe malnutrition, DIABETES and even organ failure, STROKE and HEART ATTACK. We live in a society that pushes the idea that we should be a certain size and shape, and there is no shame or blame if this is impacting you.

Treatment

It's difficult to wholly recover from an eating disorder – it has some similarities with ADDICTION in the sense that those recovering may relapse a number of times. Treatment is about learning to manage the condition, for which you will need help.

Your GP is your first port of call if you think you or someone close to you has an eating disorder. Be as open as possible with them. They will refer you for further assessment by a specialist eating disorder service. Treatment usually begins with talking therapies, but the approach will depend on the type of eating disorder and the root causes (of which there are many). Beat (www.beateatingdisorders.org.uk) and the National Centre for Eating Disorders (www.eating-disorders.org.uk) offer advice and support.

Take each day as it comes; things don't need to be perfect. Think of each meal or snack as a tiny step in your recovery.

Personality disorders

Someone who has a personality disorder thinks and feels very differently to a person who does not. This affects their emotions, which they may have difficulty controlling, and their social interactions. Borderline personality disorder was previously the most commonly diagnosed kind. Although, rather than trying to distinguish between the formerly identified types, the guidance in the UK is now to figure out if someone has a personality disorder and to categorise it as 'mild', 'moderate' or 'severe'.

SYMPTOMS

Emotions:
+ Intense, overwhelming, changeable emotions.
+ Going from feeling very happy to very sad quite quickly.
+ Emotions are easily destabilised (known as affective dysregulation).

Disturbed thinking patterns:
+ Feeling uncontrollably paranoid or angry in moments of stress.
+ Feeling like everyone else knows how to behave 'normally' and you don't.
+ Unstable sense of who you are and what you want.

Impulsive behaviour:
+ Might be reckless with safety – such as driving dangerously, substance abuse or unsafe sex – or go on unplanned spending or gambling sprees.
+ Impulsive behaviour around food, which can lead to EATING DISORDERS.

Difficult relationships with others:
+ Very intense friendships and romantic relationships that end suddenly.
+ Terrified of being abandoned.
+ Find it hard to understand that not everyone feels things as intensely as you do.

Diagnosis

Lots of people don't like the term 'personality disorder' because they think it implies there is something wrong with their personality. That is perfectly reasonable but it's important to understand that this is a MENTAL HEALTH CONDITION and it's not anyone's fault. So see a GP if you are struggling with these symptoms.

An assessment will be carried out on your feelings and behaviour, to try to rule out other MENTAL HEALTH CONDITIONS, and to identify any other factors, such as ANXIETY or DISORDERED EATING.

Treatment

Usually, therapy is carried out by trained professionals from the community mental health team. An effective treatment may last a year or more but can be really effective in helping to manage emotions and make the patient feel much better. After treatment, the community mental health team will develop a future crisis plan so the patient knows who to call if needed. There are also pop-up cafes available for patients to chat with members of the community mental health team when needed.

Bipolar disorder

Bipolar disorder is characterised by extreme mood swings, from energetic and sometimes euphoric highs to feeling very low. This is disorientating, as someone with bipolar can feel and seem like a very different person depending on whether they are experiencing a high or low.

SYMPTOMS

Highs:
+ Intense happiness.
+ Agitation.
+ Irritability.
+ Emotional intensity.
+ Higher than usual sex drive.
+ Making plans.
+ Speaking too quickly.
+ Impulsive.
+ More likely to spend money.

Lows:
+ Feelings of sadness or hopelessness.
+ Low self-esteem.
+ Withdrawal from friends, family or colleagues.
+ Lack of interest in sex.
+ Trouble sleeping (or sleeping too much).
+ Lack of appetite or overeating.

There are often periods in between where symptoms mostly go away and mood is stable.

Psychosis

Someone with bipolar disorder may experience psychosis during a manic episode (although not everyone does). Psychosis means that their perception of reality changes and is very different to those around them. For example, they may find hidden meaning or patterns in words or events, or believe they have the answers to a global problem.

Diagnosis

Bipolar disorder is difficult to diagnose. A blood test may be done to rule out other conditions (such as HYPOTHYROIDISM) but a GP will then need to make a referral to a psychiatrist. Diagnosis is by carefully assessing previous experiences of extreme highs and lows. Because the onset of the condition is often marked by a depressive episode (and these also tend to happen more often thereafter), it can be misdiagnosed as DEPRESSION.

Some people with bipolar disorder might not recognise it as an issue if they have systems in place to contain manic episodes, as they might feel very creative and productive during these times.

Treatment

There is no cure for bipolar disorder, but the severity and the frequency of episodes can be reduced or prevented with the right combination of medication and therapy.

- People with bipolar disorder generally find regular exercise very helpful.
- It's important to avoid illicit drugs and limit or stop drinking alcohol.
- Most people will have triggers – such as stress or overwork, or anything that disrupts circadian rhythms like travel across time zones – which they can learn to identify and develop strategies to manage.

Schizophrenia

Schizophrenia is a lifelong chronic MENTAL HEALTH CONDITION with serious symptoms. It can be managed with the right treatment, allowing for a normal and fulfilling life. It is often misrepresented – it does not involve having a 'split personality' and does not mean someone is violent.

Causes

We don't yet know what causes schizophrenia. However, we think that some people are more vulnerable to it and that there may be a genetic cause. Drug and alcohol misuse, along with high stress and trauma (especially childhood trauma) can trigger an episode.

SYMPTOMS

Schizophrenia affects the way you think, feel and behave. It can manifest in the following ways:
+ Hallucinations and hearing voices.
+ Unusual beliefs not based on reality (see psychosis on page 110).
+ Muddled thoughts and speech.
+ Seeming sleepy and out of it or excessively emotional.
+ Withdrawing from and avoiding people.
+ Ignoring your own needs, such as hygiene and meals.

Left untreated, it can lead to severe, compounding problems, such as declining physical health through self-neglect, social isolation and lack of support, and other MENTAL HEALTH CONDITIONS like ANXIETY and OCD, and even attempted suicide.

Diagnosis

Schizophrenia tends to be diagnosed at a late stage, when someone is already experiencing psychosis. However, it is of course easier to help someone if the condition is caught early. There is no single test; rather a diagnosis is made by a psychiatrist, following a referral by a GP.

Treatment

This is usually antipsychotic medications and cognitive behavioural therapy. If someone is unwell to the point where they are refusing or forgetting to take medication, antipsychotics can be given as injections or implants. There should also be day-to-day support available from a community mental health team.

Many people 'recover' from schizophrenia by getting the right help and learning to understand and manage the condition, although occasional relapses are likely. Friends and family knowing the signs and symptoms to look out for can be a big help.

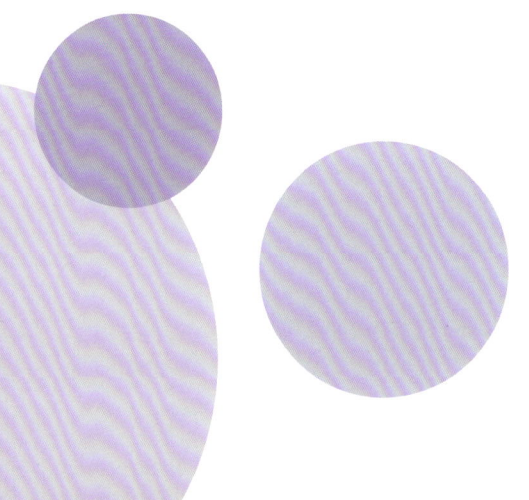

Depression

We don't know what causes someone to suffer from depression, but we believe it comes from a chemical imbalance in the brain – a lowering of dopamine (the happy, motivational hormone) and an increase in cortisol and noradrenaline (the stress hormones). It came come on after a difficult or life-changing event, or there may be no identifiable single cause. It can come and go, and affects how you feel and the way you think as well as physical health. It's a serious condition that should not be made light of.

Symptoms

You don't have to be unable to get out of bed or be constantly crying to be suffering from depression. Most people will have a combination of some of the following symptoms that persists for at least two weeks.

Psychological	Cognitive	Physical
Feeling emotionally numb	Difficulty focusing	Regular HEADACHES
Feeling bleak or empty	Poor memory, brain fog	Digestive issues, such as stomach pains, diarrhoea or constipation
Lack of motivation	Struggling to make decisions	Poor sleep/insomnia or early wakening
Low self-esteem, feeling worthless	Extreme/unusual procrastination	Dry skin
Feeling constantly guilty	Decrease in energy	Thinning hair
Filling your day with constant tasks and distractions to avoid having time to think	Decreased interest in sex	Constantly picking up bugs and feeling under the weather
Catastrophising		Twitching muscles
Tearfulness		
ANXIETY, nervousness, feeling 'on edge'		
Thoughts of suicide		

Diagnosis

Your GP will conduct a screening questionnaire (PHQ9) as well as a blood test to rule out other conditions that could be causing your symptoms. The PHQ9 questionnaire is available online but I'd discourage you from self-diagnosis as it's important to see a medical professional. They will also advise symptom-tracking for at least two weeks to look out for key behaviours.

Treatment

For mild depression

Everyone suffering from some degree of depression should try to do the following, as far as they are able, as these things will support the mind and the body.

- Stay in touch with people who care about you; try not to withdraw.
- Remind yourself that feeling this way does not make you 'weak' or a 'failure'. It happens to lots of people and it can't be cured by 'pulling yourself together' or 'toughening up'.
- Talk about how you feel to those you trust (you may even help someone else who is struggling by being open about your feelings).
- Find a form of exercise you enjoy and try to do it regularly.
- Spend time outside in nature – even ten minutes will increase your dopamine hormone.
- Ideally avoid, or limit, alcohol. It's tempting to want to numb negative feelings but for many reasons this will make things worse.
- Don't take illicit drugs.
- Don't smoke, or cut down as much as you can.
- Eat a nutritious diet – 90–95 per cent of serotonin (that vital 'happy hormone') is made in the gut.
- Try to get good, regular sleep to stimulate your melatonin hormone.
- Limit social media use to what is genuinely beneficial, like checking in with friends. Avoid 'doomscrolling' or comparison traps.
- Try to keep up hobbies and interests that you ordinarily enjoy – don't give up on something because you find it unsatisfying on a couple of occasions.
- Consider exploring therapy by self-referral to NHS Talking Therapies or privately if you can afford to do so.

For moderate or serious depression

- Speak to your GP and tell them how you are feeling.
- If you are registered with a GP in the UK, you can refer yourself to talking therapies.
- Cognitive behavioural therapy (CBT) is usually the starting point for someone suffering from depression, although there are other types that will benefit different people.
- Selective serotonin reuptake inhibitors (SSRIs) may be prescribed. We don't know how exactly they work on the brain, but they can be helpful for people suffering long-term depression.

Caring for someone with depression

When someone has depression, it can have a big impact on the lives of those around them, who may feel worried, frightened, frustrated, even angry and powerless to help. It can also affect relationships. If your partner, parent or child is suffering from long-term depression, you may need support to cope. If you are caring for someone with the disease in the UK, you may be eligible for carer's support.

Red flag symptom

If you feel that you are in crisis and you may harm yourself, tell someone you trust and/or in the UK contact the Samaritans on 116 123, or text SHOUT to 85258. If you're under 35 you can also call Papyrus on 0800 068 4141.

Phobias & post-traumatic stress disorder (PTSD)

Phobias and PTSD are different but related as they are often triggered by a stressful or traumatic experience.

Phobias can be portrayed as amusing, but having an uncontrollable fear of something your rational mind knows to be harmless can be debilitating and have a big impact on your life.

We throw around the term 'PTSD' a lot but there is a specific criteria for diagnosing someone's symptoms. However, there is no measure of trauma that you must have been through – it's about the effect it has had on you.

Types & treatment

	Phobia	PTSD
Definition	A specific uncontrollable fear or ANXIETY around a particular object or situation.	An ANXIETY disorder with ongoing symptoms resulting from a traumatic experience.
Types	**Social phobia:** Deep discomfort in specific social situations for fear of being embarrassed, e.g. eating in public or public speaking. **Bodily phobia:** For example, of being sick or losing control of bowels. **Specific phobia:** Of an object or situation, e.g. fear of heights or spiders.	**Delayed onset PTSD:** When symptoms appear six months or more following trauma. **Complex PTSD (C-PTSD):** When someone has suffered repeated trauma over a period of time, rather than one terrifying event. **Birth trauma:** This can come on even years after a woman has been through a difficult birth.
Symptoms	Strong bodily fear response, e.g. shaking, sweating, increased heartrate. Sometimes dizziness, nausea or diarrhoea.	Flashbacks, feeling jumpy or on edge, having trouble sleeping, feeling alone, losing interest in activities, feeling overwhelmed, irritable or angry, emotional outbursts, low mood.
Cause	Often unknown, although in some cases brought on by a frightening experience or learned behaviour. Phobias are often related to a fear of not being in control.	Develops in the aftermath of living through a shocking, scary or dangerous event.
Treatment	Most people don't seek treatment for a phobia unless it starts affecting how they live their lives. Counselling and CBT can be effective. Exposure or desensitisation therapy gradually introduces the object of the fear. In serious cases, medication like beta blockers can be prescribed to treat symptoms.	PTSD doesn't often 'just go away' – it will usually require treatment or it can lead to many other issues. Medication such as paroxetine, sertraline and venlafaxine can help. Therapy is effective, particularly eye movement desensitisation and reprocessing (EMDR). It's one of the most studied and widely recommended treatments and is available on the NHS.

Neurodivergence

ADHD, AUTISM, dyslexia and dyspraxia are forms of neurodivergence. 'Neurodivergent' is a general, non-medical term which means someone's brain processes information and learns differently from what is considered to be 'typical' or 'usual'. Importantly, neurodivergent conditions are not mental illnesses. Some people who are neurodivergent feel they struggle because the world is not set up for how they think. Many also feel that seeing the world differently can be an advantage. It's currently thought that one in seven – although it may well be more – people are neurodivergent.

Neurodivergence exists on a spectrum. And because we are complex, multifaceted humans, it interacts with our personalities, what has happened to us in our lives, and all the other things that make us who we are. This all means that one person's experience of a neurodivergent condition is very different from another's.

Attention deficit hyperactivity disorder (ADHD)

There are three categories of ADHD, to describe people who are more generally hyperactive, inattentive, or who combine elements of both. You do not have be hyperactive to be diagnosed with ADHD.

ADHD in children

Boys who are disruptive in class, displaying clear signs of hyperactivity, are most likely to be diagnosed, whereas girls are often better at masking their ADHD traits. It's only recently that the way ADHD shows up in different genders has started to be properly examined. This is partly why a lot of women with ADHD are being diagnosed in adulthood.

SYMPTOMS
- **Struggling to concentrate on one thing at a time.**
- **Impulsive or reckless behaviour.**
- **Restlessness and sometimes uncontrollable energy.**

Diagnosis
You can speak to your doctor, who will need to refer your child for assessment by a specialist. They will want to know:
- Behaviours or traits that are concerning you.
- How they impact your child's day-to-day life.
- Any recent significant events or life changes.
- Any other health conditions (your doctor may want to do a physical examination to rule out other causes).

Your doctor may suggest a period of 'watchful waiting' to monitor your child before referring them for an assessment.

Treatment
This depends on the age of the child and how their ADHD is affecting them. A combination of therapy and medication is thought to be best.
- The most commonly prescribed drug is methylphenidate, although there are others.
- Behaviour therapy can help a child learn how to control the elements of the ADHD that cause them problems.
- Parent training/education can be very useful for learning how best to help and encourage your child.

ADHD in adults

It is believed that it is not possible to develop ADHD as an adult; you have to have had it since childhood. ADHD traits in adults are also harder to define for a number of reasons, and there may be crossover with OCD, PERSONALITY DISORDERS and BIPOLAR DISORDER.

SYMPTOMS

- Difficulty concentrating.
- Constantly starting new tasks but not finishing them.
- Restlessness and/or impatience.
- Regularly losing and forgetting things.
- Poor organisational and prioritising skills.
- Mood swings and getting easily annoyed.
- Taking risks.
- Difficulty maintaining relationships.

Diagnosis

Your GP may refer you for an assessment with a specialist if your symptoms are causing you difficulties, you do not have another MENTAL HEALTH CONDITION that is a likely cause, and you have had similar symptoms since you were a child.

Treatment

A combination of therapy and medication is thought to be best.

- Drugs like methylphenidate are found to be effective by many. You do not have to take it forever; in consultation with your doctor, you can see how it helps you and decide if you want to continue. Bear in mind that it is not a cure.
- Therapy to learn coping skills and address emotional and behavioural issues.
- Exercise is hugely beneficial for many as it improves focus and mood.
- Getting enough sleep is particularly important for people with ADHD.

You are not broken if you are neurodivergent. It could be your superpower.

Autism

The full medical term is autism spectrum disorder (ASD) and the autism spectrum is wide and varied. There is a huge variation in how autistic people present. Some autistic people are non-verbal and may need help with day-to-day tasks; others may show little or no obvious traits and live completely independently with little or no support. Just like neurotypical people, those with autism can have any level of intelligence.

SYMPTOMS

It's worth noting that not every autistic person will demonstrate these traits, as many become adept at masking in social situations or at work or school.
+ Difficulty socialising and communicating, particularly reading tone of voice and body language.
+ Intense, limited interests.
+ Finding bright, crowded or noisy places overwhelming.
+ Stimming, or 'self-stimulating behaviour' – such as hand flapping, making a sound or fiddling with an object – as a way to soothe or manage excess energy and ANXIETY.

Diagnosis

Symptoms usually appear by age two, but autism can be diagnosed at any age. This can be the first step to understanding what support a person might need so that they can get on well at work, school or university, so early diagnosis is useful. An early diagnosis can also be important for the individual's self-esteem, allowing them to understand a little more about how their brain functions and how this might differ from the neurotypical people around them.

Diagnosis is via a series of assessments and observations carried out by an autism specialist. You can be referred for an assessment by your GP or, in the case of a child, your health visitor, a school special education needs co-ordinator or another health professional, such as a therapist. It is very useful to pre-prepare a list of all the signs of autism you have noticed in yourself or your child.

Treatment

Many different therapies are available to support an autistic child or adult to live their life as fully as possible, such as:
- Cognitive behavioural therapy to manage ANXIETY.
- Speech and language therapy to develop communication skills.
- Physical therapy to help with movement and balance.

Autism & mental health

Studies and clinical experience have shown that individuals with ASD are four times more likely to experience DEPRESSION in their lifetime, compared to neurotypical individuals. According to the National Autism Society (UK), approximately three in ten autistic adults in the UK also have ADHD and 28 per cent of autistic children are diagnosed with ADHD. According to Epilepsy Action UK, the risk of developing EPILEPSY could be as high as 40 per cent in people with autism who have severe learning difficulties.

This does not mean that having autism can cause these conditions, but it is suggested that having such conditions is likely due to the fact that similar genetic, neurobiological and environmental factors can cause them to develop. Because of this, individuals with ASD should be regularly screened and offered treatment for DEPRESSION, ADHD and EPILEPSY as there are management plans that could be put in place to support them.

Debunking myths

Vaccines do not cause autism – this is a conspiracy theory based on a long-debunked study.

Dementia & Alzheimer's Disease

Dementia is an overarching general term to refer to a range of symptoms relating to a decline in memory and thinking skills. Alzheimer's Disease is the most common cause of dementia, present in over 60 per cent of cases.

Different types & causes of dementia

There are a number of different types of dementon, all caused by damage to brain cells. These include:

- **Dementia with Lewy bodies:** one of the most common types of dementia, caused by clumps of protein forming inside brain cells. Individuals with dementia with Lewy bodies are less likely to experience memory loss as an early symptom than with other types.
- **Vascular dementia:** caused by a reduction in blood flow to the brain, due to vascular disease.
- **Frontotemporal dementia:** covers a range of less common dementia types, caused by changes in the brain's frontal and temporal lobes.
- **Young-onset dementia:** covers dementia of any cause in which symptoms develop before the age of 65.
- **Alzheimer's Disease:** the most common cause of dementia. It occurs when a build-up of proteins in the brain damages nerve cells. We don't yet fully understand why this happens, although we now know that the APOE4 gene increases your risk of developing Alzheimer's.
- **Mixed dementia:** more than one type of dementia

Symptoms of dementia often come on slowly over time, so they may be attributed to the natural aging process. Importantly, becoming more forgetful doesn't automatically mean you have dementia, although it's important to see your GP if you notice changes to your memory or thinking abilities, or if people close to you notice a difference in your character or behaviour.

There are a number of underlying conditions that could be responsible, such as THYROID CONDITIONS. Opposite are some of the early symptoms of different causes of dementia.

SYMPTOMS OF DEMENTIA WITH LEWY BODIES

Movement issues:
+ Lack of coordination.
+ Poor balance.
+ Stiffness.
+ Shaking.

Cognitive issues:
(Note that memory loss is less likely to be an early symptom with this type of dementia.)
+ Occasional confusion.
+ Changes to sense of smell and taste.
+ Sleeping in the day (if this isn't usual).
+ Sometimes hallucinations.

SYMPTOMS OF FRONTOTEMPORAL DEMENTIA

Social issues:
+ Struggling to recognise the emotions of others.
+ Strange or inappropriate behaviour.
+ Less interest in socialising.

Cognitive issues:
+ Symptoms depend on which specific part of the brain is affected first but memory is less likely to be an issue early on.
+ Difficulty with words, such as recalling the correct word or using the wrong words.
+ Unable to recognise people.
+ Lack of concentration.
+ Unable to make decisions.

SYMPTOMS OF YOUNG-ONSET DEMENTIA

People who develop dementia young (under the age of 65) may have more unusual symptoms, such as:
+ Mood, behaviour and personality changes.
+ Confusion.
+ Memory problems.
+ Difficulty with speech and movement.

SYMPTOMS OF VASCULAR DEMENTIA

Cognitive issues:
+ Problems following instructions.
+ Difficulties with learning new information.
+ Finding it hard to find the right word.
+ Difficulties with reading, writing and following conversations.

Emotional issues:
+ Changes in behaviour.
+ Getting upset easily.
+ Lacking interest in others.

Movement issues:
+ Loss of balance.
+ Weakness on one side of the body.

SYMPTOMS OF ALZHEIMER'S DISEASE

Cognitive issues:
+ Short-term memory loss.
+ Repeating oneself.
+ Losing things.
+ Feeling disorientated.
+ Forgetting words.
+ Poor judgement.

Emotional issues:
+ Feeling low, anxious or wound-up.
+ Loss in confidence or interest in others and/or activities.

Diagnosis

There is no test for dementia. The doctor will do tests to rule out other causes and will want to know about your symptoms, and in particular what changes you have been experiencing. It's very useful to prepare a list and keep a symptom diary. They may carry out a memory test and refer you to a specialist. Sometimes you will receive a 'possible' or 'probable' diagnosis, when they can't know for sure and need to monitor you.

Even if dementia is unconfirmed, it is still very beneficial to receive an early diagnosis if possible, because:
- Some drugs and treatments, if started early, will slow down the progression of the disease.
- Lifestyle changes – such as improving your diet, exercise and therapy to help with memory and mood – will be more effective in the early stages before the disease progresses further.
- You will be able to make plans and decisions for your future while you are able to think clearly.

Treatment

There is a lot of research being done in this area but at the moment there is no cure for any form of dementia. We can treat the symptoms but we can't fix the damage that has and is being done to brain cells to stop it getting worse. Some people will find that the medication available allows them to get on with their day-to-day activities for a while, and some will find it makes little difference. Everyone with dementia will experience a decline and will ultimately require progressively more care. The life expectancy varies greatly between individuals and depends on many factors. The average life expectancy for someone diagnosed with Alzheimer's in the UK is currently eight to ten years.

Preventable causes of dementia

A recent study found as much of 45 per cent of dementia is caused by factors preventable on either an individual or societal level. These include education standards, social isolation and air pollution, as well as high CHOLESTEROL, physical inactivity and smoking.

Parkinson's disease

Parkinson's is a neurological disease that gets worse over time. It's caused by a loss of dopamine-producing nerve cells in a particular part of the brain. We don't know why this happens, and research is ongoing. It can run in families and slightly more men are diagnosed than women. It is possible to develop symptoms under the age of 40, but most people are diagnosed in their 50s.

SYMPTOMS

As Parkinson's develops gradually, it's often not picked up until someone is already quite badly affected. There are over 40 symptoms, and they vary between individuals, and from day to day.

Early symptoms:
+ Muscle tremors, stiffness, slowing movement.
+ Insomnia.
+ Restless legs syndrome.
+ Change in handwriting, particularly becoming larger or smaller.
+ Needing to go to the toilet more often.
+ DEPRESSION and/or ANXIETY.
+ Feeling occasionally very TIRED for no apparent reason.

Further symptoms as the disease progresses:
+ Speech changes, such as slurring.
+ Difficulty swallowing.
+ Feeling unbalanced, difficulty walking.
+ Pain throughout the body.
+ Involuntary movement caused by painful muscle contractions (dystonia).
+ Difficulty controlling bowels and/or bladder.

Diagnosis

There is no singular test for Parkinson's. A doctor will perform an examination and carry out an assessment while you complete some physical tasks and then send you for tests – often blood tests, MRI and a SPECT scan – partly to rule out other causes. A DaTscan measures dopamine levels, which can indicate the disease, although it is not conclusive by itself. It is very useful to keep a symptom diary.

Treatment & prognosis

There are medications that can slow the progress of the disease. Complementary therapies like physiotherapy, acupuncture and yoga, to keep muscles active, can be very beneficial. Some people will find talking therapy useful after receiving their diagnosis.

Some people will be made progressively more disabled by Parkinson's. However, others respond well to medication and will be able to carry on living active lives for some time. Parkinson's is not fatal, but as the disease progresses, it makes people vulnerable to life-threating illnesses.

Parkinson's disease & dementia

These two conditions are closely linked; people who have Parkinson's disease are more likely to develop DEMENTIA. A particular kind of DEMENTIA, called DEMENTIA WITH LEWY BODIES (DLB), causes Parkinson's symptoms. **If you've noticed changes in your thinking and memory, you should talk to your GP.**

Headaches & migraine

A headache is a symptom, not a diagnosis. There are over 150 different types that can be caused by something as simple as mild dehydration. While it's helpful to know the cause, headaches are the commonest symptom that we know the least about, which can be frustrating for regular sufferers.

Tension headache

This common headache can be caused by FATIGUE, stress, issues with the muscles or joints of the neck (often exacerbated by poor sleeping position) or dehydration.

SYMPTOMS
+ A dull, squeezing pain on both sides of the head.
+ Lasts 20 minutes to 2 hours.
+ Can also cause pain in the shoulders and neck.

Treatment
- Over-the-counter pain relief such as paracetamol, ibuprofen and aspirin for those over 16.
- Heat pads or warm showers.
- Having something to eat and drinking water.
- Relaxation techniques, such as yoga and massage.
- Wearing a mouth guard if you grind your teeth.

See a GP if you get a lot of tension headaches. They may be able to prescribe tricyclic antidepressants or naproxen.

Medication overuse headaches
Corticosteroids (anti-inflammatories), opioids and other painkillers can trigger headaches if used too often or for too long. Migraine sufferers can be vulnerable to a vicious cycle of taking pain relief, becoming addicted, then the withdrawal making the headache much worse. Keep a record of your painkiller intake and speak to your GP if concerned.

Cluster headaches

These are uncommon but severe, and men have them far more than women.

SYMPTOMS
+ Sudden intense headaches on one side of the head.
+ Occurs multiple times in a day, regularly over a period of weeks or months.
+ Occurs at the same time of day or year (as changes in seasonal light and barometric pressure can influence the timings of a cluster headache).
+ Watery red eye on the same side as the headache, the eyelid may droop.
+ Runny or blocked nose.
+ Restlessness and agitation.
+ Nausea.
+ Hypersensitivity to light and sound.

Treatment
Over-the-counter painkillers will not work for cluster headaches. Prevention is key, for which verapamil or lidocaine nose drops may be prescribed. Once a cluster headache has started, if the pain is unbearable, it will need to be treated in hospital with oxygen and an injection of triptans.

Red flag symptoms

It's unlikely that a persistent headache is the sign of something serious, but these are the signs that you should get checked out by a doctor:

- You are over 50 and suddenly start to get sudden, severe 'thunderclap' headaches.
- You also have brain fog or memory issues, or there's been a change to your personality.
- You also have a FEVER, stiff neck, confusion and are feeling 'out of it' (see MENINGITIS).
- You also have neurological symptoms, such as vision changes, slurred speech, weakness or numbness.
- You have a SEIZURE.
- You also have a sore red eye or pain at the temples.
- You've had a blow to the head (see HEAD INJURY).
- You regularly have a headache when you wake up in the morning.
- You can't do your daily activities because of a persistent headache.
- You have, or have a history of, cancer.

Migraine

This is an inflammatory genetic condition. It often runs in families and is caused by changes to the brain's blood flow and nerve cell activity. Migraines come on suddenly and are much more common in women.

SYMPTOMS

- A throbbing pain, increasing in intensity.
- An 'aura' – seeing a sort of halo, sparkles or flashing lights, wavy lines, or even temporary vision loss.
- Numbness or tingling in one side of the body.
- Nausea.
- Watery eyes, runny nose.

Causes

Migraines often have specific triggers:

- Stress or ANXIETY.
- Changes in the weather.
- Lack of or too much sleep.
- Bright or flickering lights, loud noises.
- Too much screentime.
- Diet, particularly alcohol (especially red wine), chocolate, nitrates in cured fish and meats, aged cheeses and Monosodium glutamate (MSG).
- An increase or decrease in caffeine.

Treatment

Start migraine treatment as soon as you feel one coming on – don't wait for it to reach its peak and then take painkillers. The best approach to stopping an attack is this combination, taken with food unless you are vomiting. This combination can be re-taken after 4 hours if necessary, up to 3 times in a 24-hour period:

- 300mg of aspirin.
- Stomach-protecting tablets like omeprazole or lansoprazole, if you're nauseous or have acid REFLUX.
- 400mg ibuprofen.
- 2 × 500g paracetamol tablets.

If that stops working for you, your doctor may prescribe the following, with all of the below except for triptans being shown to reduce the frequency of migranes:

- Triptans to treat the migraines.
- Tricyclic antidepressants.
- Anti-seizure medication.
- Beta blockers, which can help prevent migraines.

There is no conclusive data regarding supplements but magnesium and vitamin B_2 in combination are thought to help by bringing down inflammation and reduce the frequency of attacks.

Sinus headache

This is caused by an infection in the sinuses (SINUSITIS) which leads to excess swelling.

SYMPTOMS

- Pain in the forehead, around the nose, eyes and cheeks.
- The pain increases if you lean forward or look up, adding pressure to your sinuses.
- Can cause dizziness or clumsiness.
- Excess mucus and bad breath.
- A feeling of pressure in the ears.
- FEVER.
- Toothache, particularly in the upper teeth.

Treatment

If it is caused by a viral infection, it will go away once the infection clears, but a bacterial infection will need antibiotics. In the meantime, a pharmacist can advise on treatments to ease your symptoms. Rest, fluids and cleaning your nose with a salt-water solution can also help. See a GP if you are still experiencing pain after three weeks or if the pain is recurrent.

Head injury (concussion)

A head injury, also known as concussion, is a mild brain injury that results from a blow to the head, such as from a fall or impact when playing sport. It's not usually serious and recovery will take one or two weeks. However, caution should be exercised with young children who can't communicate well how they feel. Bear in mind that there may be minimal visible damage but there could be bleeding or swelling in the brain that you can't see. Repeated concussions can cause permanent damage to the brain.

SYMPTOMS

Straight after a blow to the head, it's normal to:
+ Have a HEADACHE.
+ Feel a bit sick.
+ Feel disorientated or confused.
+ Have a ringing in the ears.
+ Have a bump on the head.

While these symptoms should clear quickly, it is possible for symptoms to develop up to three weeks later. Look out for changes to personality, mood and behaviour, or ongoing difficulty concentrating.

Diagnosis

Diagnosed by physical examination: getting someone to walk in a straight line heel to toe, as you would to test if they were drunk, can be a good way to check their balance. If their balance is off, then take them to A&E.

Treatment

It's a good idea to have someone stay with you for 24 hours after sustaining a minor head injury, and if you are caring for someone who has had a concussion, ensure their other caregivers are aware of what has happened and when. Normal activity can usually resume two days after a head injury if you no longer have any symptoms but you shouldn't particpate in sports for at least two weeks.

Red flag symptoms

Go to A&E if:
- You lost consciousness when the injury happened.
- You fell from a height.
- You have a persistent HEADACHE that painkillers don't touch.
- You take medication to thin your blood.
- You've been sick.
- You've ever had brain surgery.
- You are having problems with your balance.
- One pupil looks bigger than the other.
- You have a prolonged feeling that the room is spinning or you have a sense of VERTIGO.

Never drive yourself to A&E if you have had a head injury. With young children, look out for behavioural signs like being off their food, disinterest in toys or crying more than usual and go to A&E if you have any concerns. It's much better to get it checked out.

Call an ambulance if:
- Someone is unresponsive or you can't get them to stay awake.
- They can't stand up without falling.
- They are having or have had a SEIZURE.
- They fell from a height of more than 1 metre (3 feet) – roughly the height of five stairs.
- They hit their head at speed, such as in a car accident.
- They have severe neck pain or can't move their head.
- They are having problems with vision or hearing, or have lost their sense of smell.
- They have an obvious head wound or dent.
- They have a black eye but that's not where they were hit.
- They are bleeding from the ears.
- They are weak or numb down one side of the body.

Epilepsy & seizures

Epilepsy is a common, ongoing condition where sudden bursts of electrical activity in the brain cause seizures (also knows as fits). The cause can be genetic, due to a new change in someone's genes (which can happen randomly or due to environmental factors), or some sort of damage, such as from a brain injury, infection, STROKE or tumour. Note that withdrawal from alcohol and illicit drugs can also bring on seizures. Sometimes it can be difficult to identify the underlying reason.

SYMPTOMS
During a seizure, someone will often:
+ Collapse.
+ Lose awareness of what is happening around them.
+ Shake and jerk uncontrollably.
+ Or stare blankly into space.

Diagnosis

It's difficult to make a diagnosis after just one seizure, but you should still see a doctor if you think you have had one for the first time. You will usually be referred to a neurologist.

People who have epilepsy often have triggers that can bring on a seizure. There are different types of seizure; how they start can tell us what treatment is likely to be most effective. The person treating you will need as much information as possible, so always keep a note of:

- How you felt before the seizure.
- What you were doing.
- How long it lasted.
- How you felt afterwards.

You will usually be given an MRI (brain scan) and an EEG to measure the electrical activity in your brain.

What do if someone is having a seizure

- Don't move the person or attempt to restrain them unless they are in immediate danger.
- Do move anything out of the way that might harm them, like sharp objects.
- Do put something soft under their head (such as a rolled-up jumper).
- Once the fit is over, roll them into the recovery position (see page 16).
- Bear in mind that it is not uncommon for someone to soil themselves during a seizure.

If someone has previously been diagnosed with epilepsy, then they will not usually need to go to hospital following a seizure that is normal for them. However, it becomes an emergency situation if any of the following apply:

- They have not been diagnosed with epilepsy.
- The seizure lasts for more than five minutes.
- They have repeated seizures in quick succession.
- They are struggling to breathe.

People who have epilepsy often wear a bracelet or carry a card to let others know about their condition if they have a seizure.

Treatment

Epilepsy can't be cured but getting the right anti-seizure medication alongside an understanding of triggers means that for many people, seizures can be reduced to the point where they are very infrequent. There may also be lifestyle considerations, such as managing stress or addressing substance abuse.

Living with epilepsy

Many people will be able to live normal lives and children can usually go to mainstream schools. The considerations to be noted are:

- You will not be able to drive until you have your seizures under control (10 years seizure-free for HGV licence holders, 12 months seizure-free for other vehicles). You can be prosecuted if you do. You should contact the DVLA if you have had a seizure or blackout.
- You can play most sports but should not swim alone.
- Anti-seizure medications can interact with the contraceptive pill and stop it working.
- If you are thinking of conceiving a child (whether you are male or female), speak to your doctor first, as they may need to alter your medication.
- Sudden unexpected death in epilepsy (SUDEP) is a very rare syndrome but the risk is higher if someone stops using their medication and their seizures get worse. It's also linked to drinking a lot of alcohol.

Strokes & transient ischaemic attack (TIA)

A stroke is when blood suddenly stops flowing to the brain or there is a bleed on the brain caused by a burst blood vessel. It damages the brain and can cause life-altering injury or death. A stroke is an emergency situation, and you should call 999.

A TIA is sometimes known as a mini stroke. This is caused by a temporary interruption to the blood supply to the brain. The symptoms are similar to a stroke, but they resolve quickly without causing lasting damage. However, this can be a sign that someone is likely to have a stroke in the future.

Strokes and TIAs may be associated with older people, but the reality is that they can happen at any age.

SYMPTOMS

In addition to FAST symptoms (see box), other, more subtle symptoms can include:
+ **Confusion and memory loss.**
+ **Loss of vision in one or both eyes.**
+ **Weakness or numbness down one side.**
+ **Dizziness, falling over.**
+ **A severe** HEADACHE.

Diagnosis

When you get to hospital, you will have blood tests and a CT scan, which will show which part of the brain has been affected.

If you have had a TIA, you will be assessed to predict how likely you are to suffer a subsequent stroke. For this, we use a tool called the ABCD2 score, that takes into account things like age, BLOOD PRESSURE and how long the TIA symptoms lasted for.

Treatment

- A THROMBOSIS or EMBOLISM (blood clot) is usually treated with medication to dissolve it.
- Blood thinners may be needed to prevent further clots (or stopped if you were taking them and have a bleed).
- Medication may be given to reduce BLOOD PRESSURE and CHOLESTEROL.
- Surgery may be needed to remove blockages, prevent further bleeds or reduce swelling in the brain.

The treatment for TIA will be medication to reduce the likelihood of further clots or bleeding, lifestyle changes and possibly surgery if a narrowed blood vessel was the cause, alongside ongoing monitoring.

> **If you are caring for someone who has had a stroke**
>
> A stroke is a sudden trauma both for the person who suffers it and those who love them. The abrupt change in ability and independence can have a big impact on quality of life, and the uncertainty of how much they will recover as they go through rehabilitation is stressful. If you are supporting someone who is recovering from a stroke, try to make sure you get the support you need too.

Rehabilitation following a stroke

Rehabilitation will depend on what part of the brain was affected and how badly. Some people will be left permanently disabled and in need of care to help them manage basic tasks following a stroke, while others may be able to return to their day-to-day life. Rehabilitation will start in hospital and continue after you leave. It will often involve occupational therapy, physical therapy, speech therapy and sometimes counselling, as people who have suffered strokes can be left with PTSD and/or need support as they adapt to permanent or temporary changes in their lifestyle.

> **How to spot the signs of a stroke**
>
> If someone is experiencing any of the following symptoms, they need emergency medical help, whether it turns out to be a stroke or a TIA. The acronym 'FAST' is useful to help remember the signs and to act quickly:
>
> **F = Face:** Has their face dropped on one side? Can they smile?
>
> **A = Arm:** Can they lift their arms?
>
> **S = Speech:** Are they struggling to get their words out?
>
> **T = Time:** Call 999 as soon as you can.

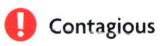 **Contagious**

Meningitis

Meningitis is the inflammation of the membrane that surrounds the brain and spinal cord, called the meninges. It can be very serious and needs urgent medical attention. Call an ambulance or go to A&E if you suspect meningitis, as it can be fatal if not treated in time. It's more common in babies, children and teenagers and it can lead to SEPSIS.

Types of meningitis

Bacterial meningitis
Rarer but more serious than viral meningitis. There is a small chance of long-term problems, such as with hearing, vision, coordination and memory, and up to 1 in 10 cases of bacterial meningitis can be fatal.

Viral meningitis
Always needs medical attention but not everyone will get very ill from it. Sometimes it can be treated at home.

Prevention
There are a number of vaccines offered to babies, children and young people that protect against different types of meningitis, so it's important to keep up to date with the vaccination programme.

Diagnosis
In hospital, the priority is to find out what kind of meningitis someone has so it can be treated quickly and effectively. A blood culture test will be conducted to diagnose meningitis and if it is bacterial or viral, and a lumbar puncture or CT scan may also be used for diagnosis.

Treatment
- Antibiotics by injection/IV drip, if bacterial meningitis is found.
- Fluids given by an IV drip.
- Oxygen.

Recovery
Once viral meningitis is established, the patient can often be discharged to treat the symptoms at home. Rest, painkillers and anti-sickness medication can relieve discomfort and you should feel better in seven to ten days.

SYMPTOMS

Symptoms for both forms of meningitis usually come on suddenly and get quickly worse.
- Non-blanching rash (the most distinctive symptom, although not everyone with meningitis will have a rash – see box below).
- FEVER.
- Severe HEADACHE.
- Stiff neck.
- Nausea and vomiting.
- Behavioural changes like confusion, sleepiness and difficulty waking up.
- Aversion to bright lights.

Bacterial meningitis, if treated quickly, should lead to a full recovery. However, some people experience long-term effects, including:
- Hearing or vision reduction or loss.
- SEIZURES.
- Problems with balance or coordination.
- Memory or concentration problems.
- Amputation of limbs may be necessary.

The glass test
Take a colourless glass tumbler and roll it firmly over the rash. If the spots do not fade under pressure, this is called a non-blanching rash. Seek urgent medical attention by calling 999. Bear in mind that not everyone with meningitis will have a visible rash.

Encephalitis

Encephalitis is inflammation of the brain tissue. It's rare but very serious. Call 999 if you suspect someone has it. We don't always know what causes it, but it can be brought on by certain other viral infections spreading to the brain. Much less commonly, it can be caused by bacterial or fungal infections or an issue with the body's immune system which causes it to attack the brain.

SYMPTOMS

- Sudden FEVER.
- HEADACHE.
- Vomiting.
- Aversion to bright light.
- Stiff neck and back.
- Confusion.

Diagnosis

It's vital someone is diagnosed as soon as possible, which needs to be done in hospital by an MRI scan.

Treatment

Someone experiencing encephalitis will need a variety of treatments to help them recover, which can take some time. These can include:

- Antivirals.
- Steroids.
- Antibiotics or antifungal medicines.
- Treatments to control the immune system.
- Painkillers.
- Seizure medication.
- Oxygen through a face mask or ventilator.

Recovery

Ongoing symptoms following recovery from the worst of the illness can include memory problems, SEIZURES, personality changes, TIREDNESS or memory and cognitive problems.

Brain tumour

A brain tumour is an abnormal growth of cells somewhere in the brain tissue. The growth might be cancerous (or malignant), or it might be benign, which means it is not cancerous. Both types cause inflammation and put pressure on the brain as they grow. This is likely to lead to symptoms which is often how the tumour is picked up.

Lots of people worry about having a brain tumour, but primary brain cancer (meaning that's where the disease starts) is very rare. Secondary brain cancer, where it has spread from somewhere else in the body, is slightly more common. Only about 6,000 people are diagnosed with a brain tumour every year in the UK, and brain tumours are not thought to run in families – only about 5 per cent are inherited.

SYMPTOMS

There are about 120 types of brain tumour, categorised according to the tissue on the brain that they penetrate. Symptoms vary depending on which part of the brain is affected, and sometimes there are no symptoms. However, common symptoms are:

+ SEIZURES or convulsions (see also EPILEPSY).
+ Language and communication difficulties.
+ Unsteadiness, weakness and lack of balance.
+ Changes to personality and behaviour.
+ Memory loss and confusion.
+ HEADACHES, particularly in the morning (although there can be many reasons for this, other than a tumour).
+ Nausea and vomiting.

Diagnosis

If your doctor thinks you have the symptoms of a brain tumour, they will refer you to a neurologist for a CT or MRI scan. You may also have a lumbar puncture. Doctors will also look at other possible causes for your symptoms.

Treatment

Sometimes, the tumour will be removed by surgery. In benign cases, a tumour may be left and monitored. You may also have radiotherapy and/or chemotherapy to treat cells left behind after surgery. Steroids may be prescribed to reduce swelling in the brain caused by the tumour.

THERE ARE OVER 100 TYPES OF BRAIN TUMOUR. HERE ARE SOME OF THE POTENTIAL SITES.

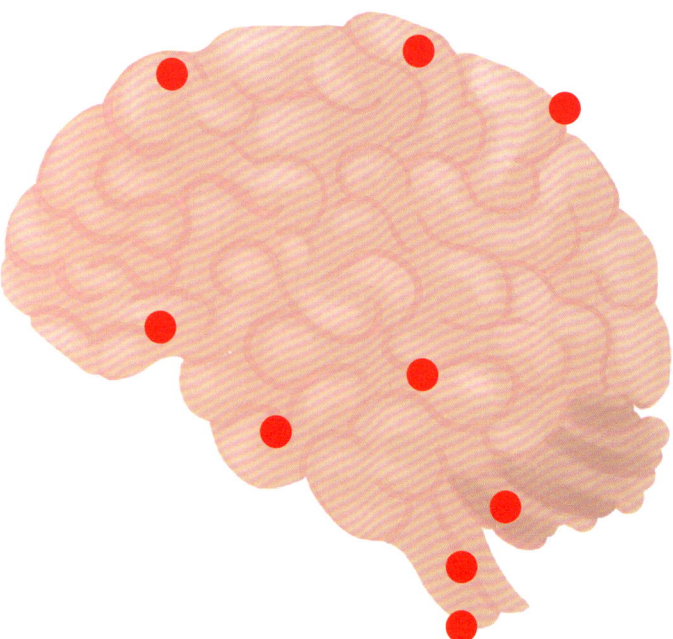

Multiple sclerosis (MS)

Multiple sclerosis occurs when an overactive immune system damages the covers of the nerves in the brain and spinal cord, stopping them from conducting electrical signals in the way they should. The disease is unpredictable: some people will go into remission and have no symptoms for long periods of time; others will have manageable symptoms and can mostly get on with their lives. Some will eventually lose their ability to speak, write or walk. Most people will be diagnosed in their thirties and forties, but symptoms can start much earlier.

Types of MS

Relapsing/remitting
There are flare-ups but then the symptoms improve.

Secondary progressive
Usually follows relapsing/remitting, when the symptoms are experienced all the time.

Primary progressive
Symptoms are present all the time, right from when you were diagnosed, and they are getting worse.

SYMPTOMS

These are the early symptoms that can help to identify the onset of MS:
+ Blurred or double vision, red or green colour distortion, pain and loss of vision caused by the swelling of the optic nerve (the optic neuritis).
+ Difficulty adjusting your vision somewhere steamy, for example in the shower or bath (known as Uhthoff's phenomenon).
+ Trouble walking, feeling off-balance, dizziness.
+ Numbness, prickling, tingling on the skin, loss of feeling.
+ Weakness in arm and legs.
+ Muscle cramps, stiffness and spasms.
+ Constant TIREDNESS.
+ Speech problems.
+ DEPRESSION.
+ Bowel and bladder problems, repeated URINARY TRACT INFECTIONS (UTI).
+ Difficulty with cognitive function: trouble focusing, memory problems.

Diagnosis
A range of tests are needed to diagnose MS, including blood tests, an MRI scan and a lumbar puncture, when a small sample of spinal fluid is taken. You will need to track your symptoms over time.

Treatment
There is no cure for MS, although treatments to manage the condition are improving.
- Disease modifying therapies (DMTs), which are medications that reduce the frequency and severity of relapses, slow the progression of the disease and potentially reduce disability, by directly targeting inflammation in the central nervous system and slowing down deterioration.
- Steroids to control inflammation.
- Plasma exchange to remove harmful antibodies.
- Treatment for your symptoms, for example, muscle relaxants and painkillers.
- Physiotherapy and other supportive therapies to help you live your life.

Spinal injuries

The spinal cord is a tube of nerves inside your spinal column. It runs from the base of your brain to your lower back. It is a vital part of your central nervous system as it carries messages to and from your brain and the rest of your body. If it is damaged, permanently or temporarily, it will have a big impact on how much you can move and what sensations you can feel. The higher up in your back the damage is, usually the more debilitating it will be.

Causes
There are many different things that can cause damage to the spinal cord, such as trauma, infection, something pushing on nerve tissue or a tumour.

Diagnosis
Because there are so many potential causes of this sort of injury, the priority is finding the underlying cause and treating the pain. Tests may include an X-ray, a CT scan and/or an MRI.

Treatment
Sometimes an operation will be needed, often followed by intensive physiotherapy. Occupational therapy can help someone figure out how best to start getting back to their normal life.

Red flag symptoms
If you have any of these symptoms, go straight to A&E as it could be a sign that you have sustained damage to your spine.
- You have suddenly lost control of your bladder or bowel, so you can't pee, you're peeing uncontrollably or you don't know when you need to poo.
- Your legs feel weak or numb and it's getting worse.
- You have lost feeling in your hands or fingers.
- You have lost feeling in the genitals, anus, inner thigh or across the buttocks.
- You have incapacitating pain that painkillers aren't touching. Particularly at night (pain from SCIATICA, or a PROLAPSED DISC, should lessen when you are in bed).
- You have SCIATICA pain on both sides of the body.
- You have a FEVER and/or a swelling in your back.
- If you have had recent trauma to the area, like a fall. If you are a man over 60, or a POST-MENOPAUSAL woman, this doesn't need to have been serious, but you may have a FRACTURE.
- You have a pain in your upper or mid back that is making it hard to breathe.

Sciatica

Your sciatic nerve is the longest nerve in your body. It starts in the lower back and runs down your legs. It transmits sensation from the bottom half of your body and controls the muscles in your lower legs. Sciatica refers to the pain felt in one side of the body when the nerve is inflamed or a structure (such as a prolapsed disc, see right) is pressing on it.

SYMPTOMS

- Pain from the buttocks down the back of the legs, sometimes also in the feet and toes.
- Numbness and pins and needles in this area.
- Mild lower back pain.

Treatment

- Try not to stay still for too long as this will make the pain worse.
- Start gentle exercise as soon as you can bear it as the body needs to move to get better. There are specific exercises to help with sciatica available on the NHS website.
- Ensure you have a good sleeping position – try a pillow between your knees if you sleep on your side or under your lower back if you are a back sleeper.
- Try heat treatment, although be careful not to burn your skin if you are experiencing numbness.
- Take over-the-counter painkillers and anti-inflammatories – your pharmacist will be able to advise.

The pain will usually subside in four to six weeks. If it lasts longer and it's stopping you from living your life as normal, see your GP. If you have any of the red flag symptoms listed opposite, seek medical advice.

Prolapsed disc

Also called a slipped or herniated disc, this occurs when the soft centre of a disc in your back in between your vertebrae leaks into the spinal canal. It can press on your nerve endings causing pain and/or irritate the sciatic nerve (see left). This can happen for various reasons, including injury or wear to the spine due to age (see ARTHRITIS).

SYMPTOMS

- Lower back or neck pain.
- Numbness and tingling.
- Difficulty bending or straightening the back.
- Muscle weakness.
- SCIATICA.

A prolapsed disc will usually resolve in four to six weeks. If the pain lasts longer, see your GP. If you have any of the red flag symptoms listed opposite, seek medical advice.

Treatment

- Over-the-counter painkillers and anti-inflammatories. It's best to take up to the recommended dose regularly rather than waiting for the pain to get very bad.
- Keep moving as much as you can – the pain will be worse if you sit still for long periods, and you need to move to heal.
- Alternate between hot and cold treatments.
- Physiotherapy and chiropractory may well be helpful, as the practitioner can show you specific exercises and help you to improve your posture, which is important for treating prolapsed discs.
- In rare cases, surgery may be required.

Motor neurone disease (MND)

Motor neurones are particular types of nerves in the brain and spine that control movement. When someone has motor neurone disease, the motor neurones gradually stop working. It's very rare and we don't know why it happens, but it leads to serious and increasing loss of movement and other symptoms, shortening life expectancy. Some studies have found that having a close relative with MND or one who has FRONTOTEMPORAL DEMENTIA may mean you are more likely to get it, but the exact correlation is still uncertain. Most people diagnosed with MND are over the age of 50.

SYMPTOMS

Early symptoms:
+ Mild weakness or muscle twitching in the lower body – you may trip or find it difficult to climb stairs.
+ Slurred speech.
+ Weak grip and loss of fine motor skills, e.g. it becomes harder to remove lids and do up buttons.
+ Unintended weight loss.
+ Feeling oddly emotional – crying or laughing in inappropriate situations.
+ Sexual dysfunction.

Symptoms as the disease progresses:
+ Spreading of muscle weakness and lack of control throughout the body.
+ Paralysis.
+ Breathing difficulties.

Diagnosis

There is no singular test for MND, plus many of the early symptoms cross over with other conditions, such as PARKINSON'S DISEASE and some types of DEMENTIA, so a GP will need to refer you for a number of tests to find out the cause.

Treatment

There is no cure for MND, but medication can slow the progression of the disease, which works well for some people. We can also treat some of the symptoms, and physiotherapists, speech therapists and occupational therapists can help someone live as well as possible for as long as possible. People diagnosed with MND and their immediate family often benefit from talking therapy as they come to terms with the diagnosis.

The Ice Bucket Challenge raised international awareness about motor neurone disease, putting much-needed global efforts into finding a cure for this terminal illness.

Tiredness & fatigue

Feeling tired all the time is commonly associated with many different illnesses and conditions, which makes a single cause difficult to pin down. There may well be a combination of issues at play, and if we are stressed and depleted, we are more likely to pick up bugs and less likely to exercise and eat well.

Common causes of fatigue

- Not getting enough or having too much sleep.
- Insomnia or SLEEP APNOEA.
- Imbalance of the sleep hormone melatonin.
- Unhealthy lifestyle, including poor diet, inadequate exercise, too much time indoors.
- Infection.
- Stress.
- DEPRESSION.
- Dehydration.
- Difficult life events, such as bereavements and relationship breakdowns (even happy periods can be exhausting!)
- Puberty, menstrual cycle, PREGNANCY, PERIMENOPAUSE.
- HYPERTHYROIDISM.
- Side effect of medications.
- Vitamin deficiencies and ANAEMIA.
- Autoimmune conditions like RHEUMATOID ARTHRITIS – particularly those that make it hard to absorb nutrients during digestion, like CROHN'S DISEASE and COELIAC DISEASE.
- Neurological conditions like PARKINSON'S DISEASE and DEMENTIA.
- CHRONIC FATIGUE and FIBROMYALGIA.
- Cancer and cancer treatments, like chemotherapy.

See your GP
- If you are constantly FATIGUED for over two weeks and the advice opposite makes no difference.
- If exhaustion stops you living your life, making it hard to go to work, for example.
- If you have unexplained weight loss, mood changes or you can sound like you are struggling for breath when you are asleep (see SLEEP APNOEA).

Diagnosis

A symptom diary over a period of weeks will be helpful if you visit your GP. Include how much sleep you are getting, your daily routine, any significant events, any other symptoms and when they occur. You may have a blood test to rule out things like infections and deficiencies such as ANAEMIA.

Treatment

The body needs rest and will not function well without adequate sleep. However, for many reasons, this may be easier said than done – particularly at challenging times such as if you have young children or go through a very busy period at work. If you are struggling with feeling tired much of the time, these are the basics to address first:

- The bed should be for sleep and sex only. Try not to work in bed or take devices into the bedroom. Buy an alarm clock rather than using your phone.
- Try to stick to regular sleep times and have a bedtime 'wind down' routine where you read, listen to a podcast or music to prepare for sleep. (No screens! The blue light stimulates dopamine, which makes it harder to sleep.)
- Make sure your bedroom is dark, cool and quiet enough.
- Avoid alcohol and don't smoke.
- Eat a healthy diet.
- Cut out or cut down caffeine. It can last for seven hours, so if you go to bed at 10.30pm, no caffeine after 3.30pm.
- Get some exercise. This might feel like a real challenge when you are feeling tired, but our bodies are built to move and this is important for good sleep.
- Small meals and light, healthy snacks work better for many people than large dinners that are hard work to digest. Do not eat less than two hours before bedtime.
- Relaxation techniques like meditation and yoga are beneficial for many people.

THE EYES

Eye health can change throughout your life, so it's important to have regular eye tests (see page 139) to diagnose if you require glasses (and often people can require glasses for specific tasks such as reading or driving). You first port of call for eye-related issues is your local opticians, where you can see an optometrist, rather than a GP. The optometrist can refer you back to your GP if necessary.

An optician: Someone who is trained to fit glasses and contact lenses based on a prescription decided by an optometrist.

An optometrist: Someone who is specially trained in eye problems – they can diagnose issues with sight and recognise eye disease and injuries. They can sometimes prescribe medication.

An ophthalmologist: A doctor who is specifically trained in the area of medicine related to the eye. They usually work in a hospital ophthalmology department or eye hospital. Your GP will refer you if necessary.

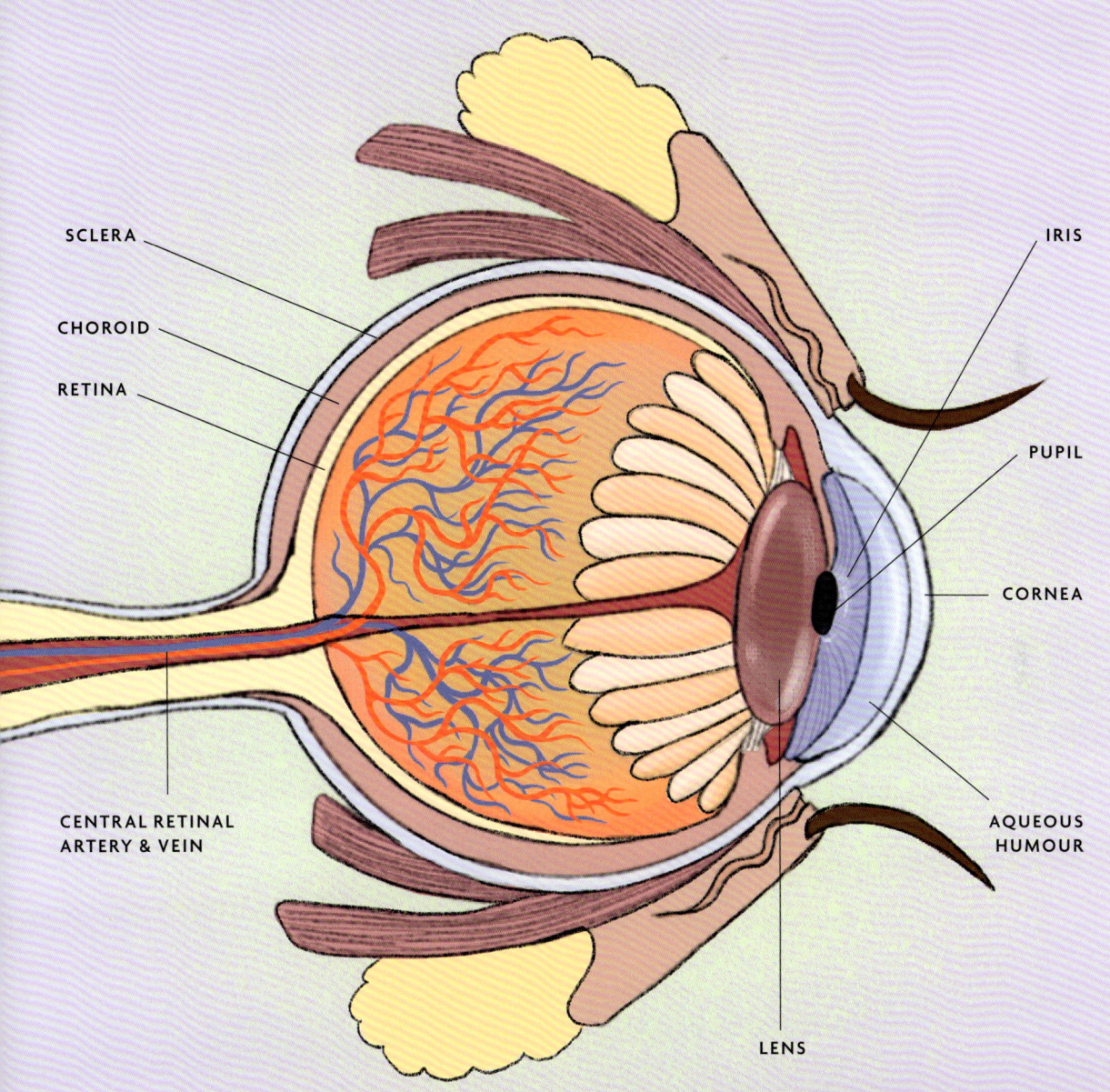

Short sightedness (myopia)

People are short sighted when the lens inside the eye focuses light that comes from objects far away in front of the retina, rather than in the correct place in the eye, which makes them appear blurry. The shape of the eye or cornea can be a factor, too. Night myopia is when you struggle to see in low light.

SYMPTOMS

If you are shortsighted and you don't have the right glasses or contact lenses, you will experience:
- Blurry vision when looking at things that are far away.
- Eye strain, 'tired' eyes.
- HEADACHES.
- Squinting to see distant objects.

Diagnosis & treatment

Myopia is diagnosed via an eye test (see page 139). While myopia doesn't cause eye problems in itself, it is linked to conditions that cause severe vision loss, so it's important to have your eyes checked regularly. Glasses or contact lenses can be worn to correct the problem – children and some adults are entitled to vouchers to help towards the cost of these. Other adults will need to pay for them. Laser eye surgery might also be an option for some adults but is not usually available on the NHS. Spending more time outdoors can stop the myopia from getting worse but you will need glasses or contact lenses too.

Presbyopia

Presbyopia is an age-related, natural loss of the eye's ability to focus, caused by a hardening of the lens. It usually occurs in people aged 40 and over, and you may notice you need to hold reading material further away to clearly see it, or that you get HEADACHES or eye strain after reading. It is diagnosed by an eye test and treated with the appropriate glasses or contact lenses.

Spotting vision issues in children

If you notice any of these signs, it is worth getting your child's sight checked, even if they are not due for an eye test.
- Their eyes are not pointing in the same direction.
- They are complaining of HEADACHES and rubbing their eyes.
- They are struggling to play ball games or recognise faces at a distance.
- They are visibly squinting.
- They are unusually clumsy.
- They seem to need to sit close to the TV and hold books close to their face.
- See also FUNDUS REFLEX.

Driving

You must be able to read a number plate from 20 metres (65 feet) away in daylight to drive in the UK. If you need glasses or contact lenses to do this, it's a legal requirement to wear them and your insurance won't be valid if you don't.

Long sightedness

Long sightedness occurs when the light coming from near objects lands on the wrong place on the retina, making them seem blurry. This is called hyperopia when it's to do with the shape of the eye (this can be hereditary), and presbyopia when it's because the lens can't flex well enough, which is a natural part of the aging process.

SYMPTOMS

- **Blurry vision when looking at things up close.**
- **Eye strain, 'tired' eyes.**
- **HEADACHES.**
- **Needing to hold things at a distance when you are trying to read or see your phone.**

Diagnosis & treatment

Long sightedness is diagnosed via an eye test. Glasses or contact lenses can be worn to correct the problem – children and some adults are entitled to vouchers to help towards the cost of these. Other adults will need to pay for them. Laser eye surgery might also be an option for some adults but is not usually available on the NHS.

Eye tests for adults

Regular eye tests are important to detect any issues early. In addition, they can pick up other health conditions, such as HIGH BLOOD PRESSURE, DIABETES, THYROID DISORDERS and even BRAIN TUMOURS.

- Most healthy adults will only need an eye test every two years.
- You may need more regular tests if you are at a higher risk of GLAUCOMA.
- Always see an optician about any eyesight concerns.
- Older people may need more regular tests.

Some people are entitled to free eye tests and a voucher towards glasses or lenses on the NHS, or your employer may offer free tests if your work is screen-based. Check the NHS website for more details.

Eye tests for children

Babies have their vision checked within 72 hours of birth and then as part of the physical examination done by a GP or health visitor when they are 6–8 weeks old. When your child has their health and development checks, which are offered in the UK until they are two years old, you will be asked if you have any concerns about their sight. They may be checked again when they first start school, or you may be advised to take them to an optician. Babies and children should have eye tests on the NHS at the following ages:

- Within 72 hours of birth.
- Between six and eight weeks old.
- Between one and one-and-a-half years old.
- At three and a half years old.
- Around four or five years old via vision screening at school, or take the child for an eye test at an opticians.
- Ongoing as advised, usually annually – children are entitled to free NHS eye tests until 16 years of age or 19 if in full-time education.

Macular degeneration

Macular degeneration is an eye disease that means you lose the ability to clearly see things directly in the centre of your vision, while retaining your peripheral vision. It doesn't usually lead to sight loss but it can cause deterioration in sight in either one eye or both. It can be a result of illness, injury or a rare inherited disease, but it is usually age-related (known as age-related macular degeneration, or AMG). We don't know what causes it although it's thought to be affected by lifestyle factors and genetics. It's the leading cause of vision loss in people over 50.

Dry (atrophic) macular degeneration

This is the most common type of macular degeneration, affecting 80 per cent of people with the condition. It occurs when parts of the macula (the middle of your retina) become thin and tiny clumps of protein build up.

SYMPTOMS

- Hazy or blurred vision.
- Reduced contrast sensitivity.
- Mild colour vision changes.
- Trouble seeing in low light.
- Blurry area at centre of vision.
- Blank spots.
- Straight lines look wavy or wonky.
- Colours may look less bright.

Diagnosis

Macular degeneration will be picked up during an eye test (see page 139). You will be referred to an ophthalmologist who may carry out more tests.

Treatment

There is no cure for macular degeneration, but treatments are more effective at preserving sight if it's caught early. Taking vitamins and some dietary changes can help to slow down the progression. There are different drugs that may be prescribed, depending on which type is diagnosed. There are new laser treatments currently being developed.

Wet (exudative) macular degeneration

Much less common than dry macular degeneration but more severe and progresses quicker, leading to a total loss of central vision. It's caused by abnormal blood vessels developing under the retina, which leak and cause a bulge.

SYMPTOMS

- Distorted area at centre of vision, e.g. when reading.
- Words 'disappear' when reading.
- Dark spots in centre of vision.
- Significant central vision loss.
- Objects may appear wavy.
- Colours fade and/or have little contrast.
- Bright lights are glaring and uncomfortable.
- Difficulty adjusting when moving from dark to light areas.

Risk factors

We don't yet know what causes either type of macular degeneration but an increased risk is associated with:

- Eating a diet high in saturated fats.
- Being overweight or OBESE.
- Having HIGH BLOOD PRESSURE.
- Having high CHOLESTEROL.
- Cardiovascular disease.
- Smoking.
- Genetics.

Cataracts

A cataract is a cloudy area on the eye's lens that can lead to vision loss. They are caused by the breakdown of proteins and are a common cause of sight loss worldwide. They develop – usually slowly – in one or both eyes. They are often age-related, but can also be caused by underlying cardiovascular disease, damage caused by UV light and injury to the eye. Some babies are born with cataracts, or they develop them soon after birth, but this is unusual and treatable.

SYMPTOMS

For many people, the first sign that they have a cataract is that they keep thinking their glasses need cleaning when they don't. Other symptoms include:
+ Cloudy, blurry or double vision.
+ Colours appear faded.
+ Seeing halos around lights.
+ Trouble seeing at night.
+ Sensitivity to light.
+ As the conditions progresses, it is like looking through a steamed-up window.

Diagnosis

An optician will refer you to an ophthalmologist if they pick up signs of a cataract in an eye test. A cataract caused by injury to the eye can develop more quickly and you will need to go to A&E.

Treatment

Not everyone needs treatment straight away. A cataract is graded from immature to mature and hyper mature depending on how developed it is. In the early stages, they are often barely noticeable, although it's still important it's picked up early so it can be monitored regularly.

The treatment is simple surgery in which the lens in the eye is replaced with an artificial one. The success rate of this surgery is very high and it usually takes two to six weeks to make a full recovery.

The fundus reflex

When light enters the eye it is also reflected back out again. You can't see this in someone else apart from in a photo taken in a dark place for which a flash has been used – it's what causes that 'red eye' effect, although the colour varies depending on ethnicity. However, if this appears white in a photo, it may be a sign of an eye issue, such as a CATARACT or even cancer.

The traditionally named 'red' reflex should more accurately be called the fundus reflex, as the reflection colour of a healthy eye varies by ethnicity (only appearing red in people with white skin). It is tested in babies by health professionals as part of the standard checks. However, if you notice that one or both of your child's eyes glows white in a photo taken with a flash, seek an urgent medical assessment at an eye clinic – call 111 if you are not sure where the nearest to you is. Note that a lot of smartphone cameras have tech to reduce the effect of 'red eye', which will hide this.

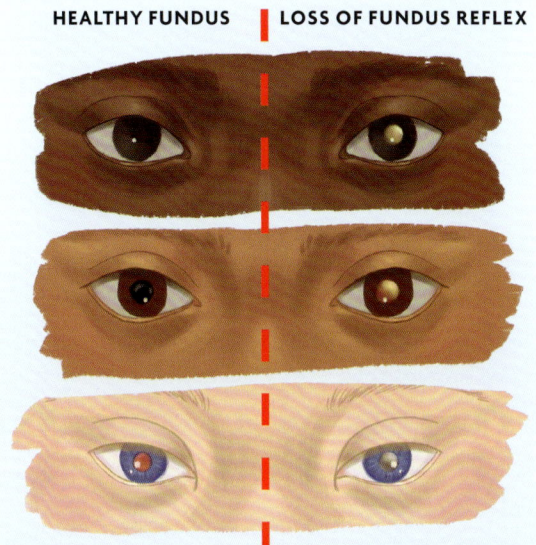

HEALTHY FUNDUS | LOSS OF FUNDUS REFLEX

Blepharitis

Blepharitis occurs when the edges of the eyelids become inflamed, and the eyelid is sore and itchy. It's sometimes known as 'eye dandruff' because it can cause dandruff-like scales in the eyelashes. There are a number of causes, including allergies or the oil glands in your eyelids becoming clogged and irritated, but it's often caused by too much of the bacteria that usually lives harmlessly on our skin. Some people have chronic blepharitis that flares up from time to time. It can also cause STYES or cysts.

SYMPTOMS
+ Inflamed, sore and itchy eyelids.
+ A 'gritty' feeling in the eyes.
+ 'Eye dandruff' in the eyelashes.

Diagnosis
Blepharitis doesn't usually need to be seen by a GP, and you can self-diagnose from symptoms alone.

Treatment
Blepharitis will usually clear up by itself. Meanwhile the following can help with the symptoms:
- Place a flannel soaked in warm water over your eyelids for five to ten minutes to relieve symptoms.
- Practise good eyelid hygiene – use cotton pads soaked in warm water or diluted baby shampoo to clean the eye area twice a day and continue once a day as it gets better, then for a few more days afterwards.
- Don't wear eye makeup or use contact lenses until it's better.

If you have recurring blepharitis, a pharmacist will be able to recommend eye drops. If this becomes severe, particularly if it's causing other eye issues, your GP may refer you to an ophthalmologist.

Red flag symptom – detached retina
The retina is a layer of tissue at the back of the eye that transmits images to the brain via electrical signals. This can start to come away, stopping you from seeing properly. This is a medical emergency as it can result in permanent loss of sight if not treated quickly. It can happen more than once.

Causes: Can be linked to CATARACTS or GLAUCOMA, caused by an injury or following eye surgery. Sometimes we don't know the cause, but it seems to run in families.

Symptoms: New 'floaters' in your vision, blurred vision, dark patch across your vision, flashing lights. These symptoms will get worse.

Diagnosis: Go to an eye hospital A&E if there is one near you. In the UK, call 111, as they will be able to advise you where to get treatment. In hospital, an ophthalmologist will put drops in your eye and examine it.

Treatment: You will need surgery to repair the retina. Most people will have their sight restored if treated quickly.

⚠️ **Transmissible**

Styes (hordeolum)

A stye is a small lump on the eyelid caused by an infection. The main cause is a blockage of one of the oil glands in the eyelids, allowing bacteria (usually Staphylococcus) to grow inside. You can get more than one stye at a time. They are not infectious but it's important to keep the area clean and try not to touch it or share makeup with other people as the bacteria can spread easily.

SYMPTOMS

- **A lump or spot on the upper or lower eyelid (although sometimes styles grow inside the eyelid, which you will feel rubbing on the eye) that looks like an acne pimple.**
- **The skin around the lump may be swollen.**
- **The lump is sore and may look red on paler skin.**

Diagnosis

A style is diagnosed by symptoms. If your vision is affected it is unlikely to be a style. Red, swollen, sore eyes with no lumps could be CONJUNCTIVITIS or BLEPHARITIS. A painless lump on the eyelid will most likely be a chalazion.

Treatment

DO NOT squeeze a stye or try to drain it yourself. You are likely to damage the delicate skin around the eye, make it worse and spread the infection. Gently press a clean flannel soaked in warm water to the eye three to six times a day. If you want to wash the eyelid, use a solution of baby shampoo on a cotton pad. Over-the-counter treatments are available from pharmacies.

Don't wear eye makeup or use contact lenses until the stye has healed. Most styes will go away by themselves over a couple of weeks (don't believe any of the 'overnight' treatments for styes you may find on the internet).

Seek medical attention if:
- The stye is weeping pus.
- Your vision is affected.
- The eye itself appears infected.
- It is very painful and over-the-counter painkillers have no effect.

Prevention

To prevent future styes, always remove eye makeup properly, don't continue to use old eye makeup and try to wash your makeup brushes regularly. I know – who has the time? But definitely do this immediately after having the stye, when it's healed and before you use the same brushes again.

Chalazion

A chalazion is a hard, painless lump on the eyelid, also known as a meibomian cyst. It's usually caused by a blocked oil gland. This can happen when you have a STYE that doesn't go away. It can make your eyelid swell and turn red. It might be sore when it first starts but is not usually painful, unless it becomes infected. It won't affect your vision unless it's on the inside of your eyelid, pressing on the eyeball.

A chalazion will often go away on its own. A flannel or cotton wool ball soaked in warm water and pressed to the eye for five to ten minutes will relieve discomfort and encourage the chalazion to drain. You can do this three to four times a day and you can then gently massage the cyst with a clean finger or cotton bud. To prevent further chalazions, keep the eyelid clean and free of grease.

❗ **Contagious**

Conjunctivitis

The conjunctiva is the membrane on the inside of the eyelid and over the whites of the eye. Conjunctivitis is a common condition that causes the eyelid to become swollen and red (on pale skin). It's sometimes call pink eye and it's usually caused by an infection. It's very contagious so it's really important not to share towels or pillows and to practice good hygiene. In the absence of FEVER or SORE THROAT, and if you feel well enough, you can still go to work or school. Sometimes it's caused by an ALLERGY.

SYMPTOMS

- Itchy, swollen and sore/uncomfortable eyes, sometimes with a burning sensation.
- Watery eyes.
- Whites of the eye appear bloodshot.
- A 'gritty' feeling in the eyes.
- Pus in the eyelashes. In cases of bacterial conjunctivitis, which causes thick, sticky yellow or green discharge, you may wake up in the morning to find your eyelids are stuck together.
- Watery discharge from the eye is common in cases of viral conjunctivitis.
- Follows a viral infection like a COLD or SORE THROAT (in cases of viral conjunctivitis).

Treatment

Viral conjunctivitis will usually get better by itself and doesn't usually need eye drops or ointment. It should clear up in seven to fourteen days but may need up to three weeks if you get reinfected. If you have bacterial conjunctivitis you will need a course of antibiotics.

- You can 'unstick' your eyes with cotton pads soaked in cooled boiled water (cooled until it feels lukewarm on the inside of your elbow).
- Try not to touch your eyes, and wash your hands regularly. Don't prepare food for others as it could spread the bacteria or virus to others.
- Wash facecloths, towels and bedding at 60°C (140°F).
- Wear glasses rather than contact lenses.
- If you think the cause is an ALLERGY, like HAY FEVER or a FOOD ALLERGY, talk to your pharmacist about antihistamines.

If it doesn't clear up after ten days, or you have very sticky discharge in your eyes, see your GP, who will take a swab to check if you have bacterial conjunctivitis. If it's a bacterial infection that isn't getting any better, they may prescribe antibiotic eyedrops – though not, of course, if it's a viral infection. Don't wear eye makeup until two days after the conjunctivitis has cleared up, and it's a good idea to wash your makeup brushes before you do.

Glaucoma

Glaucoma is a common eye condition where the optic nerve which connects the eye to the brain becomes damaged. This is caused by pressure building up when fluid in the eye isn't able to drain properly. It's usually possible to stop vision getting worse – particularly if the condition is caught early (a good reason to have regular eye tests) – but not to reverse any damage already caused. Without treatment, it will lead to sight loss. It's most common in people over 70, and we don't yet know what causes it.

SYMPTOMS
Symptoms are slow onset and include:
+ Blurred vision.
+ Seeing rainbow-coloured circles around bright lights.

Diagnosis
Glaucoma is picked up by an eye test and your optician will refer you to an ophthalmologist.

Treatment
For early stage glaucoma, eye drops may be enough to stop further degeneration. You may need laser treatment or surgery to remove blockages that are causing the build-up of pressure in the eye. You will likely need regular check-ups, and it's very important to keep these up so the condition is properly monitored.

> **Red flag symptoms**
> Rarely, glaucoma can come on suddenly and cause the following symptoms:
> - Intense eye pain and/or tenderness around the eyes.
> - Red eye in the usually white area (the conjunctiva).
> - HEADACHES.
> - Nausea and vomiting.
>
> If you have these symptoms, go to A&E or contact your GP immediately, who will be able to refer you for an urgent eye appointment at hospital.

Astigmatism

Astigmatism occurs when the eye shape is slightly irregular, causing light to focus in more than one place.

SYMPTOMS
+ Blurry vision.
+ Eye strain or 'tired' eyes.
+ HEADACHES.

Diagnosis & treatment
Astigmatism is diagnosed via an eye test and treated with glasses, contact lenses or laser eye surgery.

THE EARS, NOSE & THROAT

The ears, nose and throat are often grouped together because although they are separate organs, they are interconnected. So if you have an infection, for example, you'll often get symptoms in all of them, such as a runny nose, sore throat and blocked ears if you have a COLD.

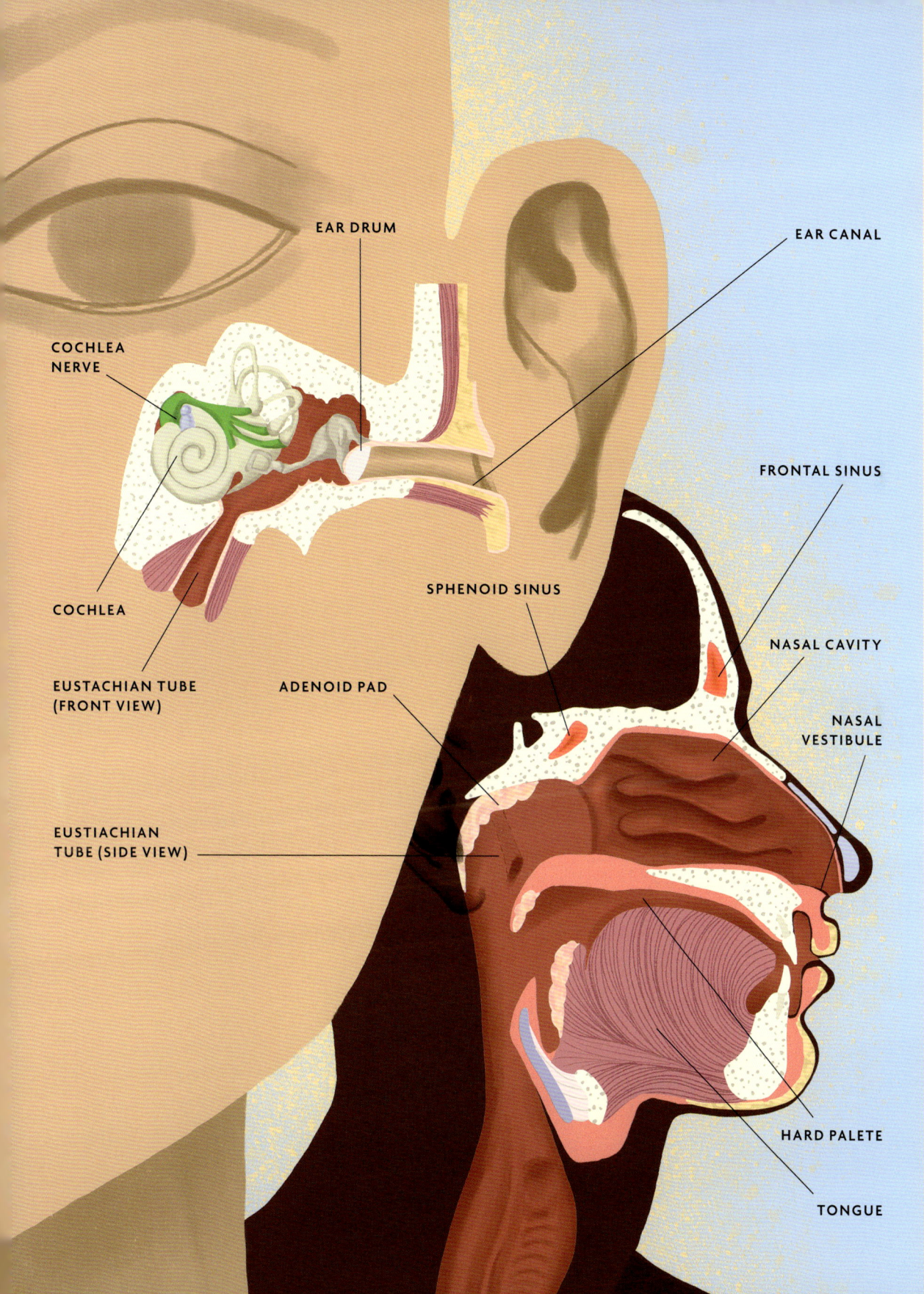

Ear

Your ears are responsible for hearing, of course, but also for your sense of balance.

Outer ear
This is the bit you can see. It's known as the pinna or oracle, and it channels sound into the ear canal.

Ear canal
Your 'external auditory canal' connects the outer ear to the middle ear and its glands produce earwax that clear dirt and prevent infection.

Middle ear
This is the area behind the eardrum. Sound waves make it vibrate and tiny bones called the ossicles move to enable the sound waves to travel to the cochlear.

Eustachian tube
The passage that connects the middle ear to the back of the throat and upper nose. It can open to make the pressure in the middle ear the same as in the environment around you (or the eardrum can't vibrate properly). You may know the feeling from when you land in a plane and everything is muffled, until you yawn to equalise it.

Inner ear
Contains the cochlear and the vestibular system. The cochlear turns vibrations into electromagnetic signals to send to your brain, which you hear as sound. The vestibular system is responsible for balance.

Nose

This is how we smell, taste and breathe, but our noses are much more than what we can see sticking out of our faces!

Nasal passages
Lined with hair and mucous membranes, to make a filtration system that traps bugs, dust, etc. They are divided by the septum.

Nasal cavity
The part of your skull behind your nose. This is where the olfactory epithelium is, which detects smells.

Sinuses
Your sinuses are actually four air pockets next to your nasal cavity. This is where mucus (snot) is made.

Throat

This is a muscular tube that houses the trachea (windpipe), oesophagus (food pipe) and larynx (voice box). It also has the following within:

Epiglottis
This is the flap that stops food getting into your windpipe, to prevent you choking.

Tonsils
Our tonsils catch bacteria and viruses before they enter your respiratory system. They also produce white blood cells that fight infection. Children also have adenoids, although they start to shrink around age seven and usually disappear. They do a similar job to tonsils.

Tongue
This powerful muscle helps you chew and swallow your food, plus it's packed with nerve endings that allow you to taste. If you burn your mouth and damage your tongue, the nerve endings will grow back. Different areas of your tongue taste different things – sweet, salty, sour, bitter and umami.

Earache

Earache is a symptom of lots of things. It may be caused by an issue with the ear itself or by something like a virus that is affecting the respiratory system. What can feel like earache can even sometimes be caused by a problem with the back teeth.

Treatment

Most cases of earache will last a maximum of five days and can be treated at home. We don't usually prescribe antibiotics for earache unless it isn't clearing up by itself or if a child is under two. If a virus is the underlying cause, they won't help anyway.

- Take over-the-counter painkillers for the pain.
- Anti-inflammatories like ibuprofen will help with inflammation.
- Antihistamines will help if an ALLERGY such as HAY FEVER is the cause.
- A pharmacist can advise on eardrops, particularly if the problem is a build-up of wax.
- Hot and cold compresses may help with the pain.
- Try not to get water in the ear – don't go swimming (and wear ear plugs if you do) and wear a shower cap in the shower unless you have to wash your hair. A chunk of cotton wool covered in petroleum jelly will also keep water out.

Some people, often children, who get repeated inner ear infections may need to have a minor operation to fit a grommet – a tiny tube – through the eardrum to allow the pus to drain. This works its way out naturally in time.

Red flag symptoms

See a doctor if:
- The pain is intense and not helped by over-the-counter painkillers.
- You or your child are getting regular ear infections.
- There is a lot of fluid coming from the ear.
- You have other severe symptoms (see also FEVER).

Wax build-up

Earwax is part of a healthy ear and serves to protect your ears from germs. But sometimes it can build up and cause temporary HEARING LOSS. This is more likely to happen if you have lots of hair in your ear canal, skin conditions or inflammation of your ear canal.

SYMPTOMS

+ **Hearing muffled sounds or similar to TINNITUS.**
+ **Itchiness around the ear.**
+ **Earache.**
+ **Repeated ear infections.**

Treatment

Don't try to remove any wax build-ups manually yourself (see below). A pharmacist can advise on ear drops. A warm compress may also help soften the wax so it can move out naturally, or you can try medical olive oil drops.

If it doesn't resolve itself and over-the-counter treatments don't work, you can be referred for (or pay privately for) ear irrigation or microsuction to remove the build-up.

Cotton buds & swabs

Please don't stick these (or anything else, including your finger) inside your ear. They are fine to use to clean around the ear – the bit you can see – but if you push them in you will push down the earwax and potentially introduce more bugs to your ear canal. The ear is self-cleaning anyway – you can't help it do this!

Tinnitus

Tinnitus is when you persistently experience noises inside your ear with no outside source. We think it's caused by a perpetual eardrum movement, a change of pressure in the ear, or the nerve endings in the ear being stimulated. It's a common condition, particularly as people get older. It ranges from mild and occasional, or temporary, to severe and debilitating. There are many things that cause it, which means that different methods to relieve it will work for different people.

SYMPTOMS

+ **Persistent ringing, buzzing, thumping, whooshing or clicking noises inside the ear.**

Causes

- Age-related HEARING LOSS, where the hair cells in the inner ear (the part that receives sound) deteriorate.
- Inner ear damage, e.g. from being at loud clubs or gigs, either as a single traumatic event or over a period of time.
- Side effect of some medications, such as BLOOD PRESSURE medication and non-steroidal anti-inflammatory drugs (NSAIDs).
- WAX BUILD-UP.
- Repeated ear infections.
- VERTIGO.
- Otosclerosis – an inherited condition that causes abnormal bone growth in the middle ear.
- ANXIETY and DEPRESSION, because the rise in cortisol and adrenaline associated with these conditions can also cause tinnitus.
- MENOPAUSE – hormonal changes affect the auditory system, potentially contributing to tinnitus.

Treatment

There is no cure as such, but the first step is identifying a cause, if there is one. For example, your GP will be able to advise about alternative medications or discuss HRT with you if you are MENOPAUSAL or PERIMENOPAUSAL and this is thought to be the cause. Other ways to manage the tinnitus are:

- Good sleep hygiene (see page 135), if tinnitus is causing insomnia.
- Relaxation techniques such as yoga, meditation and/or cognitive behavioural therapy (CBT) if stress or ANXIETY is a factor.
- Sound therapy uses low-level noise to distract from the tinnitus at night or in quiet environments.
- Hibiscus supplements have anecdotally been found to be helpful.
- Avoid loud environments.
- Laser therapy is available privately, but the evidence of effectiveness is inconclusive at present.

If the cause is otosclerosis you will usually need a diagnosis from an ear, nose and throat (ENT) specialist, and in some cases it's possible to have an operation to correct the abnormal bone growth.

Prevention

To avoid getting tinnitus, it's important to look after your auditory health by wearing the right ear protection when in loud environments. Reusable earplugs can be worn at gigs, clubs and other loud environments that offer some protection against hearing damage.

Otitis externa

Otitis externa is the inflammation of the outer ear or ear canal.

> **SYMPTOMS**
> + Pain in or around the ear, sometimes more noticeable when you move your jaw.
> + Itchiness.
> + Scaly skin around the ear and/or redness.
> + Discharge.
> + Some HEARING LOSS.
> + Mild HEADACHE.

Causes
- Bacteria.
- Fungi.
- Viruses.
- Allergies.
- Irritation caused by cleaning the ear too frequently, poking things into the ear, or by earplugs.
- Inflammation caused by getting water, which can carry germs, into the ear (hence otitis externa is sometimes called 'swimmer's ear').
- WAX BUILD-UP.
- Infection from a piercing.

Treatment
Often otitis externa will get better over two to three weeks without any treatment. To help manage the symptoms:
- Avoid wetting the ear and swimming.
- Avoid ear plugs and earrings and, if you wear a hearing aid, consider removing it from the affected ear.
- Pain relief such as paracetamol or ibuprofen.
- Ear drops from the pharmacist or your GP.

Otitis media

This is an infection in the inner ear, when the fluid can't drain away.

> **SYMPTOMS**
> + Pain inside the ear.
> + A feeling of the ear being 'blocked' or 'full'.
> + Discharge from the ear.
> + Nausea or being sick.
> + FEVER.

Causes
- Bacteria.
- Viruses.
- Allergies.
- A build-up of catarrh (snot) behind the eardrum, backed up from the sinuses.
- Pressure changes from altitude and not being able to 'equalise'.

Treatment
Often otitis media will get better over three to five days without any treatment. To help manage the symptoms:
- Take pain relief medication such as paracetamol or ibuprofen.
- Place a warm cloth over the affected ear.

> ### Burst/perforated eardrum
> This sounds much worse than it is. If the pressure from OTITIS MEDIA builds up behind the eardrum, it may rupture resulting in some temporary HEARING LOSS, but it will heal itself in about 12 weeks.

Hearing loss

It might seem like something that just happens as we get older, or something to make light of, but not being able to hear properly – and feeling unable to participate properly in social occasions – can be very isolating and lead to DEPRESSION. What's more, studies suggest a strong link between age-related hearing loss and DEMENTIA.

Prevention

It's important to look after your auditory health throughout your life as declining hearing is often irreversible.

- Wear ear protection around loud noises – in the workplace, when doing DIY and at loud events like gigs.
- Be careful with the volume of headphones – you should always be able to hear people speaking. Some apps will alert you to prolonged use at high volume; check the settings.
- Get your hearing checked just as you do your eyes.
- Many modern headphones have volume protection to protect hearing; ensure it is switched on, particularly for children.
- Ringing ears after a loud event that persist the day after are a sign of hearing damage and that you should limit exposure to such loud noises.

SYMPTOMS

Because it usually happens gradually, not everyone notices straight away when their hearing starts to decline. Here are some warning signs:

+ Struggling to make out speech, often worse in a noisy environment.
+ Finding it hard to understand people on the phone.
+ Turning up the TV or radio to the point where it's uncomfortable for others.
+ Getting TIRED and/or stressed as a result of trying to listen to others for long periods – this may also result in HEADACHES.
+ Friends and family comment on your hearing (others often notice changes before we do).

If you experience sudden severe hearing loss, always see a doctor. This may be the result of a virus that needs to be treated as soon as possible so your hearing comes back.

Hearing tests

Pharmacies and opticians often offer hearing tests (there are also basic hearing tests available online). Some people are entitled to free hearing tests on the NHS. Adults not experiencing HEARING LOSS should get their hearing checked every five to ten years unless you are over 60, when you should get checked more often – an audiologist will be able to advise.

Types of hearing loss

Hearing loss can be separated into two broad categories, depending on why you are experiencing it:
- **Conducive hearing loss:** sound can't pass from the outer to the inner ear, where nerves transmit it to the brain. It's usually due to a blockage or infection and is most often temporary.
- **Sensorineural hearing loss:** occurs as a result of damage to the inner ear, which means that sound is being received but not transmitted to the brain.
- **Mixed hearing loss:** the term used if hearing loss is caused by issues in both the inner and outer ear.

Treatment

This very much depends on the cause. Infections and blockages will often go away on their own. See EARACHE for home treatment and when to see a doctor.

Hearing & children

Newborn babies will be screened for hearing issues, and children will often be tested at school. Early signs that a child may be having trouble hearing are:
- They are unresponsive to sound (e.g. they don't turn around or look in the direction of the sound).
- They are slow learning language.
- They struggle to pay attention.
- They watch faces or lips intently, or they don't seem to realise when someone is speaking.

Not being able to hear properly does of course have a big impact on learning and development if it is not diagnosed and addressed, and the proper support given. Children who are hearing impaired or have HEARING LOSS will lead full lives with the right support.

If you have sensorineural hearing loss you will usually need to see an audiologist for assessment, and depending on the type and severity, the following may be advised:
- Hearing aids.
- Implants are devices that are fitted inside your skull during an operation (suitability and the type of implant will depend on the cause).
- Hyperbaric oxygen therapy is sometimes recommended for sudden hearing loss.
- People with permanent hearing loss will often need support in the form of aids to help them use the phone, for example, and sometimes with help to learn sign language or find other ways to manage their condition.

Hearing loss & dementia

Left untreated, severe hearing loss can increase chances of DEMENTIA by up to five times. So always consult a doctor if you are concerned or notice changes in your hearing.

Vertigo

Vertigo is a symptom of a number of conditions rather than a condition itself. It's characterised by a feeling that things are spinning or moving around you, even though you know they are still. This might make you feel slightly unsteady or completely unbalanced and unable to do everyday tasks. It can come on suddenly as an attack or be a chronic condition that lasts for weeks or months.

SYMPTOMS

Vertigo symptoms may come on suddenly:
+ Balance problems/dizziness (women may find this gets worse during their period).
+ Nausea or vomiting.
+ Feeling of pressure inside the ears.
+ HEADACHE.

Labyrinthitis symptoms also include:
+ HEARING LOSS.
+ Often TINNITUS.

Vestibular neuritis symptoms include:
+ Vertigo symptoms.
+ TINNITUS but with no hearing loss.

Causes

Vertigo can be brought on by illness, infection or MIGRAINE, or as a possible side effect of some medications. Labyrinthitis and vestibular neuritis are the most common conditions with vertigo as a major symptom.

- **Labyrinthitis** is an inner ear infection caused by a virus such as COLD or flu, or bacteria, or by jetlag.
- **Vestibular neuritis** is an inflammation of the vestibular nerve which connects the inner ear to the brain, usually caused by an infection.

Treatment

Symptoms often lessen after three or four days, once the inflammation goes down. You might feel slightly off balance for a couple of weeks. To help with the symptoms:
- Lie in a dark room if you feel very dizzy.
- Avoid being tired and practise good sleep hygiene.
- Avoid bright lights and loud noises.
- Spend time outside, with company if you feel unsteady.
- Drink plenty of water and don't drink alcohol.

Driving and vertigo symptoms

DO NOT cycle or drive with vertigo. You need to tell the DVLA if you are regularly having vertigo symptoms as you could be fined if you continue to drive, and you will put others at risk – check www.gov.uk/dizziness-and-driving.

Benign paroxysmal positional vertigo (BPPV)

This occurs when calcium carbonate particles from the inner ear get trapped in the ear canal. It's not medically serious and is fairly common, but it can be very unpleasant – some people feel like they're having a STROKE or a TIA. Different people experience different triggers but it's almost always brought on by a change in head position.

SYMPTOMS

+ Slight to severe dizziness or vertigo, bringing risks of falls.
+ Erratic or uncontrolled eye movements.
+ Neausea or vomiting.
+ Feeling sweaty and/or panicked.

Treatment

- Brandt-Daroff exercises have a good success rate (available online). They will initially cause dizziness (do them with someone close by in case you fall) but over time should reduce attacks.
- Your doctor may carry out an Epley manoeuvre: turning your head in a specific way to dislodge the crystals.
- Avoid alcohol, eat and sleep well and try not to lie down for too long as this can make it worse.

Nosebleeds

Getting a nosebleed can be distressing and, if you are swallowing the blood, it can make you feel quite sick. But they usually look more dramatic than they are and so long as they are not caused by a serious HEAD INJURY, they are rarely anything to worry about. They are very common in young children.

Causes

The tiny blood vessels inside your nose are easily damaged by a variety of factors, particularly:

- Having a COLD.
- Blowing your nose too hard or picking your nose.
- Dry air that makes the nasal passages dry and cracked.
- Blood-thinning medication, particularly when used alongside alcohol.
- ANAEMIA.
- More unusually, damage to the blood vessels deeper in the nose or the condition ATHEROSCLEROSIS.

Treatment

- Sit with a bowl in front of you to spit the blood into.
- Lean forward rather than back; don't lie down.
- Pinch the soft part of the nose above the nostrils and stay like that for 10–15 minutes. This is important even if the bleeding stops as you need to give time for the blood to clot properly. Set a timer.
- An ice pack or frozen vegetables on your forehead or the back of your neck will reduce the blood flow.

Prevention

- Don't pick your nose.
- If you are congested, avoid blowing your nose too hard or too often.
- Don't overuse nasal decongestants.
- A home humidifier can be helpful when the weather is dry and cold.

Red flag symptoms

Go to hospital if:

- The bleeding is heavy, you have lost a lot of blood, it shows no signs of stopping after 20 minutes or you are becoming weak and dizzy.
- If the nosebleed is as a result of a head injury.

See your GP if:

- If you are on blood-thinning medication and are getting regular nosebleeds.
- If you have symptoms of ANAEMIA.
- Your child under two has a nosebleed.

I've found the best way to stem a nosebleed is a tampon up the nose. There's even a brand now, called Nampons, specifically for this purpose!

Rhinitis, hay fever, sinusitis & post-nasal drip

These conditions all have the potential to make you feel like a snotty, streaming mess. One way to tell the difference if you are unsure is by the colour of the mucus – disgusting but true. They can almost always be managed by over-the-counter medications, so long as you don't have a FEVER and they resolve within a couple of weeks (although hay fever will persist according to the season).

	What is it?	Causes	Symptoms
Rhinitis	An inflammation of the nose's mucous membranes.	Irritants like dust, smoke or overuse of decongestant nasal sprays. Sometimes there's no obvious cause.	Blocked nose, clear mucus, sneezing, cough.
Hay fever	Also called 'allergic rhinitis'. Very similar to rhinitis but caused by an allergic reaction to something you are breathing in.	Pollen, dust, animal dander.	Sneezing, runny or itchy nose, clear mucus, itching or watery eyes, itchy/dry skin or ECZEMA flare up. Symptoms can last weeks or months.
Sinusitis	An infection of the sinuses (the air pockets either side of your nose). It's common after a COLD or FLU.	Usually a virus.	Facial pain or pressure HEADACHES, nasal congestion, thick yellow or green nasal discharge, inner ear pain.
Post-nasal drip	Also known as upper airway cough syndrome. Excessive mucus produced by the nasal mucosa accumulates in the back of the throat. It drips down and makes you cough as your gag reflex kicks in.	Viruses, infections or allergies.	Persistent cough, bad breath, build-up of catarrh. You'll likely feel worse at night when you're lying flat in bed, allowing a build-up of mucus. Can last for months.

Treatments

It's best to treat hay fever as soon as possible; pay attention to the pollen count and avoid outdoor activity or drying your clothes outdoors when it is high. A pharmacist can recommend specific treatments, but the treatments below help all these conditions listed:

- Antihistamines treat symptoms caused by inflammation.
- Corticosteroids in the form of nasal sprays.
- Painkillers.
- A humidifier or vaporiser with eucalyptus oil may help.
- Drink plenty of water.
- Avoid cigarette smoke.
- Reduce or avoid alcohol.

When to see your GP

If you are really struggling and over-the-counter remedies are not helping even when used consistently, see your doctor. Acute, unresolved SINUSITIS may be the result of a bacterial infection for which you may be prescribed antibiotics.

Snoring & sleep apnoea

Snoring is common, and many of us will snore if we fall asleep in a certain position. It's a problem for the people who share a bed (or a house!) with us, but snoring is also linked to an increase in risk of heart issues like HIGH BLOOD PRESSURE, STROKE and HEART ATTACK, particularly if you briefly stop breathing while asleep. This is called obstructive sleep apnoea and needs medical attention.

Snoring

Causes
Snoring is the sound of vibrating tissues in the throat and the mouth when you breathe while sleeping. It can be a soft whine, a whistle or a loud snort. It's affected by a number of factors, including:

- **Anatomy:** A low, soft palate (roof of the mouth) or extra mouth tissue can narrow your airway and cause snoring.
- **Weight:** Being overweight or OBESE leads to extra throat tissues that narrow your airway.
- **Alcohol consumption:** Alcohol consumption can increase the likelihood of snoring because it relaxes the upper airway muscles, which can lead to more noise.
- **ALLERGIES, COLDS or nasal congestion:** All these can cause snoring or make it worse by reducing space in the nasal cavity that air can pass through.

Treatment
- Sleep on your side – arrange your pillows or bedding to keep you in position.
- Elevate your head in bed with extra pillows.
- If you have a blocked nose, rinse with warm salty water before bed.
- Avoid alcohol before bed.
- Don't take sedatives or sleeping pills as they often make snoring worse.
- Some people find nasal strips, mouthpieces or mouth guards help.
- Lose weight if you are overweight or OBESE.
- Quit smoking.
- Research has shown that certain mouth exercises may help. The Sleep Foundation (www.sleepfoundation.org) has good recommendations for these.

Sleep apnoea

Causes
When you are asleep, the muscles in your head and neck relax. If your soft tissues land onto your windpipe they can obstruct your breathing, which becomes noisy and laboured. For short periods, you stop breathing. It's quite scary as you jolt yourself awake and so never feel like you have slept properly. You may nod off during the day, feel 'out of it' and have mood swings.

Diagnosis
The Epworth Sleepiness Scale is a useful tool you can find online to measure whether your level of sleepiness in the daytime is normal or not, as this a good sign of how much your nighttime sleep is being affected. If you score highly, your GP will send you for a sleep study, which involves being monitored while you sleep at a hospital or a sleep centre or using a device at home.

Treatment
Lifestyle changes: Losing weight (if necessary) is the first step – you will feel much better. Exercise is also beneficial. Avoid alcohol, sleeping pills and anti-anxiety medication if you can. Sleep on your side or stomach.
Mandibular advancement device: A bit like a gum shield, this holds your airways open while you're asleep.
CPAP machine: This is the most effective treatment for severe cases. You wear it while you sleep and it sends air up your nose to keep your airways open.
Surgery: This is a last resort but an operation, e.g. to realign your jaw or remove your tonsils, can address the physical cause of the obstruction to your windpipe.

⚠ Contagious (depending on cause)

Sore throat & hoarse voice

Having a scratchy, dry or painful throat happens when the vocal cords become irritated, inflamed or coated in mucus. It often comes with a dry cough and feeling like you need to clear your throat a lot, although it can also be linked to digestive issues.

Causes

Sore throats and hoarse voices are symptoms of many common illnesses rather than an illness itself. These can include:

Laryngitis: Often a result of a COLD or FLU and usually characterised by a sore throat, croaky voice and dry cough. It will go away by itself in one to two weeks and you are unlikely to need antibiotics.

GASTROESOPHAGEAL REFLUX DISEASE (GORD): This is when stomach acid gets up into the oesophagus and irritates it.

Throat cancers: Rare in non-smokers. Other potential symptoms are unexplained weight loss, a lump somewhere in the neck, changes to the voice and difficulty swallowing.

TONSILLITIS.

COLD and **FLU.**

Treatment

- Adults can gargle with salt water or dissolvable aspirin (don't swallow it).
- Try to rest your voice as much as possible.
- Stay well hydrated – avoid caffeine and alcohol, which will dehydrate you.
- Avoid hot, dry, dusty (or smoky) places. To keep your throat from becoming dry, try a humidifier and avoid having the heating on full blast.
- Take painkillers if needed but be aware that some people – particularly those with ASTHMA – find that non-steroidal anti-inflammatory drugs such as ibuprofen or aspirin make their cough or wheeze worse.
- Alternating warm lemon tea with honey and iced drinks can help.

Red flag symptoms

See a doctor if a sore throat doesn't improve after a couple of weeks or is combined with more worrying symptoms, such as a rash, difficulty breathing or a high FEVER. Check with your GP or call 111 if:

- Your child is making high-pitched wheezing noises and has a barking cough and difficulty breathing – this will likely be croup (see below).
- Your child has been off their food for three to four days, with a muffled voice or they are drooling.
- You see blood in your or your child's saliva.

Croup

Croup is a common childhood infection usually caused by viruses, like parainfluenza and the common COLD. It mainly affects children aged six months to three years and is more prevalent during late autumn and early winter. It is a symptom, not a diagnosis, so you can get it more than once. It is recognisable from a distinct barking, seal-like cough and a raspy sound when breathing, accompanied by COLD-like symptoms. It will usually get better after 48 hours but symptoms can be managed by staying hydrated and taking paracetamol. Beware that ibuprofen can make the cough worse and cough syrups or decongestants don't tend to help; they can also make children drowsy, worsening breathing difficulties. Warm honey and lemon can soothe the cough if needed and your doctor may give a single dose of corticosteroid. Croup is not usually serious but go to A&E if your child shows difficulty breathing, their lips go grey, white or blue or they become floppy.

🛑 Contagious (depending on cause)

Tonsillitis

Tonsillitis can make you feel quite unwell. Occasionally, it can be serious, but more often it will resolve itself with rest, good hydration and over-the-counter medication. Anyone can get it, but it's more common in children. It's caused by an infection like COLD or FLU – usually a virus but bacterial versions do exist. It's not contagious in itself, but of course COLD and FLU is, so it's important to wash your hands regularly, dispose of tissues straight away and avoid preparing food for others.

SYMPTOMS
+ **Red, swollen tonsils.**
+ SORE THROAT.
+ **Difficulty swallowing.**
+ TIREDNESS.
+ HEADACHE.
+ **Earache.**
+ **Bad breath.**
+ FEVER.
+ **Nausea and/or vomiting.**
+ **Spots or a yellowish coating on the tonsils.**

Diagnosis

You will usually start to feel better after three or four days, although full recovery can take two weeks (and it's normal to feel fairly rotten at the start). See a doctor if:

- Your symptoms are not improving after one week.
- You keep getting tonsillitis.
- You have white spots or yellow coating on your tonsils.
- You have difficulty eating and drinking.
- You have swollen glands and saliva is pooling in your mouth (also see QUINSY).
- See also FEVERS.

Treatment

A pharmacist can give advice on how to treat your symptoms with painkillers, throat lozenges and throat sprays. A doctor may take a swab to find out if the infection is bacterial or viral, or they may conclude the former and prescribe antibiotics, such as penicillin. However, most cases are viral and antibiotics won't help with this.

Tonsillectomy

If you have returning, chronic tonsillitis – more than seven episodes a year – and it's affecting your work or your schooling, then you may need to have an operation to remove your tonsils.

Complications of tonsillitis

Quinsy

A rare but serious complication where a pus-filled abscess grows between a tonsil and the side of your throat. It's caused by a bacterial infection and is more common in children and young adults, although anyone can get it. It can come on after the main illness has passed or at the same time. It causes your throat to narrow and so can affect your breathing. It needs to be treated urgently in hospital. Other symptoms include:

- Severe sudden SORE THROAT, often concentrated on one side.
- Pain and difficulty opening your mouth and swallowing, sometimes causing you to drool.

Septicaemia

A very rare but potentially life-threatening complication of tonsillitis, so it's always worth being on the lookout for the signs just in case, so you can act swiftly (see page 27).

SLEEP APNOEA

Tonsillitis might be more serious if you have SLEEP APNOEA, as it will make it more difficult for you to breathe when asleep. Talk to your doctor if you are concerned.

Dental problems

In the UK it is recommended you have a dental check-up every six months, although this can be extended as long as two years if you are an adult with very good teeth and gum health, or annually for people under 18. Most adults will need to pay a fee for NHS dental check-ups and treatment but those under 18 (or under 19 and in full-time education), who are PREGNANT or receiving certain benefits are entitled to free check-ups and treatment.

The dentist will check your teeth, gums and tongue to see your general mouth health, checking for cavities in the teeth and signs of possible gum disease. Your dentist will advise whether you should also visit a dental hygienist, who can provide a regular deep clean of your teeth to keep plaque (which causes gum disease and tooth decay) at bay.

Gum disease

Gum disease can take the form of gingivitis or peridontitis, with gingivitis describing its early stages, and periodontitis being more advanced.

SYMPTOMS

+ Swollen or bleeding gums (such as when flossing, brushing or eating hard foods).
+ Receding gums
+ Bad breath, or a bad taste in your mouth.

Treatment

Gingivitis can be reversed by a good oral hygiene routine and your dentist or dental hygienist will advise you on how to achieve it. Periodontitis can advance to loosening teeth and will need careful dental hygiene to avoid symptoms getting worse.

Tooth decay

Tooth decay can be a result of poor dental hygiene or too much sugary food and drink.

SYMPTOMS

+ Toothache.
+ Sensitivity to hot and cold food.

Treatment

The dentist will advise on fluoride treatments for early tooth decay, or whether you need a filling, root canal treatment, or removal of the tooth.

Maintaining healthy teeth & gums

The biggest risk factors for gum disease are age, genetics, smoking, stress, poor oral hygiene, clenching or grinding of the teeth, poor nutrition or OBESITY. Prevention is straightforward, however, by controlling the amount of plaque and tartar building up on your teeth. For good dental hygiene:

- Floss daily and brush twice daily – the dental hygienist can show you good techniques.
- Use a fluoride toothpaste for your regular brushing, and don't rinse the mouth after you have brushed at night-time.
- Get regular scale and polish treatments with the hygienist – these remove plaque and tartar from the teeth and below the gumline.
- Ensure you attend regular dental check-ups.
- Stop smoking and limit alcohol intake.

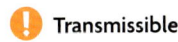 Transmissible

Headlice

We often use the words 'headlice' and 'nits' interchangeably, but they refer to slightly different things: headlice are the creatures themselves and nits are the tiny egg cases they kindly leave behind in our hair. The idea of it might seem unpleasant but in reality it's a very common part of childhood (and potentially adulthood, if you are in contact with kids), nothing to worry about and easy to treat at home. It has nothing to do with having dirty hair.

SYMPTOMS
+ Itchy scalp.
+ Tickling sensation.

Diagnosis

The only way to know for sure is to find a louse. Do this by combing the hair carefully with a special fine-toothed headlice comb that you can buy at pharmacies. Headlice are about 3mm (⅛ inches) long and brown in colour. The tiny eggs are brown/white.

Treatment

Treat headlice as soon as you spot them. The most efficient strategy is to treat everyone in the house, or whoever the person with headlice has been in close contact with recently. Headlice can't live for long if they are not on a head, so there's only a minor risk of re-transmission from bedding, towels, etc. and pets can't get headlice. You can buy medicated shampoos (containing permethrin) if the following approach doesn't work, but it often will.

- Wash your hair with normal shampoo and apply conditioner so it's easier to get the detection comb through the hair.
- Before washing out the conditioner, carefully divide the wet hair into sections and, using the headlice comb, systematically comb through each section looking for and removing the headlice and eggs. You might need to wipe the comb on white kitchen paper so the lice are easier to spot.
- Repeat the process every four days until you haven't found any lice for three consecutive sessions.

A single treatment for headlice will not kill all nits. You need to repeatedly check hair every four days when you're aware of an outbreak.

THE UPPER & LOWER BODY

THE RESPIRATORY SYSTEM

The respiratory system includes the nose, trachea (windpipe), the muscles that allow us to breathe, the lungs and all the tissues that help us get oxygen into our bloodstream.

When we breathe in, the diaphragm – a big, flat muscle under your lungs – contracts, pulling in air through your nose and mouth. Your lungs expand and the tissues inside them take in oxygen and release carbon dioxide. When you breathe out, your diaphragm and the muscles in between your ribs relax, making your chest cavity smaller, and air is exhaled back out again. Imagine a foot pump – you squash it down to make air come out.

The larynx (voice box) is also part of the respiratory system. Air vibrating the vocal cords is what allows us to make a noise, which is why it's hard to speak when you're out of breath. We also smell by breathing in air – the olfactory nerves behind the top of your nose send signals to your brain which then interprets what that smell might be.

The respiratory system has a lot of clever techniques it uses to stop bugs getting into the body. One of these is mucus (phlegm), which traps germs. So while it might feel gross to be snotty when you are ill, that's the respiratory system working hard to get rid of the bacteria or virus.

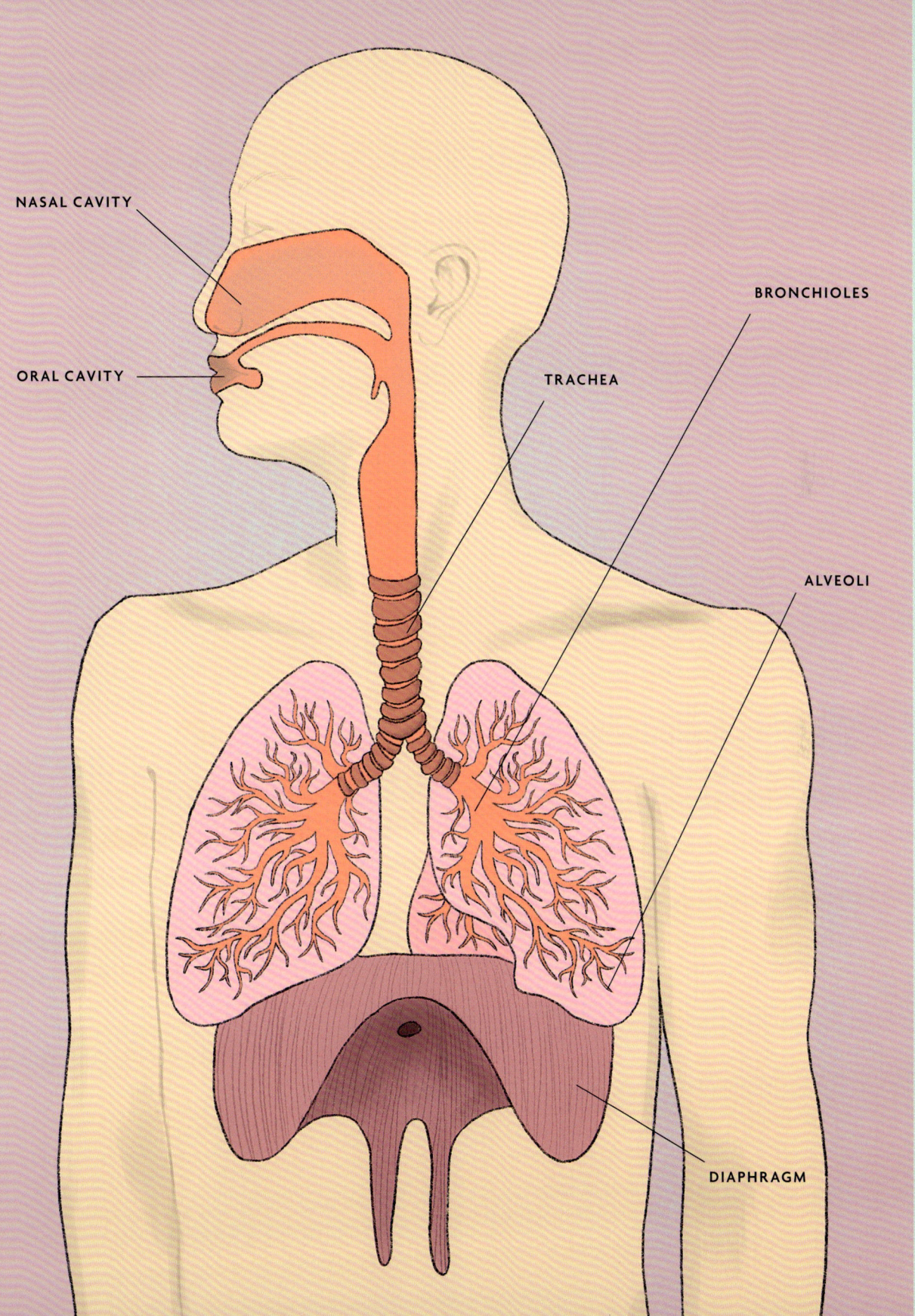

> ❗ Contagious

Colds & flu

Colds and flu are caused by many different types of viruses (but not bacteria, so antibiotics don't help). Covid-19 is just one type of coronavirus and many other types of coronaviruses also cause what we'd usually term 'the common cold'. Rhinoviruses are another frequent cause of colds, while influenza viruses cause flu. They are all airborne or 'aerosol' viruses, which means they are spread by tiny droplets in the air from coughing and sneezing.

The main difference between cold and flu is the severity – how ill it makes you. Flu is generally worse although some people can become very ill with a cold, such as those who are immunocompromised, have an underlying health condition like ASTHMA or heart problems, are very elderly or are generally in poor health. These groups need to be more careful over cold and flu season. Many people in these groups are eligible for the flu vaccine free on the NHS.

Flu

Symptoms can come on suddenly (though not always) with a feeling of extreme FATIGUE and a raised FEVER.

You are more likely to have a FEVER along with chills, aches and nausea.

Other symptoms include a SORE THROAT, loss of appetite, feeling 'out of it' and difficulty sleeping.

It can take two weeks to get over the flu, particularly the FATIGUE that comes with it.

What we call 'stomach flu' – vomiting, diarrhoea, FEVER, cramps, not wanting to eat – is actually gastroenteritis. This can be caused by a FOOD-BORNE BACTERIAL INFECTION or a virus and it will usually get better by itself within a week.

Cold

Symptoms come on gradually over a few days and often start with a SORE THROAT.

You are more likely to have a stuffy or runny nose.

A cough often comes on around the fourth or fifth day of being ill.

For those of us in good health, a cold will usually clear up in a week.

A cough that lasts for three weeks and follows a cold may be BRONCHITIS.

How to avoiding getting & passing on colds & flu

You are most infectious when you first get the virus, although this might be before you're aware you're ill. If you start to develop a SORE THROAT or feel very run down and tired, it's a good idea to stay home and limit social contact, particularly with people who are in vulnerable groups.

Get the flu and Covid-19 vaccines if you can (both can be purchased at pharmacies if you are not eligible for a free NHS vaccine). Covid-19 is still around and probably always will be. Having a vaccine reduces the severity of your symptoms should you get the virus, and helps prevent you from passing the illness onto others.

If you are ill, cover your mouth when you cough, dispose of tissues straight away and wash your hands, or cough into your elbow rather than your hands. Avoid sharing cooking and eating utensils and open a window for ventilation if you are sharing your space with others.

Treatment

The best way to deal with a cold and flu is plenty of rest and fluids. Over-the-counter medicines and treatments may help.

- Painkillers like ibuprofen, paracetamol and aspirin (take ibuprofen with food and don't give aspirin to under 16s).
- Branded cold remedies like Night Nurse or Lemsip, or a generic 'Cold & Flu Relief' drink – bear in mind that these contain painkillers so make sure you are not exceeding the recommended dose.
- Decongestants like nasal sprays and vapour rubs or burning eucalyptus oil in an oil burner can help you feel less stuffed up.
- Constant coughing will inflame your air passages so cough syrups are useful to prevent this.
- Drink warm drinks like lemon juice mixed with hot water to soothe the throat and keep the airways more open.
- Steam inhalations are helpful for SORE THROATS and coughs to keep the airways moist and open (this isn't suitable for children as they can burn themselves).
- Eat healthy foods to support the immune system as it fights to get you better.

Most of us will recover from a cold or flu within about two weeks, even when we have felt really unwell. Although there are so many bugs around in the winter that it's possible to get almost back-to-back colds, making you feel like you have been ill for weeks or even months.

Red flag symptoms

For some people, these illnesses can develop into something much more serious, requiring hospitalisation.

- What people sometimes called the 'hundred-day cough' is actually whooping cough. Vaccination against whooping cough is part of the NHS vaccination programme but unvaccinated children often get it. A low-grade FEVER is accompanied by coughing fits that end with a 'whooping' sound. You may need antibiotics. It's dangerous in young children and those who are PREGNANT, so both children and PREGNANT women are eligible to receive a whooping cough vaccination on the NHS.
- If you are over 65, have other health complications, are PREGNANT or are worried about your young child speak to your GP.
- Go to A&E or call an ambulance if you or someone else has sudden chest pains, is struggling to breathe or is coughing up blood.

See advice for FEVERS.

> ⚠️ Non-contagious

Asthma

Asthma is a chronic, lifelong autoimmune condition. Sufferers sometimes struggle to breathe because the airways swell up, extra mucus (phlegm) is produced, narrowing them further, and muscles around them contract. This produces a wheezing sound when breathing. It is usually diagnosed in children but can affect all ages. It can be managed effectively with medication and lifestyle, so those who have it can lead a normal life. It sometimes appears to go away or reduce in severity, but it cannot be cured.

Causes

Genetics, exposure to cigarette smoke and pollutants are possible causes. Children born prematurely and those who have a family history of the condition are more likely to suffer from asthma. Some people get it through exposure to certain airborne substances at work. There's growing data that it could be linked to poor gut health.

Asthma symptoms are triggered by different things for different people. It's usually a reaction to dust mites, pollen, foodstuffs, pet hair or mould spores. For some, it's cold or humid weather, exercise, being unwell or even strong emotions or stress. Others say it seems random.

SYMPTOMS

Symptoms come and go and include:
- Coughing (especially at night).
- Wheezing and shortness of breath.
- Chest tightness or pain.
- Persistent nasal congestion.

Diagnosis

Your GP can diagnose you with asthma, using a FeNO monitor, which measures nitric oxide when you breathe out, or give you a peak flow monitor to take home to check your breathing at different times of the day.

Treatment

You will be given one or two inhalers.
- A **blue** reliever inhaler is used to stop symptoms when they occur. You should always have this with you.
- A **brown** preventer inhaler contains steroids to reduce inflammation and stop you from getting symptoms.
- A **combination** inhaler contains both medications.

Try to identify what triggers your symptoms. You should also get an action plan so you know what to do if your symptoms get worse. Get your annual FLU and Covid-19 vaccines and do not smoke.

Antihistamines and decongestants can sometimes help too. Exercise and physiotherapy to improve lung capacity is also beneficial.

Red flag – asthma attacks

It's important to understand how asthma affects you and to always carry an inhaler to avoid an asthma attack, as this is a medical emergency.

SYMPTOMS

- Wheezing, coughing, struggling to talk or becoming silent.
- Muscles in the chest and neck contract.
- Feeling panicked and clammy.
- In extreme cases, fingernails and lips go blue.

What to do

In the first instance, take six to ten puffs of the blue inhaler, 30–60 seconds apart. If you do not feel better, call an ambulance. Repeat the process with the inhaler while you wait for the ambulance to arrive. If you do feel better still call your GP for an urgent appointment to check your medication as an attack could happen again.

🟢 **Non-contagious**

Pleurisy

This is when the thin lining between the lungs (pleura) and the ribs becomes inflamed. There are many different causes, including bacteria, viruses and trauma to the ribs. Pleurisy itself is not contagious, however some of the conditions that can cause pleurisy can be infectious. For example, with PNEUMONIA, which is caused by a virus or bacteria, leads to pleurisy, the PNEUMONIA itself is contagious rather than the pleurisy.

SYMPTOMS
+ Sharp chest pain when breathing, that can spread to the back and shoulders.
+ Short, shallow breathing.
+ Cough and/or FEVER.

Diagnosis
Any sort of chest pain needs investigating, especially a sharp chest pain when you breathe in or out as it is similar to what someone might experience if they have an EMBOLISM (blood clot) on the lungs, which is very serious and needs ruling out.

A blood test, chest X-ray and ultrasound scan can look for inflammation of the lung and see if there is anything else going on. You may have a CT scan or lung tissue biopsy.

Treatment
Painkillers and anti-inflammatories, such as ibuprofen, will relieve the discomfort. Then it's a case of treating the underlying cause – whether that's bacteria or a virus. Sometimes excess fluid will need to be drained to help with breathing. It can take six to twelve weeks to recover from pleurisy.

 Genetic

Cystic fibrosis

Cystic fibrosis is a chronic, inherited disorder that causes the lungs and digestive system to be clogged with a thick sticky mucus, resulting in inflammation.

SYMPTOMS
+ Thick mucus.
+ FEVER.
+ Shortness of breath, coughing, wheezing, breathing difficulties.
+ Repeated chest infections.
+ Difficulty digesting food, particularly fatty foods, leading to malnutrition, poor growth in height and diarrhoea.

Diagnosis & treatment
All newborn babies in the UK are tested for cystic fibrosis in their 'heel prick test' (newborn blood spot test), so it is usually diagnosed at birth. If this has not been the case then diagnosis is by chest X-ray or MRI scan. There is no cure for cystic fibrosis and treatment will involve a daily regime of medication to help breathing and digestion, as well as chest and breathing physio. Organ transplants (most commonly lungs) are also used as treatment, but when people start treatment from birth the condition can be managed successfully, with the majority of babies diagnosed with cystic fibrosis aging well past middle-age.

> Non-contagious

Chronic obstructive pulmonary disease (COPD)

This is a common lung disease that makes it difficult to breathe. It's caused by damage to the airways over a period of time, leading to inflammation and blocked air flow. The symptoms worsen over time and seriously impact quality of life unless treated.

Causes
- The biggest cause is smoking. The more and longer you smoke, the greater your risk. It is also caused by second-hand smoke.
- Long-term exposure to air pollution, especially from indoor heating fuel.
- Toxic fumes, such as from chemicals in the workplace.
- A genetic deficiency in a protein that protects the lungs.
- Frequent severe chest infections in childhood and beyond.

SYMPTOMS
- Coughing and wheezing.
- Mucus (phlegm).
- Difficulty catching your breath.
- Low mood.
- Fatigue.
- Blocked or runny nose.

Emphysema
This is a type of COPD with the same causes and similar symptoms. The small sacs of air in the lungs – called alveoli – have been damaged and can't transfer oxygen into and carbon dioxide out of the cells properly, leading to low blood-oxygen levels. The condition can be managed with the right treatment and lifestyle factors. Stopping smoking is by far the most important course of action.

Diagnosis
It's important to get a diagnosis as soon as possible for a better long-term outcome. The doctor will listen to your chest and give you a spirometry test to see how much air you can exhale. You may have a blood test and be sent for an X-ray to rule out other conditions. You may have a CT scan and other tests to measure the oxygen levels in your blood to determine what stage COPD you have (stages are one to four). Your stage isn't always linked to how severe your symptoms are.

Treatment
It is possible to improve lung function and have a much better quality of life with the right treatment. Early-stage COPD can be reversed if someone stops smoking or ceases exposure to the harmful substance causing the damage.

The treatment is similar to that for ASTHMA, with inhalers to relax the airways. Lifestyle changes like exercise can increase lung function. You may need a course of corticosteroids to reduce inflammation. Those with severe COPD, which causes low oxygen levels in the blood, may need home oxygen therapy.

If you are diagnosed with COPD you will have a yearly review with your doctor to monitor its progress and your treatment. You will be more susceptible to complications from COLDS and FLU so will need to ensure you get vaccines for FLU and Covid-19 when they are offered.

⚠️ Contagious

Bronchitis

Acute bronchitis is an inflammation of the bronchi, the two main tubes that go into each lung. It can happen after having a COLD or FLU. Anyone can get it but it's common in children under five. If you don't have any underlying health conditions, then it will usually get better by itself. The virus that leads to it is contagious. Chronic bronchitis is a different condition (see below).

SYMPTOMS

These are similar to COLDS and FLU:
- Hacking, productive cough.
- Coughing up clear, white, yellow or green mucus (phlegm).
- Chest pain when coughing.
- Shortness of breath.
- SORE THROAT.
- Runny nose or congestion.
- FEVER.

Chronic bronchitis

This is an ongoing CHRONIC OBSTRUCTIVE PULMONARY DISEASE resulting from long-term damage to the bronchi, rather than a virus. The symptoms are very similar to acute bronchitis but do not resolve. It's usually caused by smoking. People with chronic bronchitis often go on to develop EMPHYSEMA if not effectively treated with medications and lifestyle changes. The treatment is the same as for COPD.

Diagnosis

Diagnosed through one or a combination of physical examination, symptom evaluation, chest X-ray, sputum analysis, blood test to check for infection, blood gas to check for oxygen levels, pulmonary function test and multiplex PCR testing.

Treatment

It can take three weeks or more to get over bronchitis. The advice is the same as for COLD and FLU in terms of over-the-counter medicines, staying hydrated and rest. Do not smoke. Less often, bronchitis can be caused by a bacterial infection, which will need to be treated with antibiotics. This is more common in young children.

Red flag symptoms

See your GP if:
- You have not recovered after four weeks.
- You are coughing up blood.
- You have chest pain that comes and goes when you're coughing or breathing.
- You're over the age of 65, PREGNANT or you have a long-term lung condition or other serious underlying health issue.
- You have a weakened immune system because you're immunosuppressed – for example, you're having chemotherapy.

Call an ambulance if:
- You or someone else can't breathe.
- A child is unresponsive.

Never drive yourself to A&E if you are struggling to breathe. A complication of acute BRONCHITIS is PNEUMONIA.

THE RESPIRATORY SYSTEM

⚠️ Contagious

Pneumonia

This is an infection in one of or both of the lungs that causes the small air sacs (alveoli) to fill up with fluid or pus. It can be caused by a bacterial infection, viruses or, more rarely, fungi. Aspiration pneumonia is when something like food or water gets into the lungs and causes an infection. It can happen as a result of another illness, like FLU, Covid-19 and BRONCHITIS. Symptoms range from mild to serious; the severity depends on someone's age and overall health, and the cause of the infection. Many people will get better in two to four weeks, but older people and those with long-term health issues require medical help and sometimes hospitalisation.

SYMPTOMS

+ Cough with or without clear, yellow or green mucus (phlegm).
+ FEVER and/or chills.
+ Wheezing, trouble breathing.
+ Chest pain when breathing or coughing.
+ Heart palpitations.
+ Low blood-oxygen levels, which can cause tiredness and sometimes confusion.

How to avoiding getting pneumonia

Smoking cigarettes and marijuana, taking illegal drugs and drinking alcohol all increase the risk of getting pneumonia. There is now a vaccine against the disease called pneumococcal vaccine that is recommended for babies and over-65s. Other vaccines, like the FLU and Covid-19 vaccines, can stop you getting diseases that can lead to pneumonia.

Diagnosis

A doctor will listen to your chest and do an oxygen saturation test (though during the pandemic, it was noted that these were less accurate on black and brown skin). A blood test will indicate if the immune system is fighting an infection.

An X-ray can show levels of inflammation in the lungs. A sample of mucus (phlegm) can be used to find out what type of germ is causing the pneumonia. A CT scan may be used to check for other complications and ocassionally, a bronchoscopy will be used to look inside the airways.

Treatment

Bacterial pneumonia requires antibiotics. Mild viral pneumonia in an otherwise healthy person will often clear up by itself, with the symptoms treated by over-the-counter medicines, rest and plenty of fluids.

If someone requires hospitalisation, they may be given oxygen to help them breathe. In some cases, fluid can be drawn from the lung using a syringe.

Going through severe pneumonia and struggling to breathe can be traumatising and result in PTSD.

> **Non-contagious**

Collapsed lung (pneumothorax)

A collapsed lung is a medical emergency that requires immediate hospitalisation. It happens when air leaks from the lung into the chest wall and the pressure created means that the lung cannot expand, seriously restricting breathing.

Causes

There are many reasons why this might happen:

- Blockages caused by lung diseases create large bulging areas that can burst, allowing air into the chest cavity.
- A traumatic injury as a result of an accident or wound, or during surgery or a biopsy if the lung is punctured.
- A rare complication of ENDOMETRIOSIS when endometrial tissue growing outside the uterus causes a cyst that bleeds in the space between the lung and chest wall, causing the lung to collapse.
- Pressure changes, such as at altitude or when scuba diving, can cause an air pocket that bursts, collapsing the lung.
- Primary spontaneous pneumothorax is when there's no underlying health condition that causes a collapsed lung. This can happen if normal air pockets in your lung break apart and release air.

SYMPTOMS

This happens very quickly, so all the symptoms have a sudden onset:

+ Pain on one side (it's very rare to have two collapsed lungs at the same time).
+ Shortness of breath.
+ Bluish colour in the lips and nails (which can be harder to see in some skin tones) due to lack of oxygen.
+ Feeling exhausted, faint and like you can barely move.

Diagnosis

A CT scan and chest X-ray will show that the lung has collapsed.

Treatment

Oxygen therapy can help to re-expand the lung or it might be necessary to puncture the chest wall from the outside to allow the trapped air to escape. A larger collapse means doctors will need to put a tube into the chest. Some people will need surgery to repair the damage caused. Most people will recover well, even from a major lung collapse, so long as they are treated quickly.

> **Non-contagious**

Lung cancer

Lung cancer is the third most common cancer in the UK and the most common cancer to cause death. The primary cause is smoking. Research has shown that risk of lung cancer starts to decrease when someone gives up smoking. After 15 years, it is almost the same as someone who has never smoked.

SYMPTOMS

Sometimes lung cancer does not have any symptoms to start with or the symptoms are mild and put down to something else. This is one of the reasons why it has lower survival rates than other cancers, as it's often caught after it has spread.

- New persistent cough for three weeks or more.
- Increasingly getting out of breath doing things that you used to be able to easily.
- Coughing up mucus (phlegm) with blood in it.
- Chest or shoulder pain.
- Repeatedly getting chest infections.
- Loss of appetite.
- Losing weight without trying to.
- Feeling TIRED a lot of the time.
- Persistent hoarse voice.
- Nausea and vomiting.
- Hypertrophic pulmonary osteoarthropathy, which causes swollen wrists and ankles, and 'finger clubbing', where your fingernails bulge out, taking on the shape of the back of a spoon.

Types of lung cancer

There are two main types of lung cancer:
- **Non-small-cell lung cancer** is the most common form of lung cancer and accounts for around 85 per cent of cases.
- **Small-cell lung cancer** is less common but also more likely to spread to other areas of the body.

In addition, lung cancer can be referred to as either:
- **Primary lung cancer** in which the cancer started in the lungs.
- **Secondary lung cancer** in which the cancer started elsewhere in the body and spread to the lungs.

Diagnosis

There are a number of other conditions that have symptoms that are similar to lung cancer, so the doctor will examine you and you may have a blood test to rule some of these out.

You will be referred for an X-ray, although it's not possible to diagnose cancer from an X-ray, so if anything shows up, you will be referred to a specialist and have a CT scan which may be followed by a biopsy.

Treatment

As part of your diagnosis, how far advanced your cancer is will be established, i.e. the size of the tumour and whether it has spread to/from other parts of your body. Along with factors like your overall health and where the tumour is in your lungs, this will inform what treatment options are best for you. You may be offered surgery, chemotherapy, radiotherapy and immunotherapy. There may be more than one option for treatment, which your cancer team will discuss with you.

Respiratory red flag symptoms

While many respiratory symptoms can usually be explained by something straightforward, there are some respiratory symptoms that you should never ignore.

Go to your GP if:

- You are regularly feeling out of breath and you don't know why. Shortness of breath is called dyspnoea. It has lots of causes, including ASTHMA, having a COLD, a PANIC ATTACK and heart problems, as the heart and the respiratory system are closely linked.

Go to A&E if you experience any of the following:

- Sudden increased breathlessness, or severe difficulty in breathing.
- Coughing up blood in sputum.
- Your sats oximeter shows declining oxygen saturation.
- Confusion and disorientation.
- Using stomach muscles to breathe.

THE CARDIO-VASCULAR SYSTEM

Your cardiovascular system is the highway and byway of your body. Oxygen, nutrients, hormones, antibodies and platelets (that stop bleeding) travel around the body via the cardiovascular system – your network of blood vessels that is powered by the heart.

THE CARDIOVASCULAR SYSTEM

AORTA

PULMONARY ARTERY

PULMONARY VEIN

SUPERIOR VENA CAVA

LEFT VENTRICLE

RIGHT VENTRICLE

Heart & blood

The heart pumps blood through the lungs where it picks up oxygen, taking it to cells as it travels through the fast-moving arteries and into the smaller blood vessels. Nutrients from food jump on when blood passes the small intestine, hormones are picked up from our glands and infection-fighting vigilantes from bone marrow. They are then taken wherever the body needs them to go.

On the way back to the heart to repeat the process, blood passes through arteries and veins, picking up the 'rubbish' as it goes – i.e. any waste product that we need to get rid of. So carbon dioxide is sent to the lungs, where it can be breathed out and exchanged for oxygen. As the blood circulates, blood goes to the kidneys to get rid of urea and control the volume of blood. Nutrients picked up from the gut are then sent into the liver to be detoxed, before the blood returns to the heart.

To keep the whole thing going, the heart beats from 50 to 90 times per minute when you're not doing anything (called 'resting heart rate'). The rate depends on a number of factors, including how healthy you are.

Your heartbeat

The da-dum double beat is the heart letting the blood in through the valves and then squeezing it out into the aorta and off round the body. Your heart gets messages from the rest of the body telling it how fast to pump. For example, if something makes you jump, your brain will release hormones to tell your heart to speed up to get oxygen and sugars to your cells in case you have to run away or fight something – this is the fight or flight response. The opposite happens when you are asleep and the heart is pumping just enough to keep you alive.

What is cholesterol?

Cholesterol is a type of fat that our body needs to carry out essential processes, but too much of it is harmful. There are two types, sometimes simply described as 'good' and 'bad' cholesterol. **LDL ('bad') cholesterol** primarily comes from the liver, which produces very low-density lipo-proteins (VLDL) which are then converted into LDL as they circulate in the bloodstream. While the liver makes most of the cholesterol, a small amount comes from the food we eat, particularly in processed foods and saturated fats that are high in cholesterol. **HDL ('good') cholesterol** clears the LDL cholesterol up by removing it from the arteries and transporting it back to the liver for processing. While high HDL levels can be genetic, they are improved by exercise and good dietary choices, such as soluble fibre, antioxidant foods and prioritising unsaturated fats over saturated fats and potentially avoiding ultra-processed foods. Not drinking alcohol or only drinking in moderation also has a positive effect.

Your cholesterol will be checked as part of regular check-ups offered to the over-40s on the NHS. You can also pay for a test at many pharmacies. High cholesterol doesn't usually cause any symptoms.

Heart disease & cardiovascular disease

Cardiovascular disease is the umbrella name given to any disease that affects the heart or blood vessels. It's the leading cause of death globally. Some heart conditions are congenital, which means they exist from birth. Some are influenced by environmental factors, particularly lifestyle, which means that by living a healthy life we can significantly reduce the risk. Sometimes the likelihood of getting a cardiovascular disease is influenced by genetics and whether someone in our close family suffered from it. Sometimes other conditions such as DIABETES can lead to heart disease, particularly if they are not managed well.

Angina

Angina is chest pain caused by reduced blood flow to the heart muscle (rather than a condition in itself). It's a warning sign that you may have an issue with your coronary arteries (the blood vessels that supply blood to the heart muscle, see ATHEROSCLEROSIS) and be at risk of a HEART ATTACK or a STROKE. It feels frightening but is not usually life-threating. Don't ignore it – treated early it's possible to control and prevent serious outcomes.

SYMPTOMS
- A tight, dull or heavy pain across the chest.
- Some people, especially women, get sharp, stabbing pains across the chest.
- Pain through the arms, neck, jaw or back.
- Breathlessness.
- FATIGUE or feeling 'fuzzy headed'.
- Nausea or a feeling similar to indigestion.

Angina is usually triggered by physical exertion and stops with a few minutes of rest. Less common, but more serious, 'unstable angina' occurs without obvious cause.

Diagnosis
A doctor will look at your medical history and symptoms, check BLOOD PRESSURE and BMI. You will probably have your CHOLESTEROL checked and be tested for DIABETES. Further tests may include an electrocardiogram (ECG), sometimes with exercise, and a coronary angiogram, where dye is injected into your veins to better see your heart and blood vessels on a CT scan.

Treatment
A variety of medicines are used to control angina, so you can live a normal life and avoid further complications:
- Glycerine sprays or tablets for use during an angina attack or to prevent or stop an attack of chest pain.
- Beta blockers to slow the heart rate and prevent attacks.
- Calcium channel blockers to relax the arteries.
- Medication to guard against HEART ATTACKS and STROKES, such as statins and aspirin.

A procedure may be required, to place a stent into the coronary artery, or in more severe cases, surgery to bypass the blocked coronary artery.

A healthy lifestyle is very important: improving your diet and increasing exercise will help to lower BLOOD PRESSURE. Lose weight if you need to and do not smoke. It can feel difficult to begin exercise but if you start slowly and take regular breaks the risk of HEART ATTACK is very low. Your GP or hospital specialist can advise on this, as well as on sex, which can be a concern for people. The British Heart Foundation website has useful information on living with angina, as well as community support groups (www.bhf.org.uk).

Seek urgent medical attention
Always call 999 if you have chest pain that doesn't go away after resting for a few minutes and taking your ANGINA medication. See page 180 for action if you think you or someone else is having a HEART ATTACK.

Heart attack

This is when a blood clot or multiple clots (THROMBOSIS or EMBOLISM) block the blood flow to the heart, depriving the body of oxygen and causing serious damage.

SYMPTOMS

Symptoms can come on gradually or suddenly.
- Pain or discomfort in the centre of the chest that feels like squeezing, which may go away and then return again.
- Shortness of breath.
- Feeling faint.
- Rapid, weak or irregular pulse.
- Additional pain in the neck, arm, back, jaw or stomach.
- Flu-like symptoms, such as nausea and aches (more common in women).
- Jaw cramping

Diagnosis

Heart attack diagnosis is made on symptom evaluation, looking at risk factors, physical examination and then an ECG, to look at electrical variations in the heart that show changes associated with a heart attack. Blood tests can also be used to detect cardiac markers like troponin, which is released into the bloodstream when heart muscle is damaged. Imaging tests, such as an echocardiogram (an ultrasound scan of the heart), assess the strength of the heart muscle and see if it is weakened after the attack. During a heart attack, or if you appear at risk of a heart attack, an angiogram can also be used to identify the blocked artery and insert a stent.

Treatment

Around half of heart attacks are fatal, but if someone gets to hospital, then treatment can be given to remove the blockage, as emergency treatment and then long-term treatment. Around 90 per cent of those who make it to hospital, therefore, will survive. Emergency treatment would be blood thinner, such as aspirin and glyceryl trinitrate (GTN), as well as oxygen. If the patient has made it to hospital, then an angioplasty (a stent, which uses a balloon catheter to widen a blocked artery) can be conducted and the patient will be given a thrombolytic such as clopidogrel.

Longer-term care includes lifelong beta blockers (to reduce the heart rate and BLOOD PRESSURE, limiting heart damage), ACE inhibitors, statins (to lower LDL CHOLESTEROL levels) and aspirin as well as clopidogrel (for a year after the attack). Lifelong cardiac rehabilitation will also include exercise, education, counselling, healthy diet, weight management and smoking cessation, to help improve lifelong heart health.

How well someone recovers depends on how much damage has been done to the heart muscle. A heart attack is a very traumatic experience, so it can take time to recover psychologically, too.

What to do if you suspect someone is having a heart attack

- Call 999 immediately if someone has HEART ATTACK symptoms (see above). It doesn't matter if it turns out to be something else.
- If they have ANGINA medicine with them, help them to take some. You can also give them one aspirin (300mg) to chew if they are not allergic.
- If they become unresponsive, start CPR (chest compressions).

Heart failure

This scary-sounding term essentially means that the heart is unable to pump blood around the body properly and needs treatment to help it work. This will be medicine, a pacemaker or some other surgery. They won't cure the problem, but it can often be managed successfully for many years.

SYMPTOMS
+ **Shortness of breath, particularly when moving around.**
+ **Fatigue.**
+ **Swelling of ankles or legs.**
+ **Feeling lightheaded, dizzy or fainting.**

Causes
- The heart becoming weak or stiff – a problem that gets worse over time.
- Problems with the heart's valves.
- HIGH BLOOD PRESSURE.
- HEART DISEASE such as ATHEROSCLEROSIS.
- Irregular heartbeat.
- Congenital heart problems present from birth.

Symptoms can come on suddenly (acute heart failure) or get worse gradually over time (chronic heart failure).

Broken heart syndrome/stress cardiomyopathy
Stress cardiomyopathy is brought about by a period of extreme emotional stress or frightening illness or accident. It's unclear what the physical cause is but it could be that having a lot of adrenaline in your system for a period of time temporarily damages the heart muscle.

Symptoms are similar to a HEART ATTACK, which can be scary. They will reduce over time, but always seek urgent medical help if you are experiencing unexplained chest pains and shortness of breath. It doesn't matter what the reason turns out to be – it needs to be checked urgently.

Diagnosis
Always see your GP if you are regularly experiencing symptoms of heart failure, or if you have been diagnosed but your symptoms are getting worse.

There are a variety of tests that can be carried out to see how well your heart is working. These include:
- Blood test.
- Chest X-ray.
- Breathing tests to check your lung capacity.
- Electrocardiogram (ECG), either while resting or you may be asked to do some exercise to see how your heart responds.
- Echocardiogram (a type of ultrasound).

Treatment
This depends on what is causing the heart failure and how severe the symptoms are. Introducing the right kinds of exercise and following a healthy diet can have a big impact on symptoms and how much they affect your day-to-day life. Good nutrition and exercise can slow the progression of the problems causing heart failure.

Medications may be prescribed, such as blood thinners, diuretics to remove excess fluid from the body (which causes swelling in the legs and ankles), medicine to relax blood vessels or slow the heart rate, and aspirin to prevent blood clots (THROMBOSIS or EMBOLISM).

In some cases, a pacemaker will be fitted in surgery. This is a device that controls an irregular heartbeat.

Red flag symptom
If you are experiencing symptoms of a HEART ATTACK (see opposite), call 999.

Thrombosis

Thrombosis a blood clot that forms in one place, reducing or blocking blood flow inside your blood vessels. It falls into two categories – venous thrombosis and arterial thrombosis – and can occur anywhere in the body where there are veins and arteries, though they most commonly occur in the lungs or lower limbs. Treatment is usually effective if it's delivered in good time, before the clot has had a chance to do serious damage to the artery, organs or tissue.

Venous thrombosis

This is where a blood clot blocks a vein. This is the most common type of thrombosis and usually occurs in the deep veins of the lower legs, which is known as deep vein thrombosis (DVT), but clots can form in your thighs, pelvis or arms.

SYMPTOMS
+ Pain.
+ Swelling and redness.
+ Soreness of the skin.

Diagnosis
Get an urgent GP appointment if you think you have deep vein thrombosis. Diagnosis is through a physical examination, ultrasound scan and/or an X-ray of the veins in the affected area.

Treatment
Treatment is usually through blood-thinning medications, depending on how established the thrombosis is. Blood-thinning medication will usually need to be taken continally for around three months.

Risk factors
Risk factors for getting a THROMBOSIS are similar to those for getting an EMBOLISM. Examples include family history, being overweight or OBESE, smoking, long periods of immobility or other health conditions.

Arterial thrombosis

Occurs when a blood clot forms in an artery. This is usually caused by ARTERIOSCLEROSIS. Symptoms will vary depending on where in the body the clot occurs.

SYMPTOMS
Arterial thrombosis in the leg or arm:
+ Numbness or weakness on one side of the body or just the affected limb.
+ Swelling.
+ Skin that's cool to the touch.
+ Blisters or sores.

Arterial thrombosis in the small intestine:
+ Abdominal pain.
+ Diarrhoea and/or vomiting.
+ FEVER.

Diagnosis
Seek urgent medical attention if you think you have arterial thrombosis as it can cause a STROKE or HEART ATTACK. Diagnosis is via one or a combination of a physical examination, a D-dimer blood test (that measures protein released when a blood clot breaks down so an elevated level may suggest a clot), checking oxygen levels or an ECG which looks at heart rhythms. If the clot appears to be in the leg, then a leg vein ultrasound scan can be conducted.

Treatment
In hospital, the priority will be to remove or dissolve the clot and allow the blood to flow, either with medication or by adding a stent to widen the vein or artery.

Embolism

Embolism is a blood clot that starts off somewhere in the body, such as in the leg, then breaks off and moves through the body, blocking a blood vessel. It can also be caused by a tumour, fat or an air bubble and is more common in the veins than in the arteries. When an embolism causes a blockage of blood flow to the brain, it can cause a STROKE, which can be life-threatening or cause lifelong consequences.

Pulmonary embolism

This is a blockage in the artery of the lungs, usually as a result of a VENOUS THROMBOSIS.

SYMPTOMS
+ Sharp pain in the chest.
+ Difficulty breathing.
+ Coughing up blood.

Causes & risk factors
You are more likely to suffer a blood clot if you:
- Have a family history of blood disorders.
- Use the combined oral CONTRACEPTIVE pill.
- Have just given birth.
- Have spent a long time being immobile.
- Have recently had surgery.
- Are overweight, OBESE or have an unhealthy diet.
- Smoke.
- Have other health conditions, such as cancer, HEART DISEASE, lung disease, CROHN'S DISEASE or another inflammatory condition.

Diagnosis & treatment
Your GP will send you to hospital where you will be given an injection of anticoagulant medicine to stop clots growing. If an embolism is confirmed, treatment by anticoagulant tablets will continue for at least three months.

> **Red flag**
> An EMBOLISM is a medical emergency. Call 999 if you have chest pain and/or trouble breathing or notice the symptoms of a STROKE.

Cerebral embolism

A cerebral embolism is a blockage in the brain, usually caused by a THROMBOSIS in the neck. In more serious cases this can cause a STROKE, in less serious cases a TIA.

SYMPTOMS
+ Blurred vision, dizziness or clumsiness.
+ Confusion or memory loss.
+ Difficulty speaking.
+ Nausea.
+ Severe HEADACHE.

If the embolism leads to a stroke, symptoms can come on very quickly. The acronyn 'FAST' is useful to help to recognise them:
+ F = Face: one side of the face might droop.
+ A = Arms: there may be weakness in one or both arms or down one side of the body.
+ S = Speech: speech can become slurred.
+ T = Time: seek help immediately if you or someone else is having a stroke. The faster you get medical treatment the better the chance of a recovery.

Diagnosis & treatment
Diagnosis is via blood test and a CT, MRI or ultrasound scan. Treatment will be by medicine or surgery to remove the blood clots, and then longer-term medicines to stop new clots forming, lower blood pressure and lower CHOLESTEROL. If the embolism leads to a STROKE, then recovery times can vary significantly. See page 127 for more.

Endocarditis

Very rarely, the heart's inner lining and valves can become infected by bacteria or fungi. This usually only happens when there is already something wrong with the heart – for example, HEART DISEASE or an inherited heart condition. It can also be a complication of rheumatic fever. People who use recreational intravenous drugs are at greater risk of endocarditis, as are those with TOOTH DECAY and GUM DISEASE (the bacteria that causes it can get into our systems via the mouth), and those who are immunocompromised. It's very serious if not caught and treated in hospital.

SYMPTOMS

Acute endocarditis: Symptoms come on suddenly.
Subacute endocarditis: Symptoms come on over weeks or even months.

- FEVER.
- Chills.
- Night sweats.
- Shortness of breath, particularly during any kind of exercise.
- Muscle and joint pain.
- Feeling very TIRED.
- Less commonly, there may be red or brown spots on the skin (which may be harder to spot on brown and black skin), narrow reddish-brown lines under the nails, or painful lumps on the pads of the fingers and toes.

Diagnosis

Diagnosis is through a blood test, echocardiogram and CT scan, to look at what's going on in the heart. It's important that it is caught as early as possible.

Treatment

Antibiotics (or antifungals if the cause is a fungal infection, although this is rarer) are given via a drip. The disease can cause serious damage to the heart, which may require surgery to treat. It can also cause clots, putting you at risk of HEART ATTACK and STROKE.

Prevention

The British Heart Foundation estimates that there are only about 1,500 cases of endocarditis in the UK each year, so it is very rare. However, if you have a condition that puts you at risk of endocarditis, it's even more important to look after your teeth and gums. To find out more about help for drug ADDICTION, you can visit the Talk to Frank website (www.talktofrank.com) to find out about services near you.

Look after your gums, look after your heart. Gum disease increases susceptibility to endocarditis.

High blood pressure (hypertension)

High blood pressure is common, especially as we get older, and often doesn't cause any symptoms. However, it is important to get your blood pressure checked regularly, as high blood pressure can increase the chance of a HEART ATTACK or STROKE and puts strain on a number of organs. Also, blood pressure is a good indication of your overall health. Low blood pressure isn't usually a problem, although it can cause you to feel dizzy or faint.

Checking your blood pressure

NHS guidelines is for adults over 40 to get their blood pressure checked at least every five years. Many pharmacies offer this for free. You should have your blood pressure taken when you are sitting down and ideally feeling relaxed. It's normal for your blood pressure to go up and down during the course of a normal day. If you are worried about your blood pressure you can buy a machine to check it at home. You should take readings two or three times a week.

What do the numbers mean?

The reading is presented as two numbers with a '/' in between. The first number is called 'systolic' – the pressure as your heart works to pump blood. The second is 'diastolic' – the pressure when your heart muscle relaxes between beats.

- **Low blood pressure:** 89/59mmHg or lower.
- **Normal blood pressure**: between 90/60mmHg and 139/89mmHg.
- **High blood pressure:** 140/90mmHg or higher (unless you are over 80, when this rises to over 150/90mmHg).
- **Severe hypertension:** 180/120mmHg – this requires urgent medical treatment.

Causes
- Being overweight or OBESE.
- Being very stressed.
- Poor diet and/or one that is high in salt.
- Smoking.
- Lack of exercise.
- KIDNEY DISEASE.
- Oral CONTRACEPTIVE pill.
- SLEEP APNOEA.

Sometimes there is no discoverable cause for high blood pressure. Older people have higher blood pressure as our arteries become more rigid with age so the heart has to work at a higher pressure to keep blood moving.

Treatment

If your blood pressure is high, most people will find that improving their diet, getting enough sleep, drinking less alcohol and exercising more will have a positive impact, as well as making them feel better overall. If you are prescribed medication, the goal is to get you on the lowest dose possible, which can be achieved with the right lifestyle.

If your blood pressure is worryingly high, you will be put on medication to help bring it down immediately. The type of medication depends on your age and ethnicity:

If you are under 55
You are likely to be prescribed an ACE inhibitor. ACE inhibitors block the enzyme that converts angiotensin I to angiotensin II. Angiotensin II is a very potent vasoconstrictor and plays a crucial role in regulating blood pressure and fluid balance. However, if your blood pressure

is high then too much angiotensin II will constrict the veins further. If this doesn't work for you (as ACE inhibitors can cause a chronic cough or impact renal function) you may be prescribed an ARB inhibitor, which will block the effects of angiotensin II at its receptors.

If you are of Black African or Afro-Caribbean heritage & under 55
It is better to start with an ARB inhibitor or calcium channel blockers, because ACE inhibitors require higher doses to be effective in these populations due to genetic variations in the kidneys.

If you are over 55
The first line of treatment is a calcium channel blocker, which reduces blood vessel contractions to open them up, or thiazide-like diuretics, which promote urination (and reduce pressure because there is less liquid in the body). ARBs may be considered if channel blockers aren't tolerated.

Keep a blood pressure diary

Once you have a blood pressure monitor, it is useful to keep a blood pressure diary to keep track of patterns, recognise how you feel when your blood pressure is elevated and note triggers. A simple table format like the one below works well for you to scribble in the details as you take your blood pressure either daily, or several times a week. Note down things such as your physical activity during the day, how well you slept, and any other physical symptoms such as FATIGUE, nausea, breathlessness, pain, life events or stress, and any alcohol or recreational drug consumption.

Date	Time	Pulse	Blood pressure	Notes

Varicose veins

These are large, twisted veins that look bumpy under the skin and may be dark blue, purplish, dark brown, grey or skin-coloured. They are common in the legs but can occur elsewhere. Varicose veins are caused by a build-up of blood that stretches the vein wall and are not medically serious but can cause complications. More women get them than men and they are common in PREGNANCY.

> **SYMPTOMS**
>
> Alongside the visible veins, you can experience additional symptoms:
> + A heavy feeling in the legs.
> + Soreness and a burning sensation.
> + Aches.

Causes

We think varicose veins are mostly caused by damage to the valves in the vein that stop blood flowing backwards. This might be from:

- Sitting or standing for too long.
- Being overweight or OBESE.
- Inactivity.
- Leg injuries.
- Smoking.

Treatment

As varicose veins are usually mostly a cosmetic issue, treatment is not usually available on the NHS unless they are impacting your quality of life or you experience complications. Wearing compression stockings during the day stops the blood from pooling, may prevent discomfort in the legs and can help stop varicose veins from getting worse. Further treatments can also lead to pressure being put on collateral veins. Treatments include:

- Sclerotherapy, where a chemical is injected to block the vein.
- Endothermal ablation, where you have a tube inserted into the vein and it's treated with radio waves or lasers.
- Surgery to remove the vein.

Prevention

- Try not to stand for long periods if you can help it.
- Maintain a healthy weight.
- Regular exercise.
- Raise your legs when sitting.
- Try not to cross your legs.
- Wear compression socks if you start to notice varicose veins.

Complications

- **Phlebitis**, when a vein near the surface of the skin becomes inflamed. The skin will be sore, warm and sometimes itchy. It's not serious unless it leads to DVT.
- **Deep vein THROMBOSIS (DVT)**, when a clot forms in the leg.
- **Varicose ECZEMA** which causes itchy, dry skin, usually on the lower leg.

> **Spider veins**
>
> Spider veins are milder versions of varicose veins. They are usually blue or red and don't bulge like varicose veins. They usually occur on the face and legs and are not serious.

Atherosclerosis

This condition is caused by a build-up of plaque – a combination of CHOLESTEROL, fat and other substances – on the walls of arteries. This narrows the gap that blood has to pass through. Clots can form, leading to HEART ATTACK, STROKE, VASCULAR DEMENTIA and ERECTILE DYSFUNCTION, among other things. The impact (and symptoms) of atherosclerosis depends on which artery is affected. For example, in the carotid artery that goes to the brain, a blockage can lead to a STROKE or brain haemorrhage; in the artery to the kidneys, there's a risk of kidney failure. It's more common in older people, as the walls of our arteries become more rigid as we age, making it easier for plaque to stick.

SYMPTOMS

+ Chest pain.
+ Pain in arms and legs, especially when exercising.
+ Shortness of breath.
+ Feeling TIRED and/or weak.
+ Confusion.
+ Sometimes people have no symptoms.

Causes

- High CHOLESTEROL.
- HIGH BLOOD PRESSURE.
- DIABETES.
- Genetic factors.
- Smoking.

Prevention

It's very important to have a healthy diet throughout our lives if we want to stay well, but particularly as we get older. To prevent atherosclerosis:

- Exercise regularly (more than two and a half hours a week).
- Eat healthily, avoiding saturated fats as much as possible.
- Don't smoke.
- Don't drink alcohol, or only drink it in moderation.
- Try to reduce HIGH BLOOD PRESSURE and high CHOLESTEROL.
- Effective management of DIABETES is also important if you have DIABETES.

Arteriosclerosis

This is often confused with ATHEROSCLEROSIS. It means the arteries thicken and lose their flexibility. The causes and consequences are very similar to ATHEROSCLEROSIS and both can occur together, increasing the risk of complications.

Raynaud's disease

When we are cold, our blood vessels constrict. This is a clever way of the body conserving heat and prioritising the core areas over our extremities. People with Raynaud's disease experience an extreme version of this which usually affects hands, feet, toes or fingers. It's very common, affecting around 10 million people in the UK, and we think it runs in families.

> **SYMPTOMS**
> + Hands, feet, toes or fingers become painful or numb and difficult to use.
> + Hands, feet, toes or fingers lose their colour, becoming white on pale skin and appearing dusky on darker skin.
> + Raynaud's can also affect ears, lips, tongue and nipples.

Diagnosis

Diagnosed by medical history and physical examination by your GP. You can do a cold challenge test to observe the effects of cold on the hands, as well as a blood test to rule out other conditions such as RHEUMATOID ARTHRITIS or LUPUS. There are two types of Raynaud's disease:

- **Primary Raynaud's** is less serious and more manageable. We don't know what causes it but triggers seem to be the cold, emotional stress and vibration, e.g. from tools.
- **Secondary Raynaud's** is caused by another condition. It needs monitoring as it can lead to ulcers or sores. Can also be caused by HIGH BLOOD PRESSURE and autoimmune conditions. Quite a few drugs can constrict blood vessels and have Raynaud's as a side effect, so it's worth checking any medication.

Treatment

There is no cure for Raynaud's and most people manage the symptoms by being well-prepared for cold conditions with gloves, handwarmers, thick socks and warm clothing. If your Raynaud's is triggered by stress, learning to manage your stress levels through breathing exercises can be beneficial.

Things that encourage good circulation are helpful – particularly regular exercise. Some people say they find acupuncture and food supplements, such as evening primrose oil (Gamma-Linolenice Acid), ginkgo biloba, omega-3 fish oil, magnesium and vitamin C, help. In severe cases, there are medications that can help relieve symptoms, although they don't work for everyone. It's important not to smoke, and alcohol and caffeine can make symptoms worse.

If you have secondary Raynaud's, it's important to keep a close watch on any skin lesion. Take pictures and even draw a ring around it with a marker so you know if it is getting bigger and turning into an ulcer. See your doctor if this is the case.

> ### Scleroderma
> For some, Raynaud's can be a symptom of the much rarer condition scleroderma. It occurs when the blood vessels shrink and don't return to their normal size as they would usually do after a Raynaud's attack. There are different types that vary in severity. If you have Raynaud's and start to develop some of these symptoms, see a doctor:
> - Hard, dry, thick patches of skin.
> - Small ulcers at the tips of fingers.
> - Swollen fingers and stiff hands.
> - REFLUX and/or heartburn.

THE DIGESTIVE SYSTEM

The job of the digestive system is pretty simple: it breaks down the food we put into our mouths into particles small enough that they can be absorbed into our bodies, giving us the energy we need to go about our day and the nutrients we require to stay healthy. Any toxins left are then removed from our system via urine (with the help of the renal system, which includes kidneys and bladder) and faeces. However, there are many processes and organs involved in this.

First, we have to grind up the food with our teeth. Saliva not only helps us chew and swallow; it also contains enzymes that kickstart the digestive process.

From here, food moves through the throat, down the oesophagus and into the stomach – imagine a strong, muscular bag filled with acid and enzymes. The gurgling you might hear coming from your stomach is the food being moved around and the bubbles of gas that are produced as the digestive system starts to do its thing.

The next stop is the small intestine, where bile released from the gallbladder breaks down fats and the absorption of nutrients begins in earnest. The name 'small' intestine is a bit misleading – it's actually up to 6 metres (20 feet) long; it's just smaller in diameter than the large intestine.

The liver – which is the heaviest organ in the body – has a big part to play, as it produces a lot of the substances needed for digestion and filters and clears out toxins from the blood.

The large intestine, also known as the large bowel, takes over from here. It reabsorbs water used in the digestive process. It includes the cecum (that connects the small and large intestine), colon, rectum and anus.

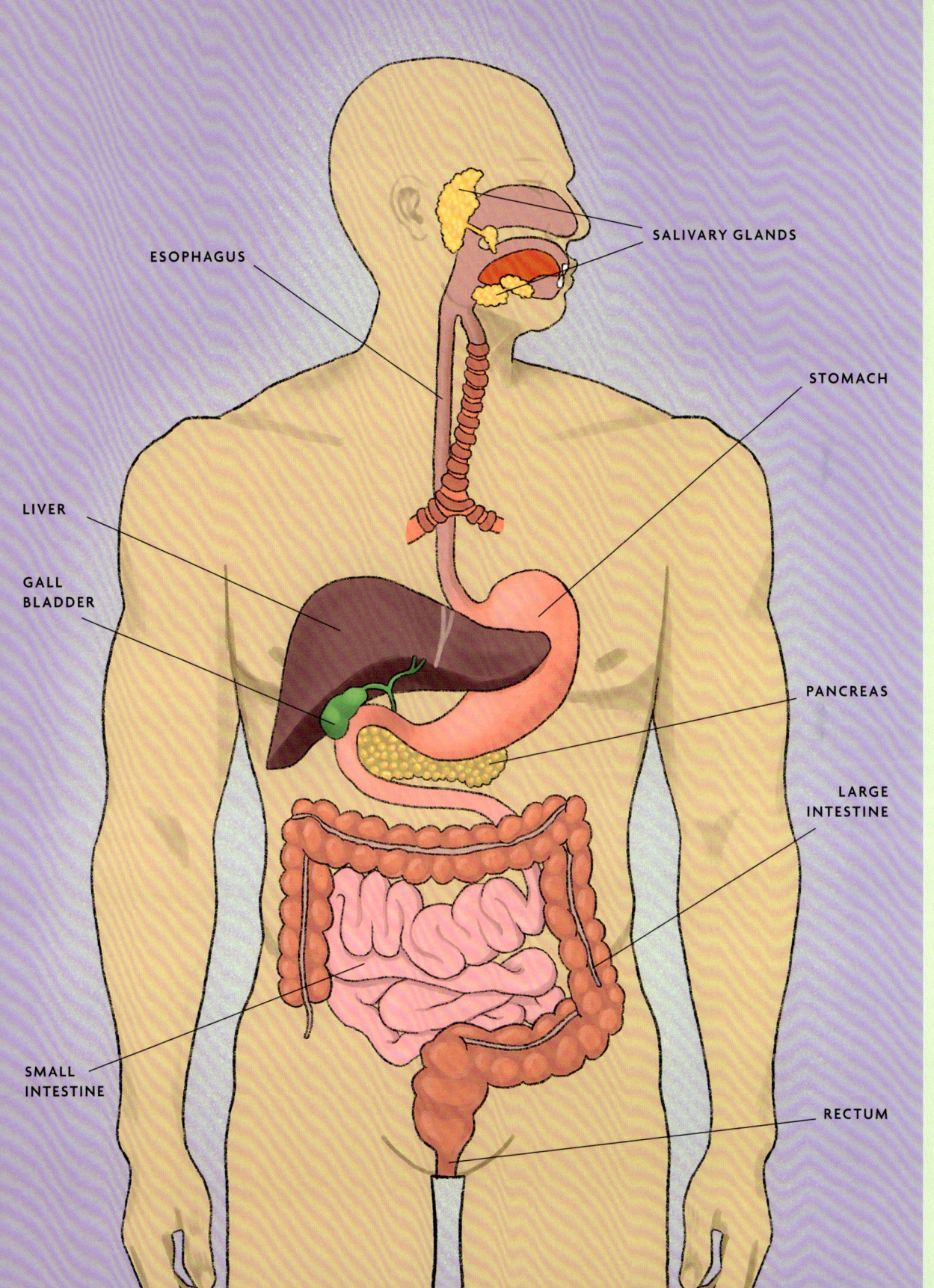

Digestive disorders

As you might expect with something as complex and clever as our digestive systems, things can go wrong or just get out of balance, causing various symptoms, discomfort or knock-on health issues.

Not only that, but this is where we really see how interconnected all our body systems are. Have you ever heard the expression 'the gut is the second brain'? It's a bit of a simplification, but our stomach, intestines and colon do have a massive part to play in our overall wellbeing. There are lots of reasons for this. For example:

- Our immune system really doesn't want toxins getting into our bloodstream via our gut. If an immune response is triggered, it causes inflammation of the gut.
- It's estimated that 90–95 per cent of serotonin, the hormone that positively affects our mood, is produced in our intestines.
- There are millions of nerves in your gut, including GABA receptors which communicate with GABA receptors in our brain. This gut–brain axis influences cognitive function via the vagus nerve, one of the most important nerves in the body.
- Lots of fungi, bacteria and viruses live in the gut to help our digestive system. We need this little ecosystem, called the gut microbiome, so if it gets out of balance for any reason, it has an impact on our health.

So when you hear medical people emphasising the importance of a good diet, it's not just about maintaining a healthy weight or getting vitamins and minerals – it's also because our digestive system has such an important part to play in our overall wellbeing, as anyone with a digestive disorder will know.

Prebiotic & probiotic
Prebiotic: A kind of plant fibre that feeds the helpful gut microbiome, found in lots of fruit and vegetables.
Probiotic: A living organism, like a yeast or bacteria, that may help maintain the gut microbiome. They are found in fermented foods like yogurt or kimchi, or in supplements. There's limited clinical evidence for how effective they are, though some people with conditions like IRRITABLE BOWEL SYNDROME (IBS) report finding them helpful.

Red flag – anaphylaxis
Severe FOOD ALLERGIES can cause anaphylaxis, a life-threatening allergic reaction. People with a known severe FOOD ALLERGY should carry two adrenaline auto-injectors (EpiPen or Jext) for emergency situations. If you or someone else have the following symptoms, use one adrenaline auto-injector and call 999 immediately:

- Sudden swelling of the tongue, throat, mouth or lips, or a tight feeling in the throat making it hard to swallow.
- Difficulty breathing.
- Sudden confusion, dizziness or drowsiness.
- Blue, grey or pale skin, tongue or lips.
- Fainting and not waking up.
- A child becomes limp, floppy or unresponsive.

Lie or sit down until help comes, and stay sitting even if you start to feel better. If symptoms persist five minutes after using the adrenaline auto-injector, then use the second one. You will be taken to hospital after anaphylaxis for observation, further treatment if necessary and medical advice.

Food allergies, sensitivities & intolerances

These are all slightly different conditions that manifest in unpleasant symptoms and discomfort after eating certain foods. Food allergies and food sensitivities are when your immune system mistakes harmless food particles for dangerous invaders and reacts to them, with food allergies, aside from COELIAC DISEASE, being fairly rare but causing severe reactions, while reactions to sensitivities are less severe. If you have a food sensitivity then you may be able to tolerate small amounts of the specific food, but if you have an allergy it should be avoided entirely. Food intolerances are not a reaction of the immune system but are caused by the lack of enzymes required to digest specific foods and so the symptoms of intolerances tend to be limited to the gut.

Symptoms of food allergies, sensitivites & intolerances

Food allergy	Food sensitivity	Food intolerance
Vomiting and/or diarrhoea		
Stomach pain, cramps, bloating and gas		
	HIVES	
Wheezing and difficulty breathing	Blood in stools	
Itchy eyes	Brain fog	
Dizziness or light-headedness	FATIGUE	
Swelling in the face	HEADACHE	
Sneezing	Joint pain	

Diagnosis

Food allergies, sensitivities and intolerances are difficult to diagnose as unfortunately there are no specific tests, although in cases where an allergy is suspected, you could be referred to a specialist who can conduct a blood test or skin-prick test. It is important to note that food allergies, the most serious conditions of this group, are pretty rare.

If you suspect sensitivity or intolerance, you may need to do your own detective work by eliminating suspected causes and keeping a food and symptoms diary. If you have a severe reaction to a common food allergen, such as nuts, peanuts, soya, cows' milk, eggs, fish, shellfish, wheat or sesame seeds, then seek advice from your GP regarding next steps, which could include referral to an allergy clinic. Allergy UK (www.allergyuk.org) also has useful resources and advice.

Treatment

Once the allergen has been identified, you will need to avoid it and learn how to manage symptoms in the case of an emergency. Antihistamines can help with mild allergic reactions and you will be given adrenaline auto-injectors to carry on your person if you have a severe allergy. It is important to check food labels and inform restaurant and catering staff if you have an allergy. You could also wear a medical bracelet and ensure friends, family, colleagues and caregivers are aware of your allergy and how to respond in an emergency.

Coeliac disease

This is a lifelong condition where your immune system attacks your gut tissue when you eat gluten. It's a severe form of FOOD ALLERGY that can stop your gut from absorbing certain nutrients. The only solution is to avoid all forms of gluten; so foods that contain any barley, rye or wheat. For some people, consuming even a trace will affect them. It's possible to have the condition and not experience symptoms, but even then you should avoid gluten as it can cause long-term complications. It has historically been underdiagnosed, partly because it can be mistaken for other conditions such as IRRITABLE BOWEL SYNDROME (IBS).

SYMPTOMS

These vary in severity between individuals but can include:
+ Bloating.
+ Diarrhoea.
+ Constipation.
+ Flatulence.
+ Nausea.
+ TIREDNESS.
+ Mouth ulcers.
+ A skin condition known as dermatitis herpetiformis (DH) – a red, raised, patchy rash, often with blisters on the elbows, knees, shoulders, buttocks and/or face.

Diagnosis

A GP can do a transglutaminase antibody blood test. You may need a biopsy of your small intestine to confirm the diagnosis, done via an endoscopy.

Treatment

Learning about foods that contain gluten, or may contain traces, so they can be avoided is vital. A dietician can advise and recommend supplements, for example, to treat ANAEMIA.

People with confirmed refractory coeliac disease – where their symptoms do not improve even when they cut out gluten – may need to take steroids.

Complications

If those who have coeliac disease do not avoid all gluten, they may be at risk of:
- Vitamin B_{12} deficiency, ANAEMIA or malnutrition, due to not being able to absorb nutrients properly.
- OSTEOPOROSIS and bone FRACTURES.
- Lactose intolerance.
- Infection if they develop problems with their spleen.
- IBS symptoms.
- Skin rashes.
- Nerve disorders.
- Complications in PREGNANCY (although this can be managed) or infertility.
- TYPE 1 DIABETES.
- THYROID DISORDERS.

People with coeliac disease sometimes develop MENTAL HEALTH issues due to suffering with their symptoms or feeling isolated because they have to follow a restrictive diet, and they may need help with this.

Non-coeliac gluten sensitivity

This means that you experience some of the same symptoms but gluten doesn't cause damage to the gut or long-term health problems. Some people with this condition may be able to reintroduce gluten into their diets or cope with small amounts.

Gastroesophageal reflux disease (acid reflux)

Your stomach produces a strong acid to help digest food. If this gets into your oesophagus it can cause a burning sensation often referred to as heartburn. This is common and not serious if it happens occasionally.

Gastroesophageal reflux disease (GORD) is an umbrella term for a number of digestive issues, including:

- **Dyspepsia** often causes heartburn, burping, nausea, feeling uncomfortable or having a sore upper abdomen (also known as indigestion).
- **Esophagitis** is inflammation of the lining of the oesophagus, usually caused by acid reflux. It causes difficulty swallowing and chest pain.
- **Silent reflux** is when you don't experience the burning sensation but you get a cough and/or croaky voice and/or post-nasal drip.

SYMPTOMS

+ Burning sensation in the upper chest and throat.
+ A bad taste in the mouth.
+ Being sick.
+ Bloating.
+ Having bad breath.
+ Symptoms may worsen when lying down.

Causes

Sometimes there's no obvious cause of acid reflux and GORD, but symptoms can be brought on by:

- Spicy, processed or fatty food.
- Caffeine.
- Red wine.
- Chocolate.
- Smoking.
- PREGNANCY.
- Medications such as aspirin, ibuprofen and steroids.
- Infection, like a stomach bug.
- A hiatus hernia, when part of the stomach pushes up into the chest through the diaphragm.

Diagnosis

If you are regularly getting severe symptoms and over-the-counter medicine isn't helping, then visit a GP. They will need to try to figure out where the problem is – e.g. the upper stomach or the oesophagus – and find the cause. Keep a symptom diary, recording when you experience symptoms and what you have eaten that day. You may also be offered a breath test, asked to give a stool sample or sent for an endoscopy, when a camera is passed down your throat. A barium swallow and meal is a test that shows up issues with your gastrointestinal (GI) tract on an X-ray. Or a test called a manometry can be done to check how well the muscles in your stomach are working.

Treatment

- Try smaller and more frequent meals. To avoid constipation, eat plenty of fibre and stay hydrated.
- Don't eat or drink alcohol in the four hours before bed.
- Check your symptom diary for patterns: is it triggered by spicy food? Coffee? Eating close to bedtime?
- Raise the head end of your bed by 20cm (8 inches).
- A pharmacist can provide over-the-counter medication, such as antacids.

If none of this helps, a GP may prescribe a proton pump inhibitor (PPI) medication, which reduces the amount of acid the stomach makes. Rarely, surgery may be needed to tighten the muscle at the top of the stomach.

Chronic GORD & Barrett's oesophagus

Chronic GORD can damage the lining of the oesophagus (esophagitis, see above) and lead to a STOMACH ULCER. A scarred and narrow oesophagus can be painful, making it difficult to swallow. Acid reflux over a long period can cause the cells in your oesophagus to change, which is called Barrett's oesophagus. Some people will then go on to eventually develop cancer of the oesophagus, although this is rare.

Obesity

This term simply means having excess body fat, but obesity is a chronic disease affecting individuals and society as a whole, and is actually much more complicated than it is often believed to be.

Risks of obesity

Obesity is the leading cause of health conditions. The World Health Organization (WHO) estimates that one in four adults and one in five children worldwide are overweight or obese. If you are overweight, you are more likely to have or get:

- HIGH BLOOD PRESSURE.
- Heart conditions.
- TYPE 2 DIABETES.
- Certain cancers.
- A STROKE.
- Joint pain.
- Sexual dysfunction.

Diagnosis

Obesity has traditionally been measured by calculating body mass index (BMI), dividing weight in kilograms by the height in metres squared. Find an online tool by searching 'Calculate your Body Mass Index' on the NHS website.

However, BMI is flawed, as it skews depending on factors like ethnicity, height and how muscular you are. People from Asian, Black African, Afro-Caribbean or Middle Eastern ethnic backgrounds have a higher chance of developing health problems at a lower BMI. But Black men and women can have a larger body size and yet a lower level of body fat. Some athletes would fall into the 'obese' category, but their weight is down to muscle mass.

Another method is to look at your waist-to-height ratio (WHtR):

- Wrap a tape measure around your waist, midway between your hips and your bottom rib.
- Divide your waist circumference (in centimetres) by your height (in centimetres).

If the result is more than 0.5 you may be overweight. The larger the number, the more likely you are to have health risks associated with obesity.

Causes

The simplest reason is that someone consumes more calories than they expend – eating too much calorie-dense food and moving too little. However, in reality, it's often more complicated than that with genetic components as well as environmental factors involved.

People in lower income brackets are more likely to suffer from obesity, as processed food high in fat and calories is often cheaper. It can be harder to access opportunities for exercise for someone in this group. Underlying physical and MENTAL HEALTH CONDITIONS can lead to obesity. For example:

- DEPRESSION.
- Chronic stress.
- HYPOTHYROIDISM.
- Certain medications, such as long-term steroid use.
- MENOPAUSE.
- POLYCYSTIC OVARY SYNDROME (PCOS).

Treatment

If you are overweight or obese, reducing your body fat will almost always make you feel better and help alleviate symptoms caused by related issues. For example, if you have ARTHRITIS and you get down to a healthy weight, you are highly likely to suffer less joint pain. Some people with TYPE 2 DIABETES will find they need less – or sometimes no – medication through adopting a healthy diet and exercising. You will reduce your risk of serious illness like HEART DISEASE by achieving and maintaining a healthy weight.

While some will find it difficult or impossible to lose weight, due to a variety of health factors, many can lose weight. To do so, it's recommended that women limit their calorie intake in the short term to 1,400 a day and men consume no more than 1,900 calories a day. The usual recommended calorie intake is 2,000 calories for women and 2,500 calories for men. But this is a guide only and the right level will vary from person to person.

Weight-loss medication & surgery

Medication
There are regular stories in the media about the latest weight-loss medication. For some people, when nothing else seems to be working, those medications that have been tested properly with clinical trials can be an important part of their treatment. However, they always go hand-in-hand with lifestyle changes, and particularly a low-fat, low-calorie diet. The only drugs currently recommended by the NHS are orlistat, semaglutide and tirzepatide (known commonly by the brand names Xenical, Ozempic or Wegovy, and Mounjaro). They work by restricting how much fat can be absorbed, by making you feel fuller more quickly and mimicking hormones that affect your metabolism. Not everyone can take these medications – it depends on factors such as other health conditions.

There are a number of side effects. They can include oily poo, oily discharge from your back passage, nausea, diarrhoea, suddenly needing the toilet and feeling gassy and flatulent. Weight-loss medication can also interfere with the effectiveness of the oral CONTRACEPTIVE pill and with oral HRT and you cannot take these medications if you are PREGNANT or breastfeeding. They are generally short-term solutions (for up to 18 months) to reduce body mass and you can't take them over a prolonged period of time. For a number of reasons, they are not suitable for people at a healthy weight or with a history of EATING DISORDERS.

Surgery
Bariatric surgery is sometimes used as a last resort to treat severe obesity accompanied by a serious health condition that is expected to improve with weight loss. There are a number of procedures that can be carried out, including making the stomach smaller, fitting a band inside the body around the stomach so it can't expand, and adding a small 'balloon' into the stomach.

Diet versus habit

As a doctor, I am not a fan of faddy diets and highly restrictive eating. They are not usually sustainable and can make people feel like they have 'failed' or even become obsessive about certain 'banned' food groups. Instead, eating healthily is about educating yourself and building good habits, sustainable in the long run. This means:
- Knowing what is good, nutritious food and what are high-calorie, processed foods that should be avoided.
- Finding a type of exercise you enjoy and doing it regularly.
- Understanding portion control – even 'healthy' food can cause you to put on weight if you don't know how much of it you are supposed to be eating.
- Knowing what can trigger you to overeat, such as stress or certain events, and developing strategies to manage it.
- Avoiding alcohol.

Obesity is a chronic medical disorder with a strong genetic component. Lifestyle is important, but it is not the only factor. Research has shown that while it is possible to lose weight with lifestyle changes, it is very difficult to normalise BMI and maintain this long term. Therefore a combination of pharmacological, surgical, nutritional, psychological and socioeconomic interventions may be needed.

Lipoedema
Lipoedema is a genetic condition that almost exclusively affects women – as much as 10 per cent of the adult female population in the UK. As there are no specific diagnostic tests, it is often a hidden condition misdiagnosed as either obesity or lymphoedema (a chronic swelling of tissue). Lipoedema causes excess fat to develop in the legs, buttocks and sometimes the arms, creating a visible difference in the size and shape of these parts of the body. The fat created can be highly sensitive and painful. Furthermore, it differs from normal excess weight so that it doesn't respond to low-calorie diets or exercise regimes. This, coupled with lack of understanding, makes lipoedema highly distressing for some. Lipoedema is a medical condition and not a failure of lifestyle.

Cancer of the oesophagus

Cancer of the oesophagus is when a tumour grows in the oesophagus (the food pipe).

Types

There are two main types of cancer of the oesophagus (as well as a few much rarer types):

Adenocarcinoma
This is the most common type, which begins in the cells of the glands.

Squamous cell carcinoma
This starts with changes to the flat, thin cells that line the surface of the oesophagus.

Causes & risk factors

- The main cause is obesity leading to chronic REFLUX, GORD and BARRETT'S OESOPHAGUS.
- It's more common in older men, particularly those who smoke and drink alcohol (it's very rare if you are under 40).
- It may run in families.
- Regularly drinking very hot liquids.
- Not eating enough fruit and vegetables.
- Smoking.

SYMPTOMS
+ **Difficulty swallowing.**
+ **Persistent heartburn/reflux that isn't helped by medication.**
+ **Loss of appetite and feeling full very quickly.**
+ **Nausea and vomiting.**

Diagnosis

If a doctor thinks there is a chance you have cancer, they will refer you for tests quickly. You will usually have an endoscopy to look inside your oesophagus and a biopsy may be done at the same time. You may also have an ultrasound, CT scan or a small operation known as a laparoscopy.

Treatment

This will depend on the type of cancer. It can be inoperable and has a poor prognosis. In other cases, treatment will involve surgery to remove the tumour, along with chemotherapy, radiotherapy, immunotherapy, medication or a combination of these treatments.

Red flag symptoms

A risk of having an undiagnosed tumour in the oesophagus is that it can suddenly start bleeding and it's difficult to get help quickly enough to stop it. Call an ambulance or go to A&E immediately if this happens. Other symptoms, which you should always get investigated, are:

- Unintentional weight loss.
- Persistant nausea for more than two weeks.
- Vomiting blood – even just a bit.
- Jaundice (yellowing of the skin and/or eyes).
- A strong metallic tarry smell to your poo.
- Severe upper stomach pain.
- Worsening REFLUX.
- Difficulty swallowing.

Stomach ulcer

You can get an ulcer – an open sore – in the lining of the stomach (a gastric ulcer) or in the lining of the top the small intestine (a duodenal or peptic ulcer).

SYMPTOMS
+ **Dull, burning pain in the stomach, usually within a few hours of eating.**
+ **Heartburn/REFLUX.**
+ **Nausea and/or vomiting.**
+ **Loss of appetite or feeling full quickly.**

Causes
The stomach or intestine lining is damaged by acid when defences are compromised, usually due to a bacteria called H. pylori or long-term use of steroids or NSAIDs. Alcohol, smoking, stress and spicy food can make symptoms worse.

Diagnosis
See a GP who can test for H. pylori bacteria. You may also have an endoscopy in hospital to see what is going on.

Treatment
Over-the-counter antacids may help for a short time, although the pain/discomfort will come back. If the ulcer is caused or partly caused by bacteria, you'll be given antibiotics. You may also be prescribed PPIs (proton pump inhibitors), which reduce stomach acid to let the ulcer heal (you may have a follow-up endoscopy to make sure it has).

> **Red flag – complications**
> Most ulcers don't cause major problems, but there can be some rare but serious complications.
> **Internal bleeding:** minor bleeding can lead to ANAEMIA; major bleeds will make you vomit blood or produce sticky, tar-like stools. Go to hospital straight away if you vomit blood.
> **Peritonitis:** a burst ulcer that causes an infection in the stomach lining. This is potentially life-threatening and must be urgently treated in hospital. Symptoms include high FEVER, vomiting, stomach pain or rapid heartbeat.

Femoral hernia

A lump or swelling in the upper thigh area, where a portion of the intestine or other tissue has pushed through, caused by a weakness in the muscle. Men can develop them but they are much more common in women.

SYMPTOMS
+ **A bulge near in the upper thigh area, below the groin crease.**
+ **The bulge will become noticeable when standing, straining or coughing, and can reduce if you press on it.**

Diagnosis & treatment
Femoral hernia is diagnosed by a physical examination. It will usually be corrected by minor surgery, so it doesn't become 'strangulated' – a serious condition where the blood flow is cut off. See also INGUINAL HERNIA.

Stomach cancer

This is when a tumour develops in the stomach's lining. According to Cancer Research UK it's the 15th most common cancer in the UK and cases are going down, so it's fairly rare. Older men make up the largest group of sufferers. Risk factors include being overweight, smoking and particularly having a STOMACH ULCER over a long period of time or chronic REFLUX leading to BARRETT'S OESOPHAGUS.

SYMPTOMS

The general symptoms (other than the red flag symptoms, see below) are very similar to other gastrointestinal illnesses and issues, so if you have these regularly and are not sure why, it's always worth getting them checked out.

+ Nausea and vomiting.
+ Loss of appetite and feeling full quickly.
+ Heartburn/indigestion/REFLUX.
+ Difficulty swallowing.
+ Feeling weak and TIRED.
+ Pain in the upper abdomen.

Diagnosis
If the doctor examining you thinks there is a chance you have a serious gastric condition, they will send you for an endoscopy to look into your oesophagus, stomach and sometimes small intestine to identify the problem. If cancer is found, you will have further tests to give more information about the nature of the tumour.

Treatment
Treatment options include surgery to remove the tumour, plus chemotherapy, radiotherapy and medication to shrink the tumour. The combination of these depends on where the cancer is, whether it had spread and how healthy you are otherwise.

Red flag symptoms
Always see a doctor if you have these symptoms:
- Unintentional weight loss.
- Vomiting blood (or dark matter that looks like coffee grounds – this is blood, too).
- Black, tarry poo.
- Lump at the top of the abdomen.

Gallstones & Cholecystitis

The gallbladder is a small organ that helps with the management and digestion of fats from the stomach. Due to the bile components that are stored and released there, gallstones can often form inside it.

Gallstones are surprisingly common, and about 80 per cent of people with them are asymptomatic. However, if the gallstones obstruct the entrance to the gallbladder, they can cause pain (known as biliary colic) or cholecystitis – inflammation and infection of the gallbladder. If the stones migrate and cause blockage of the larger bile ducts, they can cause a more serious infection: cholangitis.

SYMPTOMS

+ Pain in the upper-quarter of the abdomen, that can spread to the upper back.
+ Nausea and vomiting.
+ Pain that worsens after eating a fatty meal or at nighttime.
+ FEVER.
+ Decreased appetite.
+ Jaundice.

Causes

Gallstones are formed from cholesterol and bile salts and are more common in Caucasian women over the age of forty, but they can affect any ethnic group or sex. Other factors that can increase the risk of gallstones are:

- OBESITY or being overweight.
- DIABETES.
- PREGNANCY.
- Rapid weight loss.
- High-fat, high-protein and low-fibre diets.
- Family history of gallstones.
- LIVER DISEASE.
- Taking the oral CONTRACEPTIVE pill.

Diagnosis

Gallstones are usually diagnosed by ultrasound, CT or MRI scan as well as blood tests, which may show abnormalities of liver function as well as infection.

Treatment

Treatment of gallstones is usually by surgery to remove the gallbladder by laparoscopic cholecystectomy (keyhole surgery). Before the surgery the symptoms can be managed with pain relief and sticking to a low-fat diet. If stones are stuck in the larger bile ducts, they may need to be removed by endoscopic retrograde cholangiopancreotography (ERCP), in which a thin flexible camera is passed through the stomach via the mouth to the bile ducts to remove the stones.

Pancreatitis

This is inflammation of the pancreas, a pear-shaped organ that helps digestion and aids the regulation of blood sugar. Acute pancreatitis is characterised by a sudden onset, but repeated attacks may lead to chronic pancreatitis – inflammation that can cause permanent damage, leading to an inability to produce insulin and/or digestive juices. Symptoms include severe stomach pain that may worsen upon eating, nausea and vomiting, FEVER, swelling in the stomach, rapid heart rate, jaundice, or smelly, greasy poos. The most common cause in adults is excess alcohol consumption, whereas in children it's CYSTIC FIBROSIS, but it can also be caused by GALLSTONES, stomach injury, tumours, high levels of calcium in the blood, certain medications, immune disorders or illnesses such as MUMPS, HEPATITIS A and B or salmonella infection. Seek an urgent GP appointment or call 111 if you suspect pancreatitis. Acute pancreatitis is treated in hospital. Chronic pancreatitis can be managed but not reversed and will be treated by looking at the cause. In some cases, surgery may be required to remove damaged parts of the pancreas, which can have knock-on effects on your digestive system, for which you may need to take insulin and supplements.

Pancreatic cancer

Pancreatic cancer can be hard to spot as symptoms overlap with those of other diseases in the bowel and stomach area, and sometimes there are no symptoms. It occurs when abnormal cells in the pancreas start to grow in an uncontrollable way, forming a tumour. It can affect anyone at any age, but most people who get it are over 65. It's the tenth most common cancer in the UK according to Cancer Research UK.

Causes & risk factors

We don't know exactly how pancreatic cancer is caused, but we think the chances of getting it go up if you:

- Smoke, as it's estimated that one in five pancreatic cancers in the UK are down to smoking.
- Have an alcohol addiction or drink alcohol excessively over a period of years (see PANCREATITIS).
- Eat a diet high in red meat and processed food, and low in fresh fruit and vegetables.
- Have this type of cancer in your family, or you carry the faulty BRCA1/2 genes (see BREAST CANCER).
- Are overweight or OBESE, particularly if you carry extra weight around your middle and you are insulin resistant (see DIABETES).

Diagnosis

It's important to get diagnosed as soon as possible as, unfortunately, this cancer can spread quickly. You will likely have a blood test followed by a CT scan – sometimes as part of an endoscopy, when a camera is used to look down your throat – and a biopsy to take a sample of the tumour. The specialist doctors will want to find out if the cancer has spread.

SYMPTOMS

- Stomach pain going into the back (the main bit of the pancreas is behind the stomach on the right, though its 'tail' goes across your spine).
- Jaundice (yellowing of the skin and/or eyes).
- Unexpectedly losing weight.
- New diagnosis of insulin-dependent DIABETES as an adult.
- Floating, greasy poo (pancreatic cancer often starts in the cells that produce digestive juices needed to process fats).
- Nausea, vomiting, poor appetite.
- TIREDNESS.
- FEVER, shivering.
- Itchy skin.

Treatment

Treatment depends on your age and state of health, as well as the extent of the cancer. Usually you'll have surgery to remove the tumour alongside radiotherapy and/or chemotherapy. Sometimes, the main focus has to be on supporting the person and managing their symptoms, allowing them to live with the cancer relatively comfortably for as long as they can.

Appendicitis

The appendix is a small tube attached to the large intestine. When I was at medical school, we were taught that it had no function. Nowadays, some researchers think it might play a part in the immune system. If it becomes infected and inflamed, it will need to be removed by surgery so it doesn't burst, so it's important to get suspected appendicitis checked as soon as possible. It's most common in children, teens and young adults, but can happen at any age. Appendicitis can be acute or chronic, depending on the speed of its onset.

SYMPTOMS

Acute appendicitis:
+ Sudden pain in the belly button that moves over to the right-hand side of the stomach.
+ Loss of appetite.
+ Nausea and/or vomiting.
+ You may also have a FEVER, and constipation or diarrhoea.

Chronic appendicitis:
+ This is rarer but still serious. The pain develops more slowly and can come and go.

Diagnosis

There is no one test for appendicitis. You will need to go to hospital. The doctor will examine you and try to rule out other causes of the pain, such as KIDNEY STONES, a URINARY TRACT INFECTION (UTI) or PANCREATITIS. It can be confused with an ECTOPIC PREGNANCY too.

Treatment

If appendicitis is suspected, you will usually have surgery to remove the appendix. There will be a biopsy to confirm appendicitis.

Complications

An infected appendix can become gangrenous and burst. This can lead to infection spreading into your gut, SEPSIS or a blocked bowel – all of which are life-threatening if not treated.

Mesenteric lymphadenitis

This is an infection of the lymph glands in the stomach. It's more common in children and often follows a SORE THROAT or FLU-like symptoms. It can be caused by a virus like gastroenteritis or sometimes bacteria.

SYMPTOMS

+ Similar symptoms to APPENDICITIS and the two can be confused.

Diagnosis

Blood and urine tests to check for infection. You may have a laparoscopy – keyhole surgery – to see what's going on.

Treatment

Antibiotics will be prescribed if the cause is a bacterial infection. It usually clears up within a few days, but it needs investigating and monitoring, not least to make sure that this is the cause of symptoms.

Irritable bowel syndrome (IBS)

IBS is a very common long-term digestive condition that causes disordered bowel movements associated with abdominal pain. Different people have different symptoms and different triggers. Both men and women can have it, but for women it can overlap alongside gynaecological issues such as ENDOMETRIOSIS and OVARIAN CANCER, which may then be missed because the symptoms are put down to IBS.

SYMPTOMS

- Abdominal pain.
- Cramping.
- Bloating.
- Changes in bowel habits, e.g. going from constipation to diarrhoea or vice versa.
- Excessive wind, feeling gassy and having a noisy gut.
- Sudden and urgent need to poo.
- Lack of energy, FATIGUE.
- Nausea.
- Heartburn or REFLUX.
- General all-over body pain.

Causes

We don't really know what causes IBS. It seems often to be triggered by factors like:

- Being sensitive to (but not allergic to) specific foods.
- Emotional stress.
- Having had a severe gut infection.

Diagnosis

It's important to rule out other conditions, particularly COELIAC DISEASE, CROHN'S DISEASE, BOWEL CANCER, inflammatory bowel disease and things like ENDOMETRIOSIS in women. A sample of your poo can be sent for testing and a blood test will show signs of inflammation, ANAEMIA and deficiencies of things like vitamins B_{12} and D.

If you think you have IBS, you need to become your own gut detective. Keep a diary of what you eat and how you feel afterwards to identify any foods that trigger symptoms.

Treatment

- Avoid foods that you have identified as triggers (wheat, sugar, beans/legumes, dairy, cabbage, caffeine, alcohol and carbonated drinks are all common ones).
- Get plenty of exercise as this helps with digestion.
- Eat plenty of vegetables (avoiding anything that triggers symptoms) and avoid processed food.
- Give up smoking.
- Try over-the-counter medicines that can help with bloating, constipation, diarrhoea and heartburn – speak to a pharmacist for advice.
- Keep well hydrated.
- Some people find taking probiotics helps.
- Manage stress triggers wherever possible.

Diverticular disease

Diverticula are small bulging pockets that form in the colon (large intestine). This can happen at any age, but it's more common when we get older. They don't always cause problems, although bacteria and poo can get stuck in them, resulting in inflammation and sometimes infection – this is called diverticulitis.

Risk factors that increase the chance of developing diverticula, and subsequently diverticulitis, include OBESITY, smoking, heavy alcohol use, lack of vitamin D, eating a lot of red meat and not getting enough fibre. Certain medication, such as non-steroidal anti-inflammatory drugs (NSAIDs), opioids and steroids, can also increase the risk.

SYMPTOMS
+ Bloating and wind.
+ Stomach pain and tenderness, particularly in the lower left side.
+ Changes to bowel habits such as constipation and diarrhoea.
+ Red blood in stools.

The infection may also lead to a FEVER and more severe pain that comes on suddenly but can decrease and return. Some of the symptoms are the same as those for BOWEL CANCER.

Diagnosis
While mild flare-ups will often go away by themselves, if you have abdominal pain, a FEVER and changes to your bowel habits, see a doctor. There are a few issues that can cause this and it's best to get them checked. You might have a blood test to check for inflammation markers and be sent for a colonoscopy or a CT scan.

Treatment
The first step is to treat the symptoms, so rehydrating and replacing salt and sugars lost through having diarrhoea and bringing down FEVER with paracetamol. A doctor may recommend a liquid-only diet for a short time and/or advise against taking NSAIDs. Antibiotics will be prescribed if there's a bacterial infection.

In more serious cases, particularly where there are complications (see below), it may be necessary to have surgery. A temporary colostomy bag can be fitted and removed once the bowel has healed.

Complications
These are rare but can be very serious, and include:
- Abnormal connection between two organs, called a fistula.
- Peritonitis (an infection in the abdominal lining).
- Blockage in the bowel.
- Abscess.
- Haemorrhage.

Bowel cancer

This is a cancer found anywhere in the colon and/or rectum. It's the fourth most common cancer in the UK according to Cancer Research UK. If caught early it can be very treatable, which is why we have a screening programme in the UK whereby people aged 50–74 who are registered with a GP are offered an at-home test every two years to check for it, before they get any symptoms. If anything shows up, they will then be sent for a colonoscopy. Most people diagnosed with bowel cancer are over 50, while about 10 per cent are under 50, but it's good to be vigilant for symptoms at any age.

SYMPTOMS

+ Blood in your poo, that looks either red or black.
+ Losing weight without trying to.
+ Stomach pain and/or a lump in your abdomen.
+ Feeling like you need to poo a lot more, even when you have just been.
+ Frequent diarrhoea or constipation.
+ Nausea and vomiting.
+ Bloating.
+ Changes in bowel habits, either becoming constipated or having diarrhoea, for four weeks or more.

Causes & risk factors

Bowel cancer is more common in men than women, and you may also be more likely to get bowel cancer if you:

- Are overweight or OBESE.
- Have a close family relative who has had it.
- Have CROHN'S DISEASE, IBS or ULCERATIVE COLITIS.
- Have bowel polyps.
- Have a diet high in red or processed meat.
- Smoke.

You can lower your risk by following a healthy diet (see page 8), remaining a healthy weight and not smoking or drinking to excess.

Diagnosis

Some people can feel embarrassed going to the doctor with symptoms related to bowel habits, but it's so important to get them checked. You can take a picture on your phone of a poo that has concerned you – it's helpful and we have seen it all before. The doctor will examine your stomach and usually give a rectal exam, where they put a gloved finger in your bottom. You will often be given a kit so you can take a sample of your poo and a blood test. If anything looks concerning, you will be sent for a colonoscopy where a biopsy can be done at the same time if anything is found.

Treatment

This depends on when the cancer is caught and whether it has spread. You may need surgery to remove the tumour, and sometimes chemotherapy, radiotherapy, immunotherapy and/or targeted drugs to attack the cancer cells.

Crohn's disease

Crohn's disease is a type of inflammatory bowel disease (IBD). It is a lifelong condition in which the immune system mistakenly attacks one part of the digestive tract – anywhere from the mouth to the anus – making it swollen and irritated. It most commonly affects the lining of the small or large intestine. It sometimes runs in families. Most people are diagnosed in their teens or twenties, although it can be missed because the symptoms overlap with other gut conditions or gynaecological issues.

SYMPTOMS

There are different types of Crohn's disease and the symptoms vary depending which part of your digestive tract is affected. You may have flare-ups where your symptoms get worse for a while.

- Abdominal pain, cramps.
- Diarrhoea, incontinence.
- Loss of appetite, unintended weight loss.
- Blood in poo.
- Rectal bleeding.
- Mouth ulcers, painful mouth or gums.
- FEVER.
- FATIGUE.
- Abscesses and infections around the anus.
- Sexual dysfunction in both men and women.

Inflammatory autoimmune conditions can have a wider impact on the body, such as ARTHRITIS or joint pain, eye inflammation, KIDNEY STONES, OSTEOPOROSIS. Because it can stop you getting all the nutrients you need, in children, Crohn's can inhibit growth.

Diagnosis
- A blood test to check for a high white blood cell count, which indicates inflammation.
- A stool sample to check for bacteria and parasites, to rule out these causes.
- You may have a CT or MRI to look at the gut.
- A colonoscopy may be carried out, when a thin tube with a camera on the end is inserted into your bottom to check the bowel and take a biopsy.

Treatment
There is no cure for Crohn's disease, but there are a variety of things that can bring the inflammation down and control the symptoms. For example:
- Corticosteroids to help with a flare-up in the short term.
- JAK inhibitors, immunosuppressants and immune modulators stop your immune system attacking the gut (though immunosuppressants can make you more susceptible to illness).
- Nutrition is very important, so having support from a dietician or a nutritionist is helpful.
- For complications of Crohn's disease, like abscesses or holes/tears in the intestine, surgery may be required.

It's important to be on the lookout for complications of Crohn's. Scarring caused by repetitive inflammation can increase the risk of bowel obstruction, BOWEL CANCER and THROMBOSIS or EMBOLISM (blood clots).

Ulcerative colitis

Ulcerative colitis is another type of inflammatory bowel disease, and an ongoing condition where ulcers form in the lining of the bowel and rectum. The exact reason for this is unknown but it's thought that the immune system attacks healthy tissue, causing swelling, because it thinks there is an infection it has to deal with. There's research ongoing into how the gut microbiome might be involved. It's similar to CROHN'S DISEASE but it only affects the bowel and rectum. There may be a genetic factor as it can run in families.

SYMPTOMS

There are different types of ulcerative colitis and they vary in their severity. Some people only experience severe symptoms during a flare-up.

+ **Diarrhoea, often with blood.**
+ **Feeling like you have to poo urgently or having to wake at night to poo.**
+ **Struggling to poo.**
+ **Mucus in the poo.**
+ **Abdominal pain.**
+ **Nausea and loss of appetite.**
+ FATIGUE.
+ FEVER.
+ **Impaired growth in children.**

Diagnosis

A doctor will want to do tests to rule out other causes. A colonoscopy – where a camera is inserted into the bottom to look at the colon and take a biopsy – is the usual method of diagnosis.

Treatment

The treatment focuses on reducing the inflammation to allow the bowel to heal and work normally. The methods are the same as for CROHN'S DISEASE. In severe cases, where someone's quality of life and health is being affected, surgery may be needed to remove the bowel. In some cases, the surgeon can join the small intestine to the anus, so you can poo normally, but in other cases someone might need a colostomy (or stoma) bag that collects poo outside of the body. However, this is rare. Though it's a lifelong condition, if it's managed effectively, most people will be able to lead a normal life.

Red flag – fulminant colitis

Rarely, ULCERATIVE COLITIS or gastroenteritis can develop into fulminant colitis, which is where the walls of the colon suddenly become swollen, rapidly worsening the condition, leading to severe abdominal pain and swelling, profuse bloody diarrhoea and high FEVER. It may then be at risk of perforation because the colon walls may weaken, leading to a complication of fulminant colitis known as toxic megacolon. This needs urgent treatment in hospital.

Further complications of ULCERATIVE COLITIS include ANAEMIA, malnutrition, bowel obstruction and increased risk of BOWEL CANCER. Some people may additionally have joint, liver, skin or eye problems.

Haemorrhoids

Also called piles, haemorrhoids are lumps caused by swollen blood vessels around and inside your anus and rectum. They are incredibly common and not usually anything to be concerned about, though they can cause pain.

SYMPTOMS

- Itching around the anus.
- Mucus when you wipe your bottom or in your underwear.
- Bright red blood when you poo.
- Pain around the anus, making it hard for you to go to the toilet.
- Feeling like you still need to poo when you have just been.

Causes

Generally things that put pressure on your anus:

- Constipation and pushing too hard when you poo.
- OBESITY.
- Pregnancy and vaginal childbirth.
- Repeated heavy lifting.

Treatments

At-home treatments

- Don't spend too long on the toilet – wait until your bowels are ready to move and let the muscles do their thing without pushing. Don't take your phone to the toilet and sit there for ages.
- Avoid constipation/hard stools – stay hydrated and avoid anything that blocks you up. Regular exercise will keep you regular!
- Take paracetamol for mild/occasional pain (don't take ibuprofen if you are bleeding).
- Have a warm bath to relieve itching.
- Wipe your bottom with damp toilet paper to clean the area properly but avoid damaging the skin (washing is much better than scrubbing this sensitive area with harsh paper).
- It's fine to gently push a small pile back inside.

Medical treatments

Most people with piles have occasional flare-ups. See a doctor if you are regularly suffering with piles or they are getting worse.

- A pharmacist can advise on creams to reduce discomfort and soften poo.
- Non-surgical treatments you can have in hospital include putting a band on a pile so it drops off or using an electrical current, infrared light or an injection to shrink the pile.
- In severe cases, you may need surgery to remove the pile under general anaesthetic.

> **Red flag symptoms**
> If there is a lot of blood when you poo or wipe then seek urgent medical attention. If the blood is dark (i.e. not bright red) see your GP as this is unlikely to be HAEMORRHOIDS. See symptoms of BOWEL CANCER and, although it's rare, always get these checked out if you have them.

Liver disorders

The liver is a powerhouse of an organ – it plays a big part in digestion, metabolism and blood function, including clearing toxins. It's resilient and it regenerates constantly, which is great, but also means that we don't always know when something starts to go wrong with it.

SYMPTOMS

There are many conditions that can affect the liver, and most have symptoms in common, although early liver damage can produce no symptoms at all, or just mild ones. Symptoms include:

+ Jaundice – when the skin and/or whites of your eyes turns yellow (though this may be less noticeable if you have black or brown skin).
+ Stomach pain/swelling.
+ Swelling in the legs and/or ankles.
+ Itchy skin.
+ Darker urine.
+ Pale, floating poo.
+ TIREDNESS.
+ Nausea and/or vomiting.
+ Loss of appetite.
+ Bruising easily.

Causes

Liver disease is generally caused by infection, toxins (particularly alcohol) and genetic autoimmune conditions. Liver damage causes scarring on the liver, called cirrhosis. This stops the liver from working properly. See page 10 for more on alcohol consumption as the most common cause is long-term excessive alcohol use.

Types of liver disease

Metabolic dysfunction-associated steatotic liver disease (MASLD, previously and informally known as 'fatty liver')

Caused by a number of conditions. Fat builds up in the liver, which can cause inflammation and then scarring, eventually leading to liver failure if not addressed. Most common in overweight and OBESE people.

Alcoholic hepatitis

A result of fatty liver disease caused by drinking too much alcohol over a period of time. The liver can often recover when someone stops drinking, if the damage isn't too advanced, but alcohol stops liver cells regenerating.

Hepatitis

Inflammation of the liver. Hepatitis A, B, C, D and E are caused by a virus, and hepatitis B and C can lead to chronic viral hepatitis. There are vaccinations available for A and B. Hepatitis can also be caused by GLANDULAR FEVER.

Haemochromatosis

A rare inherited disorder that means the body absorbs and stores too much iron over time, which can cause damage. Treatment can adjust the levels.

Primary biliary cirrhosis

A progressive autoimmune disease where the body attacks the bile ducts, causing a build-up of bile and eventual liver damage. It predominantly affects middle-aged women and presents with FATIGUE and itching.

Galactosaemia

A rare inherited condition where the body can't produce an enzyme to break down milk sugars, damaging the liver and other organs.

Wilson's disease

A rare inherited condition where copper – which we do need – builds up in the liver (and brain and eyes), causing scar tissue on the liver and potentially eventual liver failure.

Diagnosis

The doctor will ask about your symptoms as well as lifestyle factors. It's important to be honest about your diet and how much alcohol you drink, not least because liver conditions have very similar symptoms, so as much information as possible is needed to make the right diagnosis. You may have a blood test to check liver function. CT scans, MRI scans and an ultrasound can be used to check for liver damage.

Treatment

Sometimes antiviral therapy will be needed to treat chronic viral hepatitis (but not alcoholic hepatitis). Lifestyle changes are key, such as losing weight and giving up drinking, so the liver can repair itself. In some cases, you may be prescribed medicine to treat the symptoms of liver disease. Acute liver failure, a medical emergency where the liver stops working suddenly – which is rarer than chronic liver failure which happens over a long period of time – may sometimes only be treated by liver transplant.

Prevention

Maintaining a healthy weight and not drinking too much alcohol are the key ways to maintain a healthy liver. For women, oestrogen protects the liver, so changes in levels of hormones (such as around MENOPAUSE) can make them more susceptible to liver damage as well as less able to process alcohol.

Liver cancer

Cancer can start in the liver or spread there from other areas of the body. It is more common in men, those who have a relative with the disease and people with other DIGESTIVE DISORDERS, like HEPATITIS and liver damage.

SYMPTOMS

In addition to the red flag symptoms below, general symptoms are very similar to a number of other LIVER DISORDERS.

Diagnosis

You will have a blood test and likely a scan. If anything shows up, you may need a liver biopsy.

Treatment

Like all cancers, treatment is much more effective if it's caught early. The treatment will depend on the size of the tumour, if the cancer has spread and your general health. It may include surgery to remove the tumour, chemotherapy, radiotherapy, thermal ablation (using heat to target cancer cells) and medication. Sometimes a liver transplant is necessary.

> **Red flag symptoms**
> Always see a doctor if you have the following symptoms:
> - Jaundice (yellowing of the skin and/or eyes).
> - Unintentional weight loss.
> - A pain and/or swelling in your stomach.
> - Vomiting for no obvious reason which continues for more than two days.

THE URINARY SYSTEM

Urine – pee – is the liquid that's left over once the body has finished processing the things we have eaten and drunk. The bowel and the urinary system are responsible for 'taking the rubbish out' – getting rid of the toxins that would otherwise cause us harm.

THE URINARY SYSTEM

KIDNEY

ADRENAL GLAND

RENAL ARTERY

RENAL VEIN

URETER

BLADDER

URETHRA

The kidneys

The process starts in the **kidneys**, two fist-sized organs below your ribs near your spine. Using a process called filtration, they remove waste products, excess salt and water from blood as it passes through them. The kidneys also produce hormones that regulate blood pressure and make red blood cells. All of your blood passes through your kidneys many times every day.

The ureter

Muscles squeeze this waste liquid through the ureter tube away from the kidneys. If for some reason this doesn't happen, that's when you can get a kidney infection.

The bladder

It ends up in the bladder – a triangular 'bag' in the lower abdomen. It can store around half a litre of urine, although you typically start to feel you need to pee when it's half full. There are two sphincter muscles that close tightly like a rubber band at the bottom to stop urine leaking out.

There are nerves in the bladder that tell the brain you need to urinate. When you pee, the brain lets the sphincter muscles relax and contracts the muscles around the bladder, pushing the urine along the urethra and out of the body.

It's hard to wee when we are anxious because our 'fight or flight' response can take over the driving seat of the muscles in our body, making it hard to relax the ones we need to so we can go!

What colour should wee be?

Straw-coloured, very pale yellow: This is the colour of healthy urine and a sign of good hydration – your body has enough water that it can do all its jobs properly.

Dark yellow, honey-coloured: This a sign of dehydration – you need more water.

Very dark yellow to a brownish: Indicates severe dehydration or a liver problem – the latter if it's accompanied by pale stools that float.

Pinkish or red: May mean blood in the urine; unless you are menstruating consult your GP.

HYDRATED

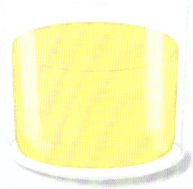

DEHYDRATED

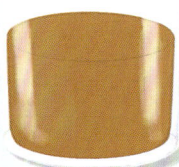

SEVERELY DEHYDRATED

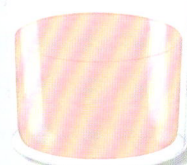

BLOOD

Urinary incontinence

Experiencing some kind of uncontrollable leak of urine is very common, possibly occurring for more than one in three women and one in four men. At the milder end, it might cause inconvenience and discomfort – though for some people it really affects their quality of life. However, it's nothing to be embarrassed about.

Types

Stress incontinence
When the muscles holding the pelvic organs in place become weak, so coughing, sneezing, bending, laughing, straining and lifting things can cause a leak.

Overactive bladder
Also called urgent or urge incontinence, when you suddenly need to pee immediately or you feel you will leak urine, or you pee frequently, including duing the night. This is common as we get older, as well as in people with DIABETES, MULTIPLE SCLEROSIS or who have had a STROKE.

Overflow incontinence
When the bladder can't properly empty, causing it to get bigger and leak. Most common in men with prostate problems.

Causes

Urinary incontinence it not considered a condition, but rather a symptom, as it can be caused by many things. Some of the most common are:

- URINARY TRACT INFECTION (UTI).
- Constipation.
- Some medicines such as diuretics, antidepressants and antihistamines.
- Long-term health issues, such as DIABETES, STROKE or MULTIPLE SCLEROSIS.
- In men, enlarged prostate or following prostate surgery.
- In women, damage from a vaginal birth or another issue with the vagina.
- Pressure on the bladder area caused by PREGNANCY, OBESITY or a medical condition.
- Bladder stones.
- Loss of muscle tone due to age.

Diagnosis

If urinary incontinence is an ongoing problem, speak to a doctor so they can check for health issues. Keep a diary over at least three days, recording what and how much you drink, how often you pee, how much and how urgently, and how many times you feel you have leaked.

There are a number of tests the doctor can do to check your bladder function. Women may have a vaginal exam to check the pelvic floor and for a prolapse. In men, the doctor may do a rectal exam to check the prostate.

Treatment

This depends on the cause of your incontinence. Treatments include lifestyle changes, pelvic floor exercises, medication and – in some cases – surgery.

Pelvic organ prolapse

This occurs when the pelvic floor muscles and tissues weaken, causing pelvic organs like the bladder, uterus, or rectum to sag or push into the vaginal space. It manifests in a feeling of heaviness or pressure in the lower abdomen or vagina, sometimes with a bulge inside (or coming out of) the vagina. You may also have urinary incontinence or need to wee more often, pain during sex or constipation. Diagnosis is usually by physical examination but you might also be sent for an ultrasound scan or urodynamic tests. If the prolapse affects your daily life, treatment can be a combination of hormonal treatments, vaginal support pessaries or physiotherapy. In severe cases surgery can be conducted to lift and support the pelvic organs.

Urinary tract infections (UTIs)

A urinary tract infection can affect any part of your urinary system. They are very common and women are more prone to them because of their hormones and anatomy – the urethra is shorter and its opening much closer to the anus, so germs can spread more easily. Children, particularly girls, can get them too.

Types of UTIs

Acute UTI (cystitis)
A sudden, short-term infection that will clear up by itself or with a short course of antibiotics.

Chronic UTI
Two or more UTIs within six months or an infection that does not clear up with antibiotics. The recurrence could be due to reinfection – the bacteria gets back in again after the first infection cleared up. Or a persistent infection that doesn't go away despite treatment.

SYMPTOMS

Lower UTI:
The symptoms of an infection of the bladder (cystitis) and/or urethra are:
+ Needing to pee suddenly, more often than usual and feeling like you can't properly empty your bladder.
+ Pain, discomfort or a burning sensation when you pee.
+ Pain in the lower abdomen.
+ Urine that's cloudy, foul smelling or contains blood.
+ Feeling generally unwell, achy and/or TIRED.

Upper UTI:
This is an infection of the kidneys and/or ureters (tubes that connect the kidneys to the bladder). You may have some of the symptoms above as well as:
+ A FEVER of 38°C (100°F) or more and/or shivering and chills.
+ Pain in your sides or back.
+ Nausea and/or vomiting.
+ Confusion, agitation or restlessness (particularly in older people).

If left untreated, an upper UTI can damage your kidneys and, in rare cases, even spread to the bloodstream, causing SEPSIS.

Causes

The root cause is almost always a bacterial infection. This can be triggered or exacerbated by:

- Dehydration.
- Sexual intercourse.
- Changes in hormones in women, so around menstrual cycles, PREGNANCY or MENOPAUSE.
- Obstructions in the urinary tract such as KIDNEY STONES.
- A weakened immune system e.g. if you've been ill or you take immunosuppressants.
- Condoms coated in spermicide.
- DIABETES.
- If you have a catheter.
- For men, an enlarged prostate can make it harder to empty your bladder.

If you have pain in the kidney area and have blood in your pee, seek urgent medical help.

Diagnosis

For a sudden, mild UTI, a pharmacist will be able to advise on your symptoms, recommend over-the-counter treatments and tell you if you need to see a GP.

If you have a recurring or chronic UTI (see opposite), see your GP. They may ask you for a urine sample and/or send you for a cystoscopy, in which a camera on the end of a thin, flexible tube looks inside your bladder and can take biopsies at the same time. You may have an ultrasound scan of your kidneys and bladder or have other tests to check your bladder function.

Treatment

Acute UTIs (cystitis)

Take paracetamol or ibuprofen if you can to ease the pain. Drink lots of fluids, ask your pharmacist for over-the-counter remedies, rest and avoid having sex.

If your symptoms are getting worse, causing you considerable discomfort or do not start to improve within three days (or earlier if you have a FEVER), see your doctor as you may need antibiotics. **Always finish the course of antibiotics.**

For chronic UTIs

Bacteria in urine can embed themselves in the lining of the bladder wall where antibiotics and the immune system can't reach them, causing recurring or constant inflammation in the bladder. The bacteria may become dormant for a while, so the antibiotics don't work on them. This sometimes doesn't show up in tests, leading to a misdiagnosis of an irritable bladder or a chronic overactive bladder.

You may need to take antibiotics for up to six months. POST-MENOPAUSAL women can benefit from topical oestrogen cream. In rare cases, surgery may be required.

Recurring, chronic UTIs are miserable, as well as causing long-term damage to the bladder and sometimes leading to stress incontinence. So be persistent in getting the right treatment and don't suffer in silence.

Prevention

- Stay hydrated.
- Pee soon after having sex (this is important for women; it's a good idea for men too, though).
- Women should wipe from front to back after peeing.
- Change nappies or incontinence pads as soon as they are wet.
- Don't try to hold your pee in; pee when you feel you need to.
- Some people find cranberry juice can prevent occasional bouts of acute UTI, although it's not recommended if you take warfarin or are diabetic as it is high in sugar.

Kidney stones

Kidney stones are clusters of crystals that form from a build-up of substances in your urinary tract. In about 80 per cent of cases they break down of their own accord or are so small that you pass them with only a little discomfort. Occasionally they are larger and need treatment. The main risk is that if they get stuck they can cause kidney damage. They are most common in men in their twenties to forties due to a combination of factors including dietary habits, fluid intake and potentially higher uric acid levels associated with a high-protein diet. Men are also more likely to develop HIGH BLOOD PRESSURE, OBESITY and TYPE 2 DIABETES, which can also lead to kidney stones, especially if there is a family history of kidney stones. If you have had kidney stones once you may get them again.

Types
- **Calcium:** The most common.
- **Struvite:** Often caused by a bacterial infection.
- **Uric acid:** Sometimes an excess is caused by eating a lot of meat, eggs and fish.

Causes
You are more likely to get kidney stones if you:
- Are often dehydrated.
- Eat a lot of food high in salt or sugar.
- Have a family history of kidney stones.
- Have a blockage in your urinary tract, e.g. if you have had a URINARY TRACT INFECTION (UTI) or kidney infection.
- Take certain medications, like calcium-based antacids or anti-seizure medications.
- Have a certain medical condition, such as CYSTIC FIBROSIS, HIGH BLOOD PRESSURE, GOUT or DIABETES.

Diagnosis
See a doctor if you have symptoms of kidney stones, and always if you have blood in your pee. Kidney stones can be detected with a blood test and urine sample. If your GP thinks the stones are large, they may send you for a CT scan.

Treatment
This depends on the size of the stones:
- For small or medium stones (under 5mm, or 5–10mm), you will be advised to drink plenty of water and take painkillers until they pass in your urine – usually in a week or two. Passing them can cause pain and discomfort.

SYMPTOMS
These symptoms may come and go.
+ Pain in the side of the abdomen.
+ Pain in the testicles.
+ Struggling to pee, needing to pee more often.
+ Blood in pee.
+ Bad-smelling pee.
+ FEVER and/or chills.

- You may be prescribed anti-inflammatories or anti-sickness drugs if you need then.
- Shock wave lithotripsy (SWL) uses shock waves to break up medium or larger stones. They can then take three weeks to pass.
- A ureteroscopy is when a thin tube is inserted via the urethra into the bladder. The stones can be removed or broken up with a laser.
- For very large stones, you may need surgery to break them apart and remove them.

If you have kidney stones and they haven't passed out through your urine after three weeks (depending on the severity of symptoms), you will need a different treatment; if they hang around, they can cause blockages, infection and further kidney problems.

Chronic kidney disease

This is when the kidneys gradually stop working, usually due to other conditions. It's serious, as the damage can't be repaired, but if it's mild and picked up in good time, it's possible to manage it to stop it getting worse. If untreated, it can lead to the kidneys not working at all. It's common as we get older.

SYMPTOMS
There are no symptoms to begin with. As the condition gets worse, you may experience:
+ FATIGUE.
+ Nausea.
+ Blood in pee.
+ Swollen feet, ankles and/or hands.
+ Shortness of breath.

Diagnosis
Always seek medical help if you have these symptoms persistently, and if you have blood in your pee. Diagnosis is by blood and urine tests. If you've had KIDNEY STONES, suffer from DIABETES, HEART DISEASE, HIGH BLOOD PRESSURE or LUPUS, or you have an enlarged prostate, among other conditions, you can get checked for chronic kidney disease, as these conditions can make you more susceptible.

Treatment
This is mainly lifestyle-based, to keep your CHOLESTEROL down and eat as healthily as possible. Medications to control other conditions — such as HIGH BLOOD PRESSURE — that put strain on the kidneys may be necessary. If kidney function is severely reduced, you may need dialysis — a life-sustaining treatment whereby the kidney's function of filtering waste and excess fluid from the blood is replicated by a machine. It involves either diverting blood to a machine for filtration (hemodialysis, typically done several times a week in a hospital setting), or using a dialysis fluid in the abdomen to filter waste (peritoneal dialysis, usually done daily at home).

Acute kidney disease

This is when the kidneys suddenly stop working. Toxins build up in the blood, damaging other organs. Many people recover but it is fatal if not treated quickly. It is usually brought on by another illness.

SYMPTOMS
+ **Passing small amounts of urine or being unable to pee.**
+ **Dark brown urine.**
+ **Swollen abdomen, legs and/or feet.**
+ **FATIGUE.**
+ **Confusion.**
+ **Nausea and vomiting.**
+ **Loss of consciousness or a seizure in extreme cases.**

Causes
- Interruption to blood flow to the kidneys, e.g. dehydration due to vomiting and diarrhoea, blood loss or HEART FAILURE.
- Severe kidney infection or SEPSIS.
- Problems affecting the flow of urine from the kidney to the bladder.
- Reaction to certain medications.

Diagnosis
This is by blood test, though the underlying cause will need to be identified.

Treatment
The priority is rehydration, identifying what's caused the condition and bringing down the inflammation so the kidneys can heal. You may need to have a catheter for a short time. In severe cases, dialysis may be needed.

⚠️ Transmissible

Sexually transmitted infections (STIs)

It's very easy to get tested for STIs and, if you are sexually active, it's something you should do regularly. Using a condom will prevent transmission of many, but not all, STIs. Many can be transmitted via sharing sex toys, too. Lots of STIs have no or minimal symptoms but, left untreated, can cause long-term damage and infertility. Most are very contagious.

Common STIs

	In women	In men
Chlamydia	**Symptoms:** Unusual vaginal discharge, pain when peeing and/or having sex, pain in abdomen and/or lower back, bleeding between periods, or in POST-MENOPAUSAL women. It can also not have any immediate symptoms but then cause infertility. **Treatment:** Cured by antibiotics but can be caught again.	**Symptoms:** Unusual discharge from tip of penis, pain when peeing and/or in testicles, itching around scrotum and penis. **Treatment:** Cured by antibiotics but can be caught again.
Genital warts	**Symptoms:** Small, flesh-coloured lumps – sometimes a cluster anywhere around the genitals or inside the vagina. May not cause symptoms, can be painful, itchy or bleed. Caused by HPV. **Treatment:** A sexual health clinic can prescribe a cream to remove the symptoms but the virus will remain in your body and can lead to subsequent flare-ups. Cryotherapy in serious cases. Avoid sex until the warts have gone.	**Symptoms:** Small, flesh-coloured lumps – sometimes a cluster anywhere around the genitals. May not cause symptoms, can be painful, itchy or bleed. Caused by HPV. **Treatment:** A sexual health clinic can prescribe a cream to remove the symptoms but the virus will remain in your body and can lead to subsequent flare-ups. Cryotherapy in serious cases. Avoid sex until the warts have gone.
Gonorrhoea	**Symptoms:** Change in vaginal discharge – sometimes greeny-yellow. Pain when peeing, bleeding between periods. **Treatment:** Cured by antibiotics but can be caught again.	**Symptoms:** Greeny-yellow discharge from penis. Pain when peeing, swollen foreskin. **Treatment:** Cured by antibiotics but can be caught again.
Herpes (type 2)	**Symptoms:** Can take a long time to appear after an infection. Small blisters around genitals and/or bottom that may burst and leave sores. Burning or itching, pain when peeing. Unusual vaginal discharge. **Treatment:** Antivirals, cream to treat symptoms, but the virus will remain in your body and can lead to subsequent flare-ups.	**Symptoms:** Can take a long time to appear after infection. Small blisters around genitals and/or bottom that may burst and leave sores. Burning or itching, pain when peeing. Discharge from the penis. **Treatment:** Antivirals, cream to treat symptoms, but the virus will remain in your body and can lead to subsequent flare-ups.

Common STIs

	In women	In men
Syphilis	**Symptoms:** Can come and go but the infection remains in your body. Ulcers around the vulva/anus. Sores around the mouth. Swollen glands, FATIGUE, aching joints, rash on palms and soles of feet. **Treatment:** Cured by antibiotics but can be caught again.	**Symptoms:** Can come and go but the infection remains in your body. Ulcers around the genitals/anus. Sores around the mouth. Swollen glands, FATIGUE, aching joints, rash on palms and soles of feet. **Treatment:** Cured by antibiotics but can be caught again.
Pubic lice (crabs)	**Symptoms:** Itching in pubic area. Tiny spots on skin (bites) and white dots in pubic hair (lice eggs). **Treatment:** Medicated lotion. More than one treatment will be needed to cure you of the lice and they can be caught again.	**Symptoms:** Itching in pubic area. Tiny spots on skin (bites) and white dots in pubic hair (lice eggs). **Treatment:** Medicated lotion. More than one treatment will be needed to cure you of the lice and they can be caught again.
Trichomoniasis	**Symptoms:** Unusual vaginal discharge, may be greeny-yellow and smell bad. Soreness and itching. Pain when peeing and/or having sex. **Treatment:** Cured by antibiotics but can be caught again.	**Symptoms:** Discharge from the penis. Soreness and itching around the foreskin and/or head of penis. Pain when peeing and/or ejaculating. Needing to pee more often. **Treatment:** Cured by antibiotics but can be caught again.

See also HIV and HUMAN PAPILLOMAVIRUS (HPV).

Diagnosis

In the UK, go to www.sh.uk where, depending on your location, you may be able to order a free, at-home test, learn more about STIs and find your nearest sexual health clinic. You can also buy tests from some pharmacies.

Testing at home

After completing a questionnaire (or speaking to a pharmacist) you'll be advised which test you need based on your symptoms and sexual behaviour. This may be a finger-prick test, a vaginal swab, a urine sample and/or a throat or rectal swab. In some regions you may be offered an online consultation for herpes, otherwise see your GP or go to a sexual health clinic (also see your GP or go to a sexual health clinic if you suspect pubic lice/crabs or genital warts).

Finger-prick blood test: HEPATITIS B and C, syphilis and HIV.
Urine sample: Chlamydia, gonorrhoea, trichomoniasis and sometimes for THRUSH and BACTERIAL VAGINOSIS.
Vaginal swab: Chlamydia, gonorrhoea, trichomoniasis and sometimes for THRUSH and BACTERIAL VAGINOSIS.
Throat swab: Chlamydia and gonorrhoea.
Rectal swab: Chlamydia and gonorrhoea.

Gonorrhoea vaccination

In recent years, some doctors have been offering a booster of the MenB vaccine, for use off-licence in adults at increased risk of gonorrhoea, which has been found to reduce risk by 40 per cent. You can self-refer to sexual health services to discuss your options.

THE FEMALE REPRODUCTIVE SYSTEM

The job description of the female reproductive system is simple on paper: release eggs and if a foetus is created, look after it until it's ready to be born. But the processes involved are complicated and super interesting.

Between the ages of 10 and 16, most females will start having a monthly period which will continue until they reach menopause, aged around 40–50. These days of bleeding are part of a cycle that lasts, on average, 28 days, although all women are different.

Reproductive hormones work as 'switches', telling the body what to do and triggering the release of the next hormone in the process. Hormones are powerful things, impacting other bodily process as well as how you feel.

Menstruation phase (days 1–4)
The lining of the uterus (womb) is shed because you haven't become pregnant during your previous cycle. The first day of proper bleeding is counted as day one of the menstrual cycle.

Follicular phase (days 4–14)
Follicle stimulating hormone (FSH) tells your ovaries to produce follicles containing an egg. Oestrogen and testosterone levels rise.

Ovulation phase (day 14)
Luteinising hormone (LH) prompts the release of the most dominant follicle (corpus luteum) into the fallopian tube. This is when you are most fertile.

Luteal phase (day 15 onwards)
The egg becomes a clump of cells called a corpus luteum, which releases progesterone and oestrogen. If it isn't fertilised, it will break down and leave your body with the lining of your uterus in your next period.

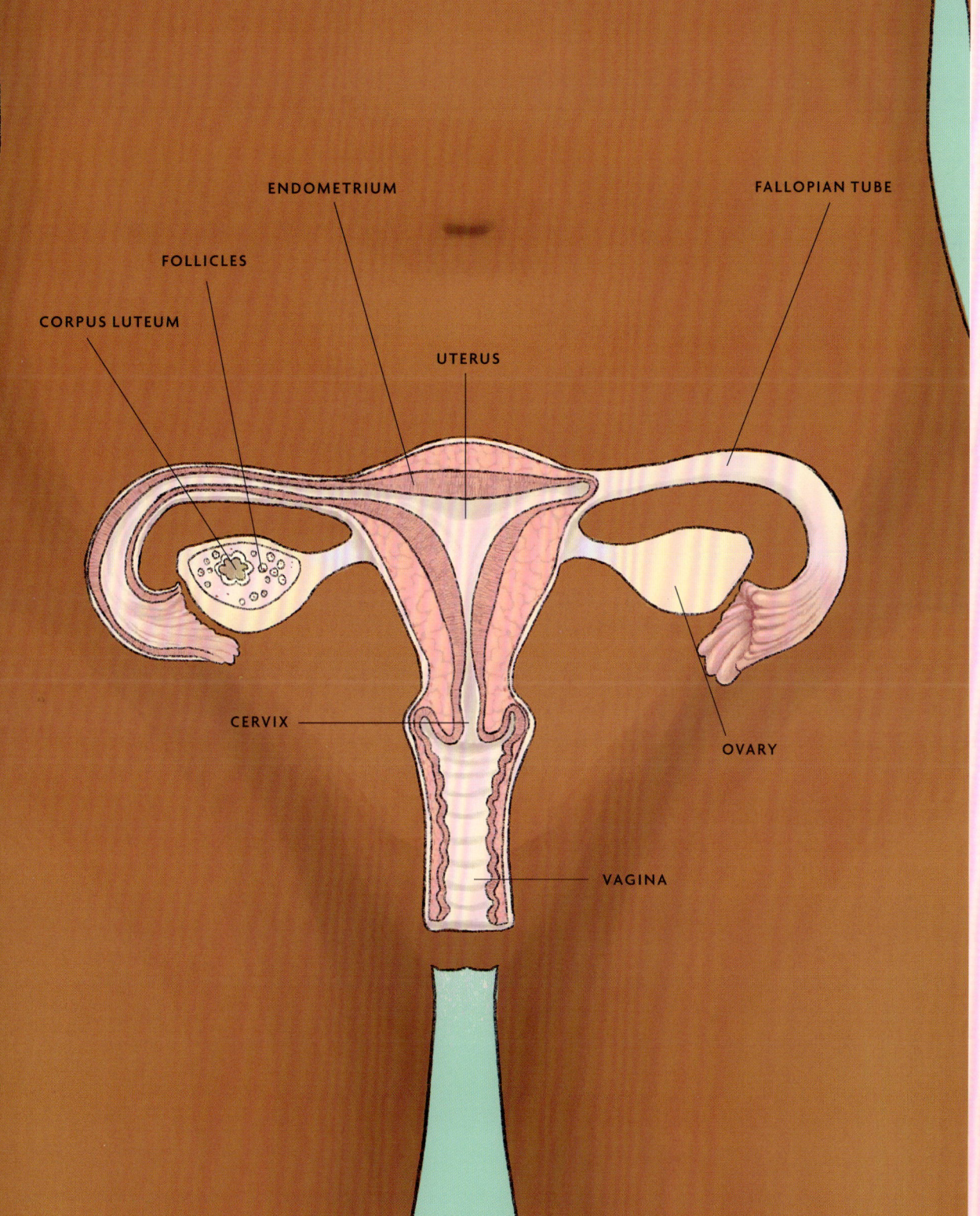

Irregular periods

There's no such thing as a 'normal' cycle, other than what is usual for you. How often and how much you bleed depends on your hormone levels, the type of CONTRACEPTION you are on, diet, lifestyle and factors like stress and underlying medical conditions.

No periods

If you are PREGNANT, breastfeeding, MENOPAUSAL or using certain CONTRACEPTION, you won't have periods. If none apply to you but you haven't had a period for more than three months, speak to your GP.

Infrequent periods

Infrequent periods are those that are more than 35 days apart. This is normal for some people and during PERIMENOPAUSE, but it can make it harder to get PREGNANT. If your periods have recently become irregular you may want to talk to a doctor or check in with the clinic where you get your CONTRACEPTION.

Irregular bleeding

Bleeding between periods can be down to CONTRACEPTION or caused by FIBROIDS, polyps or a SEXUALLY TRANSMITTED INFECTION (STI). In rare cases, it can be a sign of UTERINE CANCER. If you have missed a period, or have pain and could be PREGNANT, get checked as it could be an ECTOPIC PREGNANCY.

Heavy bleeding

When you need to change your highest-absorbency period pants, pad or tampon every hour, you have flooding, large clots or your period has lasted longer than eight days. This can be caused by a number of things, but get it checked if it's not normal for you, it's affecting your quality of life and/or you have other symptoms like feeling faint or severe cramps (also see ENDOMETRIOSIS).

Premenstrual syndrome (PMS) & premenstrual dysphoric disorder (PMDD)

Premenstrual syndrome (PMS) is a wide range of physical and emotional symptoms that occur five to eleven days before a menstrual cycle and stop after a period begins. Mild symptoms are very common, but some people suffer from a severe form called premenstrual dysphoric disorder (PMDD). Neurotransmitters in the brain are affected by the rise and fall of oestrogen, causing intense physical, emotional and psychological distress, impacting daily life. We don't know what the cause is and there has historically been a lack of research in this area. However, there are things that can be done, so track your cycle and your symptoms and speak to a doctor.

Don't suffer in silence

Many women experience minor cramps and bloating that can be solved by a hot-water bottle and some painkillers. But if you are worried about anything to do with your menstrual cycle and/or you are in pain that painkillers don't touch, see a doctor.

How to track your periods

It's great to have an idea of not just when you bleed, but how you feel throughout your cycle. You can use an app or a good old-fashioned diary. Tracking means you know what is normal for you and can be useful at any future medical appointments. Keep a note of:

- Starts and end dates.
- Blood flow and consistency.
- Physical and emotional symptoms.

Contraception

Do your research to understand potential side effects before choosing the best contraception for you.

- Are you having sex with one or multiple partners? Do you need protection from STIs?
- Are you thinking of getting PREGNANT soon?
- Ease of use and lifestyle, e.g. will you remember to take a pill at the same time each day?
- What are the possible side effects?
- Do you have existing health conditions that may affect which hormones you can take?
- Do you want to address any issues with your menstrual cycle, such as HEAVY BLEEDING?

Hormonal contraception

These add hormones into your body to stop it preparing for PREGNANCY. They can have side effects, particularly at first. Some are also used to help ease heavy or painful periods. No hormonal contraceptives protect against STIs.

- **Combined pill:** Contains oestrogen and progesterone and is taken for three weeks of your cycle followed by a break week when you will usually bleed. It's very effective when taken consistently. Note vomiting or diarrhoea can stop it being absorbed properly.
- **Progesterone-only pill:** Must be taken at the same time each day. Again, it's very reliable so long as you follow the directions and do not have vomiting or diarrhoea.
- **Contraceptive implant:** A small piece of plastic containing progesterone inserted under the skin of your upper arm. It lasts three years then needs to be removed and replaced. May cause fewer or lighter periods.
- **Contraceptive injection:** A progesterone-only injection given every three months. May stop you having periods.
- **IUS coil:** A small device inserted by a doctor or nurse into the uterus that releases a small amount of progesterone, usually for five years. The procedure, while not pleasant, is quick and you can't feel it once it's in.
- **Vaginal ring:** A soft plastic ring inserted into the vagina for 21 days that releases progesterone and oestrogen. Once removed, you will have a period and then must insert a new ring after seven days.

The withdrawal technique

Removing the penis from the vagina before ejaculation is *not* a reliable method of contraception.

Non-hormonal contraception

These methods tend to act as a barrier to stop sperm meeting an egg and can have fewer side effects because they are not changing the hormones in your body.

- **IUD coil:** Similar to the IUS coil (see left) but it contains copper rather than hormones which weakens sperm so they can't reach an egg. Can be kept in for ten years. The IUD coil does not protect against STIs.
- **Female and male condoms:** These do protect against STIs. Female condoms are harder to buy and trickier to use but can be inserted before you start intercourse and there's no need for the penis to be withdrawn immediately afterwards, as with male condoms.
- **Diaphragm:** Inserted into the vagina to cover the top of the cervix, usually with spermicidal gel. It can be washed and reused but must stay in place for six hours after sex. Does not protect against STIs and is less effective than other methods.
- **Sterilisation:** A permanent operation involving ligation of the fallopian tubes. Does not lead to chemical or surgical MENOPAUSE. See also VASECTOMY.

Red flag – emergency contraception

This is available from most GPs and some walk-in centres and pharmacies. You need to take it within three (sometimes five) days of having unprotected sex (the sooner the better), or when CONTRACEPTION has failed. Its hormones prevents or delays egg release, and impacts the cervical mucus and uterine lining, making it more difficult for sperm to reach an egg and embed in the uterine lining.

Pregnancy

Pregnancy signifies a big life change, and can affect your overall sense of wellbeing in many ways.

Preparing to get pregnant

- Get up to date with CERVICAL SCREENING TEST and vaccines.
- Consider your overall health, including your weight, diet, how active you are and your mental health.
- Reduce alcohol intake and quit smoking.
- Consider taking supplements like folic acid.
- Review any medications you take.
- Track your periods.
- Check if there are any genetic conditions that run in your or your partner's family.
- Many people have healthy pregnancies despite having serious health conditions, but it's vital to talk to your doctor first.
- If you are the sperm-supplying partner, it's equally important to review your health – unhealthy lifestyles have a big impact on fertility.

If you are struggling to get pregnant

If you are under 35 and you have been trying for a year, or six months if you are over 35, see a doctor. Provide as much info as you can about your cycle and how often you have sex. Both partners will need to be checked as fertility issues affect both sexes equally.

Red flag symptoms

Speak to your doctor or midwife if you experience any bleeding during PREGNANCY. In early PREGNANCY, this could be implantation bleeding, spotting often mistaken for a light period, that is caused by the embryo implanting in the uterus lining. Other forms of bleeding can be common in PREGNANCY too but it is always safest to get it checked out if you are concerned.

SYMPTOMS

Some people have no symptoms at all, but early symptoms typically include:
- Vaginal bleeding.
- Pain in the lower abdomen.
- Tender or swollen breasts.
- Nausea or vomiting.
- Needing to pee more often.
- Diarrhoea or constipation.
- Feeling really TIRED.

Diagnosis & antenatal care

The best time to take a pregnancy test is after your first missed period, or 21 days after you had sex – although some tests claim to be accurate just 10 days after conception. If you get two solid lines, this is 99.9 per cent accurate that you are pregnant. It's a good idea to do another three to four days later. You can self-refer to your local antenatal care team via an online form or speak to your GP. Do this as soon as you can so you can get booked in for your first scan, usually at 11–13 weeks.

Termination

If you are PREGNANT and don't want to be, make an appointment as soon as you can with your doctor, sexual health clinic or British Pregnancy Advisory Service (BPAS) in the UK. You can also pay to see a medical professional privately. After 24 weeks, termination can only take place in extreme circumstances (12 weeks in Northern Ireland). Some people find this to be a traumatic experience – try to get the support of someone you trust if you are going through this.

Miscarriage

Sadly, some pregnancies will end in miscarriage, defined as the end of a pregnancy during the first 23 weeks; an early miscarriage is the end of a pregnancy during the first 12 weeks. It is important to remember that the majority of miscarriages are one-off occurrences, and it is often possible to have a completely healthy pregnancy afterwards.

SYMPTOMS

While the main symptom of a miscarriage is vaginal bleeding, please note that light bleeding is fairly common during the first three months of pregnancy. But it is always wise to consult your GP or midwife if you are concerned about bleeding in pregnancy.
+ Vaginal bleeding.
+ Pain in the lower abdomen.

Diagnosis
Usually an ultrasound scan will be undertaken in hospital to determine if you are having a miscarriage. Occasionally, no bleeding will be experienced but your first pregnancy scan can show with no heartbeat; this is known as a missed miscarriage.

Treatment
If a miscarriage is confirmed, your doctor and midwife will discuss your options to help the pregnancy tissue leave your body, though often this will happen naturally over a week or so. Miscarriage can be extremely distressing and your midwife or GP can connect you to counselling services if you need them. You can request a baby-loss certificate after any pregnancy loss, including ECTOPIC PREGNANCY, miscarriage and TERMINATION, no matter when in your pregnancy you experienced it. These optional certificates can be used as a way of remembering your baby if this feels appropriate to you.

Ectopic pregnancy

Ectopic pregnancy is when a fertilised egg has implanted outside the uterus, commonly in the fallopian tube, ovaries or cervix. This can cause life-threatening complications such as rupture of the fallopian tube and internal bleeding.

SYMPTOMS

A positive pregnancy test or missed period accompanied by the following:
+ Abdominal pain, often to one side.
+ Vaginal bleeding/spotting.
+ Severe lower back pain.
+ FEVER.
+ Nausea or vomiting.
+ Shoulder tip pain, which occurs when the diaphragm is irritated by blood leaking from a ruptured or leaking fallopian tube.
+ Dizziness or fainting, which also indicate internal bleeding or shock.

Diagnosis
Ectopic pregnancy is diagnosed by a combination of pregnancy test, symptoms and ultrasound scan.

Treatment
Dependent on severity of the symptoms but involves hospital care with active monitoring. In very early stages, if symptoms are mild and the individual is medically stable, careful monitoring will see if the pregnancy resolves on its own. Alternatively, an injection of methotrexate is used to dissolve the pregnancy tissue. If symptoms become life-threatening, keyhole surgery is performed to remove the pregnancy tissue, often along with the fallopian tube.

> **Red flag**
> An ectopic pregnancy is an emergency requiring urgent medical attention. Call 111 or visit A&E.

THE FEMALE REPRODUCTIVE SYSTEM

Perimenopause & menopause

If you have a female reproductive system, once you reach the end of your fertile years you will go through a biological change where your hormone levels decrease. For some, this is a relatively easy transition. Others, however, can experience a range of symptoms, from unpleasant to debilitating. This used to be a taboo subject and something women were expected to put up with. But do not grin and bear it – there is help and effective treatments available.

Stages of menopause

Perimenopause
This is the time leading up to your final period when you can start to experience menopausal symptoms. You still menstruate but less often or the flow may vary. Generally this begins from age 40 onwards.

Menopause
Simply defined as 12 consecutive months without a period. This usually happens between the ages of 45–55.

Post-menopause
When you haven't had a period for one year and one day. You are then post-menopausal for the rest of your life.

Surgical menopause
When the ovaries are removed, e.g. as part of a hysterectomy.

Early menopause
When periods stop before the age of 40.

In Japan, menopause is known as 'konenki'. It literally means 'rebirth' or 'the season of renewal of years'. It is seen less as a loss, and more as a natural transition into a new stage of life.

SYMPTOMS

These vary hugely in severity and from person to person. Not everyone will experience symptoms, or they may have a few that come and go.

Emotional/psychological:
+ Lack of concentration.
+ DEPRESSION/low mood/feeling tearful.
+ Low self-esteem/confidence.
+ Irritability.
+ Lack of libido.
+ Sleep issues.
+ Forgetfulness/brain fog.

Physical:
+ Irregular periods.
+ Needing to pee more.
+ Dry, itchy skin.
+ Night sweats.
+ Achy, heavy legs.
+ Heart palpations.
+ Pain during sex.

Keep a diary of all your symptoms. It will help you understand what is changing for you and be invaluable if you need to talk to a doctor. And remember that it's fine to ask for a GP specifically trained in women's health when you book your appointment.

Diagnosis

Perimenopause is diagnosed via symptoms, age and ruling out other causes for your symptoms. Below the age of 45 years old perimenopause can be diagnosed with a follicle stimulating blood test to check the person isn't in early menopause.

Treatment

Oestrogen is a hugely important hormone that affects many bodily processes. When this declines in perimenopause, some people will choose to have hormone replacement therapy (HRT). HRT can be taken in the form of systemic oestrogen, which is traditionally viewed as a synthetic preparation, but we now have body-identical oestrogen preparations in the form of gels, patches and sprays, which are taken through the skin, and are therefore safer in regards to clot risk than synthetic oral options.

If you have ENDOMETRIOSIS and have a uterus, taking progesterone alongside your oestrogen supplement is vital to protect the endometrial lining in your uterus from endometrial hyperplasia. If you have ENDOMETRIOSIS but have had a hysterectomy, the progesterone stops any progression of ENDOMETRIOSIS that's left behind from growing elsewhere in the body. This can be taken orally in the form of body-identical micronised progesterone or progestin (which is synthetic) or via a 52mg levonorgestrel IUS coil.

There are other options, such as topical oestrogen cream. Lifestyle changes, particularly exercise, can make a big difference, as well as setting you up to have a good older age. Some excellent books have been written about this subject and there are good online resources too (see page 252). No two perimenopause/post-menopause experiences are the same so please do educate yourself and listen to and care for your body.

⚠️ **Transmissible**

Gynaecological infections

A gynaecological infection is any kind of infection of the vagina, vulva, cervix, uterus or fallopian tubes. Some are caused by SEXUALLY TRANSMITTED INFECTIONS (STIS), while others aren't categorised as STIS. They are usually very easy to treat and nothing to be embarrassed about.

Bacterial vaginosis (BV)

This occurs when the bacteria that usually live in the vagina without causing problems grow too numerous, usually due to a change in the pH balance.

SYMPTOMS

- Thin, watery, white/grey discharge, sometimes with a fishy smell.
- Can be symptomless.

Diagnosis & treatment

Your GP or sexual health clinic can test you using a swab and prescribe antibiotics. You can pass this infection on to a sexual partner if you are having unprotected sex, so ensure that any partners (including male partners) are treated too, to prevent reinfection.

Thrush/candida

This is caused by a yeast that usually lives harmlessly on our skin. It's common in PREGNANCY and can be triggered by stress and poor diet.

SYMPTOMS

- Thick and lumpy white discharge.
- Itching and/or soreness.

Diagnosis & treatment

A pharmacist can supply a cream, pessary or oral tablet, though it may take two weeks to completely clear. Sexual partners of all genders should be treated if you are having unprotected sex, as they can reinfect you.

Pelvic inflammatory disease (PID)

An uncommon but serious complication of an infection that spreads to other areas of the reproductive system, sometimes as the result of an STI. It can cause infertility and scarring of the fallopian tubes, increasing the chances of ECTOPIC PREGNANCY if untreated.

SYMPTOMS

- Pain in lower abdomen and/or back.
- Green/yellow discharge that smells bad.
- Vaginal irritation.
- Pain when peeing and during sex.
- Heavy/painful periods and/or bleeding between periods or after menopause.
- Sometimes nausea, vomiting and FEVER.

Diagnosis & treatment

Your GP or a practitioner at a sexual health clinic will examine you and take a swab to try to find out the cause. They will then prescribe antibiotics.

Maintain good health in your vulva

- Wash with mild soap and water.
- Avoid using perfumed washes or sprays.
- Wear cotton underwear.
- Don't stay in sweaty gym clothes or wet bathing suits.
- Wipe from front to back after peeing.
- If you feel irritation in this area, avoid sex until it subsides.

Breast conditions

Any unusual or worrying changes to your breasts should be checked by your GP. However, it's worth knowing that there are non-cancerous conditions that cause issues in this area of your body.

Cysts

A cyst is a fluid-filled lump that may cause pain. They're common in younger women and affected by the menstrual cycle. They usually go away by themselves, but sometimes larger ones need to be drained.

Fibrocystic breast changes

A thickening or lumpiness to both breasts caused by hormonal changes before a period that then goes away again. Your breasts may feel swollen and you may have cloudy nipple discharge. It's not usually anything to worry about but always get it checked.

Fibroadenoma

A solid, round, rubbery lump that moves easily when pushed. It is more common in younger women and change with the menstrual cycle, but should be checked by a GP if it's new to you.

Intraductal papilloma

Wart-like growths in the ducts near the nipple which can be sore. The doctor will do a biopsy. Multiple papillomas slightly increases your risk of developing BREAST CANCER.

Atypical hyperplasia

A non-cancerous growth of cells in the milk duct (called atypical ductal hyperplasia, or ADH) or glands (known as atypical lobular hyperplasia, or ALH). It can increase the risk of developing BREAST CANCER.

Adenosis

This is when the milk-producing glands are larger than normal. It can cause painful lumps that change in size during your menstrual cycle. You may have scar tissue in the area. It doesn't usually need treatment but usually requires a biopsy to make sure it's not anything else.

Mastitis

An infection in the breast that's common when breastfeeding and has led to blocked milk ducts, which may cause pain, a burning sensation in the breast, red, bluish or darker colour swelling (dependent on your skin colour) and a yellow, crusty discharge, as well as FEVER and FLU-like symptoms. It's treated with antibiotics and you can ease the symptoms with paracetamol or ibuprofen, and a warm (to aid milk flow) or cold (to soothe pain) compress. As with many infections, drinking plenty of fluids and resting where possible should help too. If you are breastfeeding, you should continue to do so and offer your baby a breastfeed if your breasts feel uncomfortably full. A lactation consultant or lactation midwife can assess your baby's latch and position to ensure they are feeding properly as poor latch or positioning can cause milk to build up and lead to mastitis.

Fat necrosis

This happens when the blood supply to breast-fat tissue has been cut off, for example as a result of injury, surgery or radiation treatment, although it can take a long time to appear. It can happen in other places but particularly the breast and may result in lumps, dimpling, puckering, skin irritation, nipple inversion, discharge and pain. It isn't serious but, as it can look a lot like cancer, it can be stressful and needs investigating.

How to check your breasts

Knowing what's normal for you means you are much more likely to spot any changes. You should perform a self-examination monthly, preferably between periods if you have them, and standing up or lying on your back. Carry out the following on both breasts, using the pads of your fingers and applying firm but comfortable pressure. Look out for any changes in the flesh or skin at each stage:

1. Feel around the fleshy breast tissue in a circular motion, moving outwards from the nipple to your ribs and armpit.
2. Feel underneath and around the nipple.
3. Feel underneath the armpit.
4. Walk your fingers up your chest to your neck, feeling as you go.

Changes you should look for include: new lumps, irritation, redness, darkening or flaking of the skin, thickening in the breast, nipple puckering, dimpling or inversion (if not normal for you), nipple discharge, pain in any areas or a marked change in breast size.

STEP 1

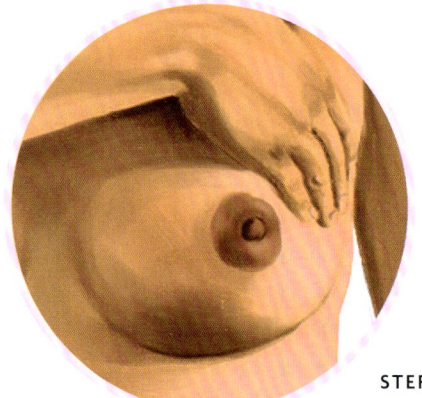

STEP 2

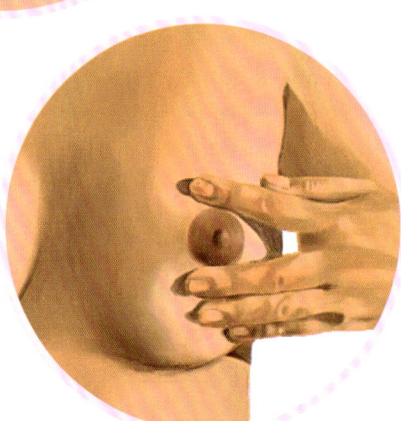

STEP 3

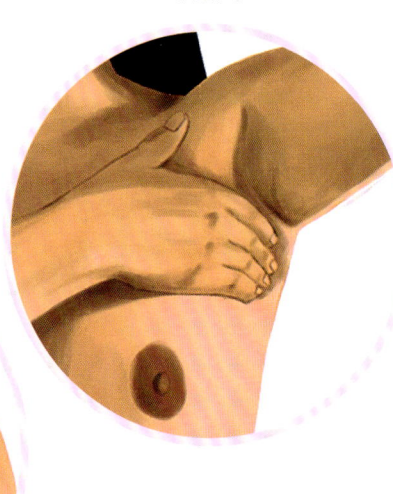

STEP 4

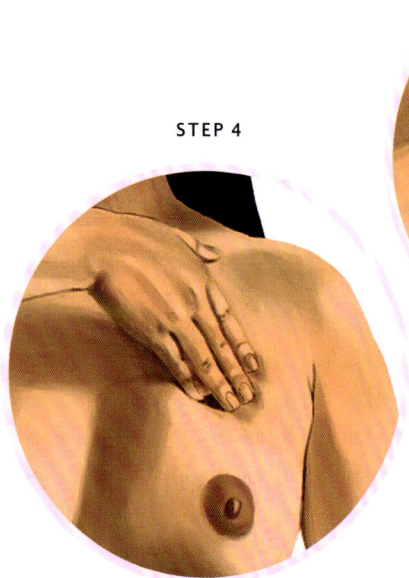

Breast changes in puberty

It's usual for developing breasts to be a bit sore sometimes, or for one to be bigger than the other. A small difference is fine but if there's a big difference it's worth getting this checked. Variation in nipple size and shape is also normal but be aware of sudden changes, such as inversion of the nipple (particularly if only on one nipple), discharge (unrelated to PREGNANCY or breastfeeding), rash, puckering or dimpling of the nipple.

Breast cancer

This is the most common type of cancer in women, and about one in seven women in the UK will be diagnosed with it. However, if it's caught early, it can be successfully treated. This is why it's so important to check your breasts once a month – if you menstruate, do this two weeks before or after your period. A lump or change in your breasts is not necessarily cancer but it's crucial to get it checked as soon as possible.

People born male can also get breast cancer. Although it's uncommon, it is still important to get any lumps checked.

SYMPTOMS
+ **Lump in the breast or armpit.**
+ **Change in size, shape or feel of one breast.**
+ **Changes to the skin, such as reddening, puckering, dimpling or 'orange peel' effect.**
+ **Changes to the nipple, e.g. it inverts or you have what looks like a rash.**
+ **Discharge from the nipple, if you are not pregnant or breastfeeding.**
+ **Constant breast pain that doesn't come and go.**

Diagnosis
This is done by breast examination, a mammogram, a breast ultrasound scan and sometimes a small tissue sample is taken from the breast, called a biopsy.

Treatment
There are different kinds of breast cancer; treatment depends on what kind you have and whether it has spread, and also whether you have been through MENOPAUSE. You will usually have surgery to remove one breast, both breasts or part of the breast. If you want to, you can often have breast reconstruction. You may also have chemotherapy, radiotherapy and/or hormone therapy, which reduces the levels of hormones that can make the cancer grow.

Follow-up care
After successful treatment, most people will have follow-up tests, sometimes yearly at first, moving eventually to five-yearly, as cancer can come back. However, many people are now living long lives with a breast cancer diagnosis and some I've met even see themselves as 'breast cancer thrivers'. You may need other support too – practical and emotional – particularly if you are having treatment to suppress hormones.

Breast screening
A mammogram is an X-ray that picks up signs of cancer cells. If you are registered with your doctor as female you will be invited for one every three years between the ages of 50 and 70.

BRCA1, BRCA2, TP53 genetic fault. If you have a family history of certain cancers, you may be eligible for a screening to see if you have inherited these, which makes you more likely to get BREAST CANCER (though it doesn't mean you will). Your doctor can advise on this. Not everyone wants to be screened – you don't have to be.

Uterine conditions

There are many conditions that can affect the uterus and most are underdiagnosed, i.e. lots of people have them without realising. They can cause issues with fertility and so are often discovered when someone is taking longer than expected to conceive. Don't put up with pain and other symptoms that impact your quality of life — make sure you are well-informed, monitor your symptoms carefully and get the healthcare you need.

Endometriosis

A lifelong, whole-body, inflammatory condition whereby cells similar to those in the lining of the uterus are deposited elsewhere in the pelvic cavity. These cells are glandular and stroma-like, whereby they behave independently to the activity in the uterine cavity and form scar-like adhesions that wrap around structures in the pelvis, thereby causing pain and can affect fertility.

SYMPTOMS
+ Pain during ovulation.
+ Heavy, painful periods.
+ Pain during/after sex and/or when peeling.
+ Pain during bowel movements and/or diarrhoea, constipation and bloating.
+ FATIGUE and leg cramps.

Diagnosis
It can take a long time and much persistence to be diagnosed. Scarring may not show up on an ultrasound, which may look normal even though you have the condition. The gold standard is to do a laparoscopy (keyhole surgery) and then a biopsy on the sample.

Treatment
Although there is currently no cure, hormonal treatment and medication can get it under control and reduce pain. Precision excision surgery or ablation can help with fertility issues and symptom management. A hysterectomy is not a cure but can help to manage symptoms.

Fibroids

Non-cancerous growths in and around the uterus that vary in size. They are common but disproportionately affect Black women and can be a cause of infertility.

SYMPTOMS
+ Heavy, painful periods.
+ Pain in the abdomen and/or lower back.
+ Pain during sex.
+ Bloating and/or constipation.
+ Needing to pee more.

Diagnosis
A doctor will perform an internal examination, feeling for fibroids. You may have an ultrasound.

Treatment
Sometimes very small fibroids resolve by themselves. Symptoms can be managed with hormonal treatment and medication. If they are impacting your quality of life or fertility, you may be offred laparoscopic myomectomy, endometrial ablation or a hysterectomy, depending where you are in your fertility journey.

Adenomyosis

Adenomyosis is a whole-body, lifelong condition, in which the inner lining of the uterus breaks into its muscle wall, causing it to become thick and stiff. It is a condition we know very little about but one in ten women are believed to have it, most commonly those in their forties and fifties who have had children. Although it is not believed to hinder fertility, the stiffened uterus lining that it causes can prevent the uterus from expanding, and increase the likelihood of miscarriage or premature birth.

SYMPTOMS

+ Severe pain/cramping in the lower abdomen.
+ Irregular periods.
+ Heavy and painful periods.
+ Pressure in the lower abdomen.
+ Bloating.
+ Pain during or after sex.
+ Severe anaemia.

Diagnosis

As so little is known about adenomyosis, it can take years to diagnose, and is often misdiagnosed as FIBROIDS or simply painful periods. A transvaginal ultrasound scan will diagnose in the later stages, or a laparoscopy or MRI scan can diagnose it in earlier stages.

Treatment

There is no cure, but you can have help in managing the discomfort through painkillers and hormonal CONTRACEPTIVES, which can help to lessen symptoms. In more severe cases, as with ENDOMETRIOSIS, precision excision surgery or ablation can help. A hysterectomy to completely remove the uterus can resolve severe cases but this is a major procedure that might not be preferable for younger women who want to start a family someday.

Uterine cancer

Most cancer of the uterus starts with a tumour in the endometrial lining of the womb. A rarer kind develops in the muscular wall. It's most common in women who have been through MENOPAUSE but can affect younger people. You may be at more risk of this type of cancer if you have higher levels of oestrogen – if you are overweight, OBESE or have POLYCYSTIC OVARY SYNDROME (PCOS), for example, or you take tamoxifen or have a family history of BOWEL CANCER, OVARIAN CANCER or uterine cancer.

SYMPTOMS

Symptoms can overlap with other conditions that affect the uterus and female reproductive system more generally.
+ Bleeding between periods.
+ Heavy and prolonged periods.
+ Post-menopausal bleeding or bloody discharge.
+ Pain/cramping in the lower abdomen.
+ Lumps or swelling between hip bones.
+ Changes in bowel habits.

Diagnosis

An ultrasound can check the lining of the uterus. If anything is found, you will have a hysteroscopy, in which a tiny camera on the end of a thin tube is inserted into the womb via the vagina to investigate and usually take a biopsy. You may also have an MRI or CT scan.

Treatment

Treatment depends on how advanced the cancer is. You will usually need a hysterectomy to remove the womb, followed by chemotherapy and/or radiotherapy. If you have not been through MENOPAUSE, this will mean you go into surgical MENOPAUSE, so you will need ongoing support to manage various aspects of your health. Many people go on to live long lives after treatment for uterine cancer – as with all cancers, it's about catching it early.

Ovarian disorders

The ovaries are the site of egg storage and an integral part of the female reproductive system, responsible for the production of hormones as well as preparing the body for PREGNANCY. Therefore, the consequences of any ovarian disorders can take effect all over the body.

Polycystic ovary syndrome (PCOS)

This is a lifelong, whole-body condition that causes the ovaries to get bigger and develop tiny cysts, which can stop eggs being released and reduce fertility.

SYMPTOMS

- Irregular or no periods.
- Excessive hair growth, particularly on the face, pubic areas, arms and legs (caused by too much of the hormone androgen).
- Weight gain and insulin resistance, which can lead to TYPE 2 DIABETES.
- ACNE.

Diagnosis
A blood test can show hormone levels and you'll have an ultrasound on your ovaries. Confusingly, you can have PCOS if you have the symptoms but not the cysts, and you can have cysts without having the symptoms of PCOS.

Treatment
PCOS cannot be cured but symptoms can be treated effectively. You may be monitored for related conditions, such as DIABETES and UTERINE CANCER. Talk to your doctor if you are trying to get PREGNANT (in my experience, many people with PCOS can).

Ovarian cyst

A non-cancerous fluid-filled sac that grows on the ovary. They are common and sometimes caused by an underlying condition like ENDOMETRIOSIS. Cysts make it harder to conceive but don't usually cause infertility.

SYMPTOMS

- Changes to periods, such as periods stopping, heavy periods, spotting or bleeding between periods.
- Swollen stomach.
- Pain in the pelvis/during sex.
- Needing to pee more often.

Diagnosis
Diagnosis is via an internal ultrasound scan using a wand inserted into the vagina.

Treatment
Some cysts go away by themselves so you may only need follow-up scans to monitor it. Surgery may be required if the cyst is large or there is a concern it could be cancerous.

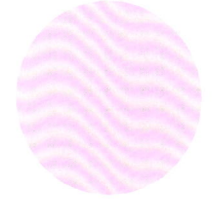

Ovarian cancer

If abnormal cells start to grow in and around the ovaries and fallopian tubes they may form a cancerous tumour. This is most common in people who are over 50, but it's possible to get this type of cancer at any age. If you have had your ovaries removed, it is still possible to get ovarian cancer in the fallopian tubes. If it's caught early, it is very treatable; however, it is not the easiest cancer to detect. There is currently no screening programme.

Causes & risk factors
You are more likely (though it's far from certain) to get ovarian cancer if you:
- Went through MENOPAUSE late (over 55).
- Have a family history of breast or ovarian cancer (if you carry the faulty BRCA genes, or those connected to Lynch syndrome).
- Have had BREAST CANCER or BOWEL CANCER, particularly if you had radiotherapy as part of your treatment.

SYMPTOMS
+ **Feeling bloated, have a swollen stomach.**
+ **Feeling full quickly, poor appetite.**
+ **Unintentional weight loss.**
+ **FATIGUE.**
+ **Lower back pain.**
+ **Needing to pee a lot more, recurrent UTIs.**
+ **Bleeding from the vagina after menopause.**
+ **Changes to your bowel habits – it is rare to never have had IBS and then develop it over the age of 50, so this should always be investigated.**

This type of cancer has symptoms common to many conditions, so don't panic if you have any of them. However, that also means it's even more important your symptoms are properly investigated.

Diagnosis
- A CA125 blood test checks the levels of certain proteins in the blood.
- You may have an internal scan, using a wand inserted into the vagina, or an external ultrasound or CT scan.
- A biopsy if anything is found.

Treatment
There are different types of ovarian cancer tumours, so the treatment will depend on this, as well as factors like where the tumour is and whether it has spread. You will usually need surgery to remove the ovaries and sometimes the uterus too. You may have chemotherapy, radiotherapy and potentially follow-up surgery after that.

Cervical cancer

This is when abnormal cell changes happen in the cervix, where the vagina meets the uterus. It's almost always caused by the HUMAN PAPILLOMAVIRUS (HPV).

SYMPTOMS

There may be no symptoms to begin with. If you have a condition like FIBROIDS or ENDOMETRIOSIS, it can be easier to miss symptoms, as they can overlap.
- Vaginal bleeding that's unusual for you e.g. between periods, after sex or post-menopause.
- Unusual, persistent changes to vaginal discharge.
- Pain in the lower back and/or lower pelvis.
- Pain during sex.
- FATIGUE.
- Unintentional weight loss.

Diagnosis

You will have an internal examination and cervical screening test, where a sample of the cells in the cervix will be taken for analysis. If necessary, you'll then have a colposcopy to look at your cervix and a biopsy.

Treatment

This depends on the type of cervical cancer you have and whether/how far it has spread. You will usually have surgery and if the tumour is small this may be to remove part of the cervix. In some cases, a full hysterectomy may be necessary. Chemotherapy, radiotherapy and/or immunotherapy may be needed.

Cervical screening

Sometimes called a smear or a PAP test, this screening procedure looks for human papillomavirus (HPV). HPV is the most common SEXUALLY TRANSMITTED INFECTION, spread by any kind of genital contact (not just penetrative sex). Many people have HPV at some point in their lives and it doesn't cause any symptoms. However, we know that sometimes it can lead to cancer in the cervix, vulva or vagina. The HPV vaccine is now part of the NHS childhood vaccination programme and is also available for people at higher risk from HPV, such as men aged under 46 who have sex with men, some transgender people, sex workers or people living with HIV.

In the UK, those registered with their doctor as having been born female, with no history of high HPV levels, will be offered a test every five years from when they are 25 up until the age of 64. A sample of cells is taken from your cervix and tested for HPV and abnormal cells. If any are found, you'll be offered a colposcopy to remove them so that they don't become cancerous. You don't have to have the test, but it is very effective at catching HPV before it becomes a problem. Speak to the clinic or your doctor if you are worried. They will have measures in place that can help you. You can take someone along with you if you want to. People in England who rarely attend their regular cervical screening can also request an at-home HPV sampling kit. This will allow you to take your own sample and return it for testing.

Note that if you use topical vaginal oestrogen, you should stop this two days before your cervical screening test or at-home HPV sample.

Other types of gynaecological cancers

Vaginal cancer
This is very rare and mostly affects women over 45.

SYMPTOMS
+ Bloody, unpleasant-smelling discharge.
+ Lump in the vagina.
+ Bleeding between periods or after menopause.
+ Spotting after sex.
+ Painful sex.

Vulval cancer
Rarely, cancer can develop in the outer part of the female genitals.

SYMPTOMS
+ Lump in the vulva or groin.
+ Urinary issues, such as stress INCONTINENCE, urge INCONTINENCE, cystitis or UTIs.
+ Itchiness/pain that feels like severe thrush.
+ FATIGUE.

How to check your genitals
It's important to regularly examine yourself for changes and get anything unusual checked out. Please don't feel embarrassed. Finding cancers early gives a much better chance of a good outcome. Use a mirror and sit with your legs slightly bent to get a good view of your genitals.

1. Examine the fleshy area of your vulva from top to bottom. Then check your clitoral hood – the fold of skin where the inner labia meets at the top of the vulva.
2. Check your labia majora – the outer lips.
3. Check your labia minora – the inner lips.
4. Prop the mirror in front of you and use one hand to gently hold open your labia minora, and look into your vagina. Finally, check your perineum (the area between the entrance to the vagina and the anus).

Changes you should look for include: moles, bumps or spots, warts, ulcers or lesions, rashes, white patches or discoloration.

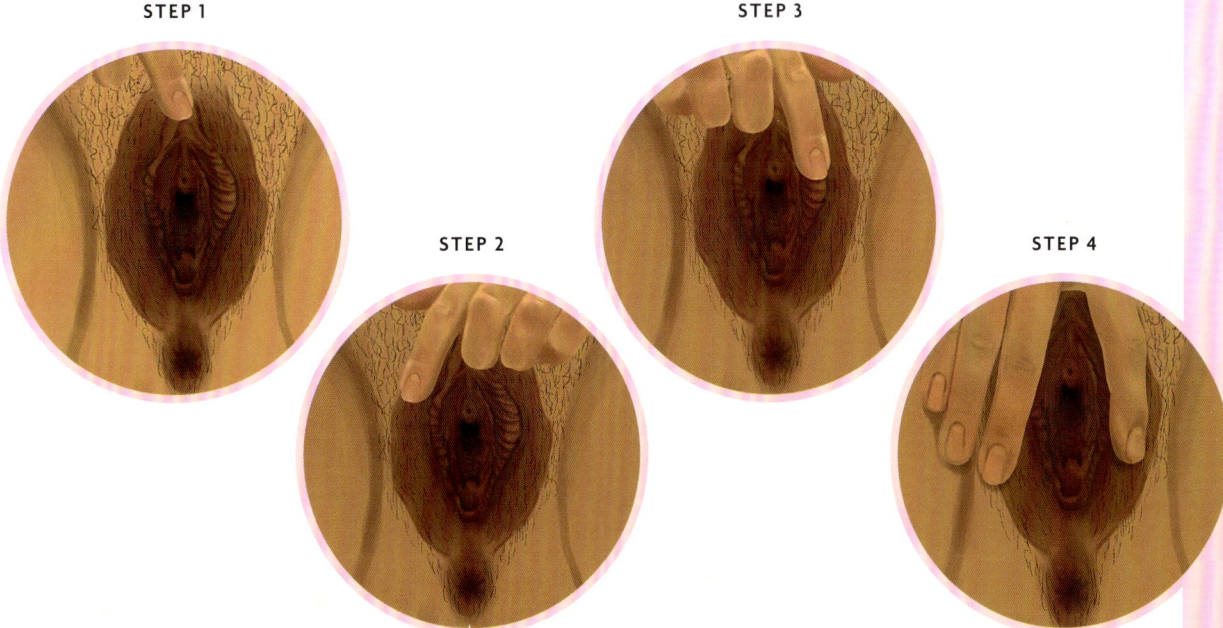

STEP 1

STEP 2

STEP 3

STEP 4

THE MALE REPRODUCTIVE SYSTEM

The male reproductive system is made up primarily of:

- **The penis**, which contains spongy erectile tissue. When you have an erection, this fills with blood, making the shaft and the glans (the head of the penis) rigid and larger.
- **The urethra** is the tube that runs up the inside of the penis. It transports pee and semen, the fluid containing sperm, when you climax.
- **The scrotum** is the skin covering the testicles. It can contract to move the testicles closer to the body.
- **The testicles, or testes** (most, but not everyone, born male have two) make the hormone testosterone and produce sperm.
- **The epididymis** is a tube at the back of each testicle that carries sperm to another tube, **the vas deferens**, then to the urethra.
- **The prostate** is a small gland below your bladder that helps make the fluid that goes into semen.

The other hormones involved in the male reproductive system are luteinising hormone (LH) and follicle stimulating hormone (FSH), both made in the pituitary gland. Men also have oestrogen, but in lower levels than women.

Testosterone levels do decrease as men get older, though gradually, and there is no equivalent to the female menopause. Low testosterone levels can cause problems though and some men will take hormone replacement. Many men carry on producing sperm into older age.

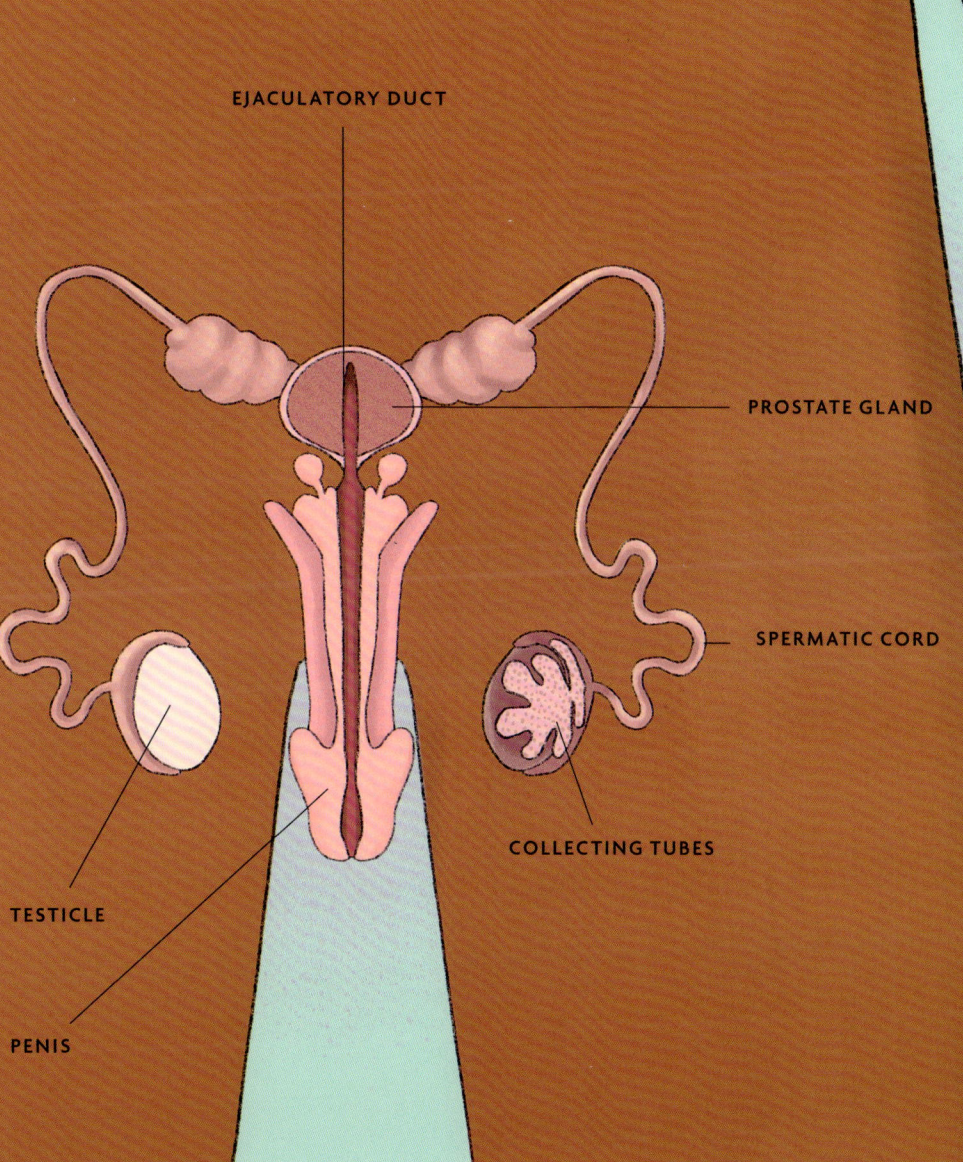

Testicular problems

There are a number of issues that can affect the testicles and the scrotum, causing pain, discomfort, inflammation and/or irritation. The one people worry about the most is TESTICULAR CANCER, although this is only the 17th most common type of cancer in men in the UK. Other problems in this area can be serious too, particularly if left untreated, so be vigilant and always see a GP if you are concerned.

How to check your testicles

Knowing what's normal for you makes you more likely to spot any changes. The best time to do a self-examination is after a bath or shower, once a month.

1. Feel around each testicle one at a time and check behind them too, as the small tubes at the back (epididymides) can become inflamed.
2. Roll each testicle between your thumb and fingers to check for lumps or swellings (testicles should feel smooth and firm, not hard).

If you notice any lumps (see bottom right picture), swelling, changes to size and shape or anything else that is not normal for you, see your GP.

Red flag symptoms

Go to A&E if you:
- Have sudden, intense testicular pain that doesn't go away.
- Have pain in your testicle, feel or have been sick, have stomach pain and there is blood in your pee.

See a doctor if you:
- Have an ongoing pain that doesn't seem to be getting any better.
- Have a lump or swelling in the testicles or groin area.
- Are experiencing ongoing discomfort that isn't improving.

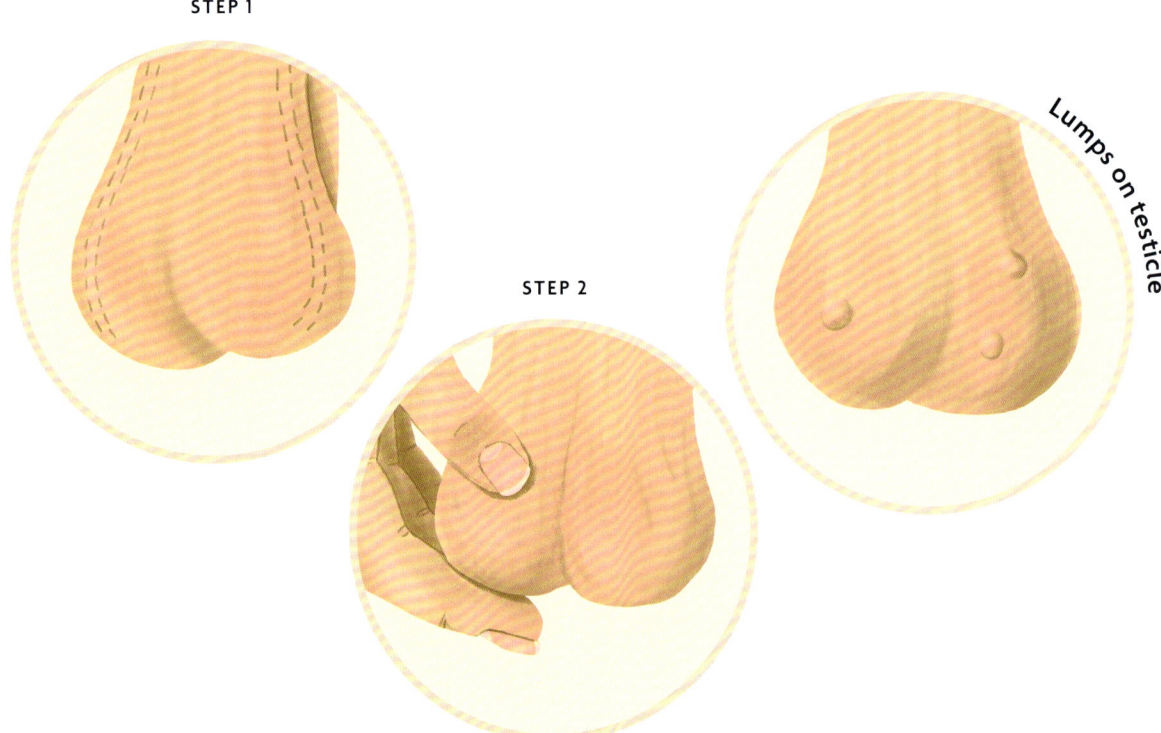

STEP 1

STEP 2

Lumps on testicle

Erectile dysfunction

This term covers a few different issues – you can't get an erection at all; you do get an erection but you can't sustain it long enough to have sex; or you aren't able to produce any ejaculate when you climax. Unfortunately, because people can feel embarrassed about it, they often don't seek help, despite the fact that it's a very common problem that will affect most men at some point, particularly once they reach 40. If it's an ongoing issue, it could be a sign of an underlying health condition.

Causes

Physical causes:
- HIGH BLOOD PRESSURE and HEART DISEASE.
- Drinking too much alcohol, illicit drug use, smoking.
- High CHOLESTEROL.
- OBESITY.
- DIABETES.
- Prostate issues (see page 249).
- Chemotherapy.
- Hormonal issues.
- Neurodegenerative diseases like PARKINSON'S DISEASE and MULTIPLE SCLEROSIS.
- Some prescription medicines have low libido or sexual dysfunction as a side effect. Discuss this with your doctor.

Psychological causes:
- ANXIETY.
- Stress.
- Past trauma.
- Relationship issues.
- FATIGUE.

If you rarely or never have an erection, it may be a physical/hormonal problem. If you can get an erection sometimes, if you can masturbate to climax and the problem only occurs when you are with a partner, the main cause may be a psychological one. It's common for there to be more than one factor at play – for example, HIGH BLOOD PRESSURE alongside stress, or drinking too much alcohol linked to ANXIETY.

Diagnosis

Don't suffer in silence with this very common issue that may be easily resolved. Seek medical help if this is an ongoing problem for you. You can go to a sexual health clinic as well as to your GP. You will be examined to identify any obvious physical cause and have your general health checked.

Treatment

Lifestyle changes
Cut out or cut down on alcohol. Maintain a healthy diet and reduce stress. Exercise and get good sleep. Lose weight if you need to (studies have found OBESITY to have a significant impact on erectile dysfunction).

Medications
Medicines like sildenafil (Viagra) and tadalafil work by increasing the blood flow to the penis. They can be bought at pharmacies but not everyone can take them, for example those with a history of HEART ATTACK or STROKE.

Vacuum pumps
A plastic device, put onto the penis and pumped to increase blood flow to the tissue. This will work for many men, where medication can't be taken or hasn't worked. Constriction rings can then be used to maintain the erection.

Therapy
If the underlying cause is psychological then therapy is an avenue to consider. There are lots of experienced, well-qualified professionals who will be able to help.

Priapism

This is a rare, little-known condition that can be dangerous, so it's worth anyone with a penis being aware of it. It means a long-lasting, usually painful erection or partial erection that won't go away. Or it goes away and repeatedly comes back, becoming more painful. It can permanently damage the penis if not treated.

Causes
- Blood-thinning medication.
- Cannabis, cocaine and/or amphetamine use.
- Blood disorders like SICKLE CELL DISEASE, THALASSAEMIA, LEUKAEMIA.
- A side effect from some other medications.
- Taking too much sildenafil (Viagra).
- More rarely, injury to the groin area.

Treatment
At hospital, the doctor will need to remove the blood that is trapped in your penis. They may give you medication or an injection into your penis, or give you a local anaesthetic and use a needle to drain the blood. Afterwards, they will usually assess if any long-term damage has been caused.

> **Red flag symptom**
> An erection that lasts longer than four hours is an emergency. Go to A&E immediately.

Balanitis

This infection of the head of the penis isn't necessarily contagious but it can be caused by chlamydia and gonorrhoea (which are both contagious). So, unless you have been checked and had balanitis confirmed, it's best not to have sex. It can be caused by a fungus, bacteria or virus and is much more common in those who have not been circumcised. Young boys are particularly susceptible and those with DIABETES. It's not serious and but it should be treated as soon as possible.

SYMPTOMS
+ Swollen, itchy and/or painful head of the penis.
+ Thick, sometimes smelly discharge from under the foreskin.
+ Pain when weeing.

Diagnosis
Balanitis is diagnosed by physical examination, either by your GP or a physician at a sexual health clinic — many of which offer walk-in services. They may take a swab to find out what is causing the infection.

Treatment
Treatment is usually an antifungal or antibiotic cream, depending on the cause. It's important to practise good hygiene — wash the penis regularly with water but avoid soap. And dry the penis afterwards to avoid creating the conditions in which fungus can thrive. Infection can be caused or made worse by poor hygiene, so it's important to always clean under the foreskin if you have not been circumcised.

Orchitis

Inflammation in one or both testicles, usually caused by a bacterial or viral infection. This might be a SEXUALLY TRANSMITTED INFECTION (STI), a URINARY TRACT INFECTION (UTI) or an illnesses like CHICKENPOX or MUMPS. You may get EPIDIDYMITIS at the same time.

SYMPTOMS
- FEVER.
- FATIGUE.
- Nausea.
- Feeling generally unwell.
- Discharge from the end of the penis.

Diagnosis
The doctor will want to find out the underlying cause by testing for STIS, UTIS and taking a medical history.

Treatment
If it's a bacterial infection you'll be prescribed antibiotics. You can use over-the-counter pain relief and icepacks to ease the symptoms. Wearing supportive underwear and trying not to move around too much while the infection clears will help.

Inguinal hernia

A lump or swelling in your groin or scrotum, caused by a weakness in the muscle wall that allows other tissue to poke through. Common in babies and older people, this can occur in women and men, but men are eight times more likely to develop them.

SYMPTOMS
- A bulge near the pubic bone that disappears or is less obvious when you are lying down.
- Soreness or pain, particularly when coughing or lifting something.

Diagnosis
By physical examination or an ultrasound scan.

Treatment
This will usually be corrected by minor surgery so it doesn't become 'strangulated' – a serious condition where the blood flow is cut off.

See also FEMORAL HERNIA.

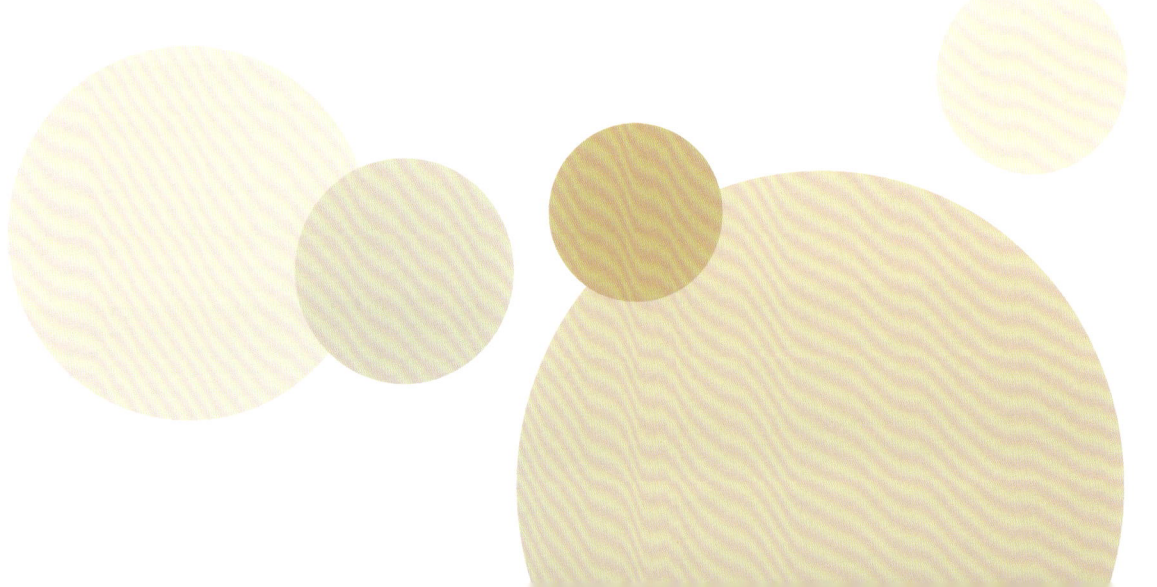

THE MALE REPRODUCTIVE SYSTEM

Male hypogonadism

A condition where the testes don't produce enough testosterone (it can also be an issue with the pituitary gland). It can increase the chances of getting OSTEOPOROSIS and affect fertility. Some people are born with this; others develop it later in life. More common in those who are overweight or OBESE and/or have TYPE 2 DIABETES.

SYMPTOMS
+ Reduced sex drive.
+ Decreased body hair.
+ Increased breast tissue.
+ Loss of muscle mass.
+ FATIGUE.
+ Mood issues such as DEPRESSION and low motivation.

Diagnosis
A blood test will be carried out to check testosterone levels.

Treatment
If blood tests reveal low testosterone levels, hormone replacement therapy, usually given as a gel or via injection, can often resolve or at least improve symptoms.

Testicular torsion

This is when a testicle twists, cutting off the blood supply. It's most common in teenage boys but can happen to anyone with testicles.

SYMPTOMS
+ Severe pain and swelling in the scrotum.
+ Pain in the stomach.
+ Nausea and/or vomiting.
+ FEVER.
+ Needing to pee more often.
+ One testicle feeling like it's in an unusual position.

Diagnosis
If you suspect testicular torsion, go to hospital straight away (don't drive). A testicle may untwist by itself but even if you have these symptoms and they go away quickly by themselves, you still need medical attention as it is likely to happen again.

Treatment
Surgery will be needed as if the blood supply is cut off or restricted for too long, it causes permanent, irreversible damage and the testicle may even need to be removed, which can reduce fertility.

Approximately 45 per cent of men over the age of 45 are thought to have hypogonadism.

Epididymitis

Usually caused by either a URINARY TRACT INFECTION (UTI) or a SEXUALLY TRANSMITTED INFECTION (STI) like CHLAMYDIA, the sperm-transporting tubes behind the testicles at the top (epididymides) swell and become painful. Can also be a complication of a VASECTOMY.

SYMPTOMS
+ Pain and swelling in one or both testicles.
+ Scrotum may feel hot.
+ Difficulty peeing.
+ Discharge from the tip of the penis.

Diagnosis
See your doctor or go to a sexual health clinic (even if you don't think you have an STI, they can still help). You will usually be examined, have blood and urine tests and a swab taken of the urethra.

Treatment
You will usually be given antibiotics and can take over-the-counter painkillers to help with the pain.

Other testicle issues

Spermatocele
A cyst that develops in the epididymides, the tubes that transport sperm. A common condition that often doesn't cause symptoms or need treatment unless it's large, in which case you can have a small procedure to remove it. However, always get any lumps, bumps or swelling checked out.

Hydrocele
A build-up of fluid in the scrotum, usually more on one side. It doesn't often hurt though may be uncomfortable if the build-up is large. More common in babies but adults can develop one, sometimes as a result of an injury. It will often go away on its own but you should always get any swelling in the testicles checked out, just in case.

Varicocele
When blood vessels in the scrotum become larger – a bit like a VARICOSE VEIN. It may feel bumpy under the skin. It's a common condition that doesn't usually cause problems but has sometimes been linked to fertility issues. Very rarely, they can be linked to other, more serious conditions so it's worth getting checked if this is a new issue, particularly if you are over 40, and always if you have any other symptoms, like pain or blood in your urine.

Vasectomy
A vasectomy is a method of male sterilisation, regarded as a permanent procedure and form of contraception. It is a day procedure conducted by a urologist with pain relief and local anaesthetic, to remove a small section of the vas tubes. The area is then stitched with absorbable stitches that disappear as they heal. It is important to note that a vasectomy is not immediately effective: post-operative semen tests are conducted 12 weeks and at least 20 ejaculations after the procedure, so alternative contraception should be used up until then. In rare cases (1 in 2,000 men) the procedure may not work due to the tubes rejoining, and one to two per cent of men can be left with chronic testicular pain. As with female sterilisation, vasectomies are not routinely offered to men who have not had any children.

Testicular cancer

There are lots of reasons why you might get a lump in a testicle. Sometimes it will be nothing at all. But if there is a tumour, so long as it's picked up early, testicular cancer has one of the best survival rates of all cancers. It mainly affects men in their teens up until the age of 49 (it's possible to get it later, but unusual). See page 242 for how to check your testicles.

SYMPTOMS

- A lump or swelling in either testicle, or a change to the shape or how firm it is.
- An ache in the testicle or scrotum.
- Unintentional weight loss.
- Ache in the groin, back or abdomen.

Diagnosis

Your doctor will examine you and send you for an ultrasound. If anything is found you will have other tests, often including an MRI or CT scan, to check whether the cancer has spread.

Treatment

You will usually have surgery to remove the affected testicle. Some people chose to have a prosthetic replacement. If it's relevant to you, you may have your sperm collected in case of future fertility issues (having only one testicle doesn't lead to infertility but can reduce fertility). You may have chemotherapy, which will temporarily make you infertile and can lower sex drive for a time. Radiotherapy may be needed in some cases but won't usually affect fertility.

Men's general health

In general, males are more likely to experience CARDIOVASCULAR DISEASE and LIVER DISEASE. And despite the change in recent years of removing the stigma around talking about MENTAL HEALTH, suicide is still the leading cause of death in men under the age of 50. Also, EATING DISORDERS are much more prevalent in males than many people realise. Studies suggest that men are still less likely than women to see a doctor about a medical issue. Which is a problem, particularly when you consider, for example, how much better outcomes are for diseases like cancer when they are discovered and treated early.

Prostate cancer

The prostate is a small gland that makes the fluid that carries sperm. It's between the bladder and the penis. It naturally grows in size as you age, but a tumour can make it larger. This will usually develop slowly, so you may not notice any symptoms until it's large enough that it presses on the urethra, the tube that carries urine to the penis. Your risk of prostate cancer is higher if you carry the BRCA 1 or 2 genes and/or you have a history of BREAST CANCER or prostate cancer in your family.

SYMPTOMS
+ Difficulty peeing – it's difficult to get started and the flow is reduced.
+ Having to pee more often and feeling like you haven't completely emptied your bladder.
+ Back pain.
+ Loss of appetite.
+ Blood in pee or semen.
+ Unintentional weight loss.
+ Pain in the testicles.

Urinary problems can be a sign of prostate cancer or other prostate conditions, like prostatic hyperplasia (a non-cancerous enlargement of the gland), or prostatitis (inflammation usually caused by an infection).

Diagnosis
This is not the most straightforward cancer to diagnose, and a number of tests are needed. Your GP will first need to examine your prostate by putting their finger in your bottom. A blood test can be conducted to check for the presence of a prostate-specific antigen, but it is not always totally accurate. You will then be sent for an MRI if it's needed, followed by a biopsy if anything is found. You may need further tests.

Treatment
This depends on a number of factors, particularly whether the cancer is just in your prostate or if it has spread anywhere else. It's usually a slow-growing cancer and sometimes no treatment will be needed, particularly for older people. The cancer will be monitored. For more aggressive tumours, it may be necessary to remove the prostate. This means that you will be able to orgasm but not to ejaculate. You may also have radiotherapy, cryotherapy, hormone therapy and/or chemotherapy.

Prostate cancer has better survival rates than any other cancer, if detected early.

Glossary

Acute Symptoms that are sudden and severe.
Anaesthetic Used to numb sensation in certain areas (local anaesthetic), or to induce sleep, for example for surgery (general anaesthetic).
Aneurysm A balloon-like bulge in the wall of a blood vessel, in areas where the wall is weak.
Antibiotics A group of drugs used to treat bacterial infections.
Antibody Proteins produced in the blood by the immune system to attack and neutralise bacteria and viruses.
Bacteria Single-celled organisms abundant in air, soil and water. Some, such as gut bacteria, are beneficial and help break down food. A few (pathogens) can cause disease.
Benign A growth or tumour that is not cancerous and which will not spread to other parts of the body.
Biopsy Diagnostic test in which a small amount of tissue or a few cells are removed from the body for microscopic examination.
Chronic A condition, illness or disease that is persistent, continuing over a long period of time or constantly recurring.
Consultant Senior physician or surgeon who has completed their specialist training.
Contusion Medical term for a bruise, caused by damage to small blood vessels under the skin.
Counsellor Trained professional who can offer talking therapies, guidance and emotional support for mental health and psychological concerns.
CT scan Computerised tomography – a medical imaging technique that creates detailed pictures of the inside of a body.
Echocardiogram A type of ultrasound scan using the 'echoes' of sound waves to create an image of the heart and its nearby blood vessels.
Electrocardiogram (ECG) A test that records the heart's electrical activity.

Fever A temporary rise in body temperature (over 38°C/100°F), usually as a result of an infection.
Fracture A broken or cracked bone.
GP (General Practitioner) Doctor who assesses and treats common medical conditions, and refers patients to other medical disciplines for more specialist treatment when necessary.
Gynaecologist Doctor or surgeon specialising in the branch of medicine that focuses on female health and the female reproductive system.
Haemorrhage Severe bleeding from a damaged or burst blood vessel.
Immunocompromised Also immunosuppressed. When the immune system isn't working as it should be, or is weakened, and therefore offers less protection from infections and illness.
Infection An invasion of the body by harmful and illness-causing germs – microorganisms such as bacteria, viruses, fungi or parasites.
Inflammation Pain, swelling, heat and redness in one or several areas of the body as a result of an injury or infection.
Inpatient A patient who is admitted to hospital, is assigned a bed, and stays overnight.
Intravenous Medicine administered into or within a vein, usually via a needle or tube.
Intubation The process of inserting a tube into the airway through the mouth or nose to support ventilation.
Invasive A medical procedure that involves entering the body, either via an incision (cut) or inserting instruments into the body.
Jaundice A yellowing of the skin and/or of the eyes, caused by a build up of bilirubin in the body.
Laparoscopy Also known as keyhole surgery. A minimally invasive surgery using small incisions to operate on the internal organs with the aid of a camera.

Lesion Any area of abnormal skin, usually as a result of disease, injury or damaged tissue.
Lumbar puncture Also known as a spinal tap. Diagnostic test where a needle is inserted into the spinal canal to remove and test a sample of cerebrospinal fluid.
Malignant Cells, tissue or tumours that are cancerous, which grow in an uncontrollable manner.
MRI scan (Magnetic Resonance Imaging) Diagnostic technique that produces cross-sectional or three-dimensional images of organs or body structures.
Nausea Feeling sick or the need to vomit.
NSAIDs Non-Steroidal Anti-Inflammatory Drugs used to decrease pain, fever and inflammation.
Nurse Trained and licenced healthcare professional who provides direct care to patients.
Obstetrician Doctor or surgeon specialising in the branch of medicine concerned with childbirth.
Oedema Swelling caused by fluid trapped in the body's tissues, often in the feet, ankles and legs.
Oncologist Healthcare professional with special training in diagnosing and treating cancer.
Outpatient A patient who is not admitted to hospital, and doesn't stay overnight – they arrive for their appointment and then are able to leave again.
Paediatrician Healthcare professional specialising in children's health.
Pharmacist A trained professional who is qualified to prepare and dispense prescription medicines.
Physiotherapist Healthcare professional who provides physical therapy treatment to help prevent or reduce joint stiffness and aid movement.
Prognosis A forecast of the likely course and outcome of a medical condition.
Radiologist Medical doctor specialising in analysing and interpreting medical imaging (through scans such as X-rays and MRIs) to diagnose and treat conditions or injuries.
Remission Period during which the body is showing little or no signs or symptoms of a disease. The disease may have abated, diminished or temporarily disappeared, but it may not mean the disease has been cured.
Sedation The inducing of a state of calmness, relaxation or sleepiness through administration of sedative drugs to help a patient feel more relaxed and less agitated during medical procedures.
Stent A small, flexible tube (often made of a metal mesh) inserted into a blocked passage in the body, such as a blood vessel or duct, to hold it open.
Steroids Synthetically produced compounds designed to replicate human hormones, usually used to treat redness and inflammation and to stop the body from attacking itself.
Surgeon Medical doctor specially trained to perform operations to remove or repair parts of the body.
Transdermal Application of a drug through the skin, typically via an adhesive patch.
Ultrasound scan Diagnostic tool in which high-frequency sound waves are passed through the body, and the reflected echoes build a picture of the organs.
Vaccine Medical preparation that is given to induce immunity to an infectious disease. Some require several doses to take effect; for others one dose provides lifelong immunity.
Ventilation The use of a mechanical ventilator that helps the patient breathe or breathes for them, keeping their airways open during surgery or if their lungs aren't working properly.
Virus Simple, small microorganisms that replicate inside cells and can cause disease.
X-ray Diagnostic tool that involves passing electromagnetic radiation of short wavelength and high energy through the body to view bones, organs and internal tissues.

Resources

Websites

Alcoholics Anonymous (www.alcoholics-anonymous.org.uk): support with finding a local meeting, for sufferers and their loved ones

Allergy UK (www.allergyuk.org): information and resources for those living with an allergy

Balance Menopause (www.balance-menopause.com): menopause-tracking app and advice

Barnardo's (www.barnardos.org.uk): information and support for children and young people, in areas such as drug and alcohol misuse, mental health, abuse, special educational needs, homelessness, foster care and being a young carer

Beat (www.beateatingdisorders.org.uk): information and support for all eating disorders, including how to support others

The British Heart Foundation (www.bhf.org.uk): information and support for heart-related conditions

British Red Cross (www.redcross.org.uk): step-by-step first-aid information and skills, and support for many health conditions

Child and Adolescent Mental Health Services (CAMHS) (www.youngminds.org.uk): information and support for young people experiencing any mental health problem

The Cystic Fibrosis Trust (www.cysticfibrosis.org.uk): help for those living with cystic fibrosis

Diabetes UK (www.diabetes.org.uk): advice, lifestyle tips, community support forums and more, for those living with diabetes

Every Mind Matters (www.nhs.uk/every-mind-matters): advice and tools for easing anxiety, managing stress, and finding support for mental health issues

Fit for Travel (www.fitfortravel.nhs.uk): information on health risks and vaccinations regarding travel to specific countries

Lipoedema UK (www.lipoedema.co.uk): information and support for those with lipoedema

The Menopause Charity (www.themenopausecharity.org): information and support for anyone who wants to learn about or who is experiencing menopause

Menopause Support (www.menopausesupport.co.uk): information to destigmatise menopause

MIND (www.mind.org.uk): information and support for anyone suffering with mental health problems

National Centre for Eating Disorders (www.eating-disorders.org.uk): information and support to help you find treatment or a counsellor

Oasis Project (www.oasisproject.org.uk): support for families affected by drug or alcohol addiction

Perimenopause Support (www.perimenopausesupport.co.uk): FAQs, checklists and advice for those in perimenopause

Planning Ahead for End of Life Care (NHS) (www.nhs.uk/tests-and-treatments/end-of-life-care/planning-ahead): information and links for end-of-life planning, such as living wills and lasting power of attorney

RNI:D (www.rnid.org.uk): support for people who have hearing loss or tinnitus

Samaritans (www.samaritans.org): statistics and support for all mental health issues, and advice for encouraging good mental health practices for workplaces and schools

SH.UK (www.sh.uk): free, confidential STI home-testing kits, contraceptives, support and sexual health care

The Sleep Foundation (www.sleepfoundation.org): information about sleep-related issues, plus tests and help for snoring, sleep apnoea and insomnia

Talk to Frank (www.talktofrank.com): information about recreational drugs

Versus Arthritis (www.versusarthritis.org): information about arthritis and supportive guides for those newly diagnosed

Helplines

Galop: phone 0800 999 5428 or use their webchat at www.galop.org.uk. Support for LGBTQ+ people who have experienced abuse or violence

NSPCC: phone 0808 800 5000 or visit www.nspcc.org.uk. Support for children or carers of children experiencing abuse

Papyrus: phone 0800 068 4141 or use their webchat at www.papyrus-uk.org. Support for young people struggling with mental health issues and suicidal thoughts

Refuge National Domestic Abuse Helpline: phone 0808 200 0247 or use their webchat at www.nationaldahelpline.org.uk. Support for women and children experiencing domestic abuse

Respect Men's Advice Line: phone 0808 8010327 or use their webchat at www.mensadviceline.org.uk for support for men experiencing domestic abuse.

Samaritans: phone 116 123 or email jo@samaritans.org. A free, safe space to talk about anything you're struggling with

Shout: text SHOUT to 85258. Free, confidential mental health support via text

Talk to Frank: call 0300 1236600 or text 82111. Support about drug abuse, addiction, peer pressure, or general enquiries about drug use

Index

acid reflux 195
acne 51–2
addiction 10, 106–7
Addison's disease 94, 95, 97
adenomyosis 235
ADHD (attention deficit hyperactivity disorder) 115–16
adrenal gland conditions 94–5
alcohol 10, 42, 106–7
Alzheimer's disease 118–19
anaemia 64–5
anaphylaxis 192
angina 179
ankylosing spondylitis 47
anti-NMDA receptor encephalitis 84
antibiotics 72
anxiety & generalised anxiety disorder (GAD) 103–4
appendicitis 203
arteriosclerosis 188
arthritis 44–5
asthma 168
astigmatism 145
atherosclerosis 188
athlete's foot 58–9
autism 117
autoimmune diseases 82–4. see also individual conditions

babies 14–15, 25
back pain 35, 132–3
bacterial infections
　bacterial vaginosis (BV) 230
　gastroenteritis 73–4
　skin 56–7
balanitis 244
bipolar disorder 110
bladder 214
bleeding, tourniquets for 40
blepharitis 142
blood 62–3, 178
blood pressure, high 185–6

BMI (body mass index) 196
boils 56
bone marrow 30, 62, 68, 69
bones 28–30, 40–3
bowel cancer 12, 206
brain tumours 130
breasts 231–3
　breast cancer 12, 233
　checking 232
bronchitis 171
bunions 38

calcium 30, 41, 42
cancer 12. see also individual types
cardiovascular disease 179
cardiovascular system 176–8
cartilage 31, 44–5
cataracts 141
cellulitis 56
cervical cancer 12, 238
chalazion 143
chickenpox 24, 55
children 14–15, 25, 26, 115
cholesterol 178
chronic fatigue syndrome (CFS) 78
coeliac disease 194
colds & flu 166–7
concussion 124
conjunctivitis 144
connective tissue disorders 85
contraception 225
COPD (chronic obstructive pulmonary disease) 170
cortisol 95, 112
Covid-19: 78, 166, 167
Crohn's disease 207
croup 158
Cushing's syndrome 94, 97
cystic fibrosis 169

defibrillators 17
dementia 118–19, 153

dengue 80
dental problems 160
depression 112–13
diabetes 11, 38, 89–91
diet 8, 30, 41, 72, 192
digestive system 190–2
diverticular disease 205
dopamine 112–13
drugs, recreational 10, 106–7. see also medicines

ear conditions 146–51
earache 149
earwax 149
eating disorders 107–8
ectopic pregnancy 227
eczema 50–1
Ehlers-Danlos syndromes (EDS) 85
embolism 183
emergency contacts 17–18
emphysema 170
encephalitis 129
endocarditis 184
endocrine system 86–8
endometriosis 234
epididymis(itis) 240, 247
epilepsy 125–6
erectile dysfunction 243
exercise 8–9, 43
eye conditions 136–45
　detached retina 142
　long sightedness 139
　short sightedness (myopia) 138
eye tests 11, 139

fascia 31
feet 38
ferritin 64–5
fevers 24–7
fibroids 234
fibromyalgia 39
first aid 7, 16–18

253

folate 64–5
folliculitis 57
food allergies/sensitivities/
    intolerances 192–3
food poisoning 73–4
fractures 40
fundus reflex 141
fungal nails 58–9
fungal skin conditions 58–9

gallstones 201
gastroenteritis 73–4
gastroesophageal reflux disease
    (GORD) 195
gender dysphoria 21
giant cell myocarditis 82
glandular fever 77
glaucoma 145
gout 46
GP and safeguarding 20
Guillain-Barré syndrome 84
gum disease 160
gut microbiome 72, 192
gynaecological cancers 235, 237–9
gynaecological conditions 234–8
gynaecological infections 230

haemoglobin 62, 64–5, 66
haemolytic anaemia 65
haemophilia 66
haemorrhoids (piles) 209
hands 30
hay fever 156
head injury 124
headaches 121–3
head lice 161
health checks 11–15
health visitors 14
health workers 6
hearing 11, 152–3
heart attack 180
heart disease 179
heart failure 181
hernias 195, 199, 245
HIV & AIDS 79

hives (urticaria) 54
HRT (Hormone Replacement
    Therapy) 43
hypertension 185–6
hyperthyroidism 92–3
hypothyroidism 92–3

ice vs heat treatment 33
immune system 82, 70–2
impetigo 56
incontinence 215
infectious diseases 73
inflammation 72
injuries. see specific body parts
insect bites 57, 81
iron 64–5
irritable bowel syndrome (IBS) 204

joints 28–9, 31, 37
    ankylosing spondylitis 47
    arthritis 44–5
    gout 46
    knees 31, 34
    shoulders 36

kidney disease 219
kidney stones 218
kidneys 214
knees 31, 34

leukaemia 68–9
lifestyle 8–10, 43, 72
ligaments 31, 32–3, 37
lipedema 197
liver cancer 211
liver disorders 210–11
long Covid 78
lung cancer 174
lung, collapsed (pneumothorax) 173
lupus 83
Lyme disease 81

macular degeneration 140
malaria 80
male hypogonadism 246

mastitis 231
ME (myalgic encephalomyelitis) 78
measles 75
medicines, over-the-counter 7
men 12, 240–1, 248
meningitis 128
menopause 42–3, 228–9
menstruation 64, 222, 224
mental health 9, 82, 102–14, 117, 248
mesenteric lymphadenitis 203
migraines 121–3
miscarriage 227
motor neurone disease (MND) 134
multiple myeloma 69
multiple sclerosis (MS) 131
mumps 76
muscles 28–30, 31, 32–3, 37

nappy/incontinence pad rash 58–9
nervous system 100–1
neurodivergence 115–17
neurological conditions 100–2
nose 146–8
nosebleeds 155

obesity 196–7
obsessive compulsive disorder
    (OCD) 105
oesophageal cancer 198
orchitis 245
organ transplants 18
osteoarthritis 44–5
osteomalacia 41
osteopenia 42–3
osteoporosis 42–3
otitis externa 151
otitis media 151
ovarian disorders/cancer 236–7

pancreatic cancer 202
pancreatitis 201
panic attacks 104
Parkinson's disease 120
paronychia 57
pathogens 73

pelvic inflammatory disease (PID) 230
pelvic organ prolapse 215
penis 240, 243–4
perimenopause 43, 228–9
personality disorders 109
pharmacists 6
phobias 114
pituitary gland disorders 96–7
plasma 62, 69
pleurisy 169
pneumonia 172
polycystic ovary syndrome (PCOS) 236
post-nasal drip 156
post-traumatic stress disorder (PTSD) 114
pregnancy 226–7
    autoimmune conditions 82
    gestational diabetes 90
    infectious diseases 13, 75, 76
premenstrual dysphoric disorder (PMDD) 224
premenstrual syndrome (PMS) 224
priapism 244
prolapsed disc 133
prostate/prostate cancer 240, 249
psoriasis 53

rashes, glass test 24, 128
Raynaud's disease 189
red blood cells 30, 64–5, 66, 67
Red Cross 16
relationships 9
repetitive strain injury (RSI) 37
reproductive system
    men 240–1
    women 222–4
respiratory system 164–5
rheumatoid arthritis 44–5
rhinitis 156
rickets 41
ringworm 59
rosacea 52
rubella 76

safeguarding 20
scabies 81
scarlet fever 77
schizophrenia 111
sciatica 133
scleroderma 189
screening programmes 12, 21, 233, 238
scrotum 240
seizures 125–6
sepsis/septicaemia 27, 159
sex/sexually transmitted infections 11, 79, 82, 220–1
shingles 55
shock 40
shoulders, frozen 36
sickle cell disease 67
sinus headache 123
sinusitis 156
skeleton 28–30
skin 48–9
    bacterial infections 56–7
    cancer 60–1
    conditions 50–4
    fungal conditions 58–9
    viral infections 55
sleep 9, 135
sleep apnoea 157, 159
smoking 10, 42, 106–7, 170, 174
snoring 157
spinal injuries 132–3
spots. see acne; rashes
sprains & strains 32–3
stomach cancer 200
stomach ulcer 199
stress cardiomyopathy 181
strokes 126–7
styes (hordeolum) 143
sunscreen 61
synovial fluid 31

temperature, taking 24
tendons 31, 37
termination of pregnancy 226
testicles 240, 242, 245–8
thalassaemia 66

throat 146–8, 158–9, 198
thrombosis 182, 187
thrush, oral 59
thrush, vaginal 230
thyroid conditions 92–3
TIA (transient ischaemic attack) 126–7
tinnitus 150
tiredness & fatigue 135
tooth decay 160
tonsillitis 159
trans health 21
travel health 19

ulcerative colitis 208
ureter 214
urethra 240
urinary incontinence 215
urinary system 212–14
urinary tract infections (UTIs) 216–17
urine 214
uterine disorders/cancer 234–5

vaccinations 13–15, 19, 167, 221
vaginal cancer 239
varicose veins 187
vasectomy 247
vasculitis 83
vertigo 154
viral diseases 75–7
vitamin B12: 64–5
vitamin D 30, 41
vulval cancer 239

white blood cells 30, 68–9, 72
women 12, 222–4. see also menopause; menstruation; pregnancy

Acknowledgements

I want to start by saying a huge thank you to YOU, the reader, for picking this book up. You will find it packed with gems of knowledge and information, and my dream is for it to become a mainstay of your bookshelf, a gift and a resource that you can share among your family.

The level of misinformation, disinformation and (let's just call it out) pure lies that we are currently seeing around health care, particularly for those in marginalised communities and lower socioeconomic groups, is vast. So in this book, I have tried to communicate my 20 years of clinical knowledge – the issues and realities that I face on a daily basis – as a counterpoint to the online noise. I hope that, through its evidence-based information, it is able to provide a reality check, and a fact check, of sorts and bring reassurance to you and your family.

Writing this book has been, by far, the hardest project of my life. It has definitely been that 'difficult second album' but it was also something that I'd carried inside me for a very long time, and never thought I'd actually see it come to fruition. I now completely understand why few of my clinical colleagues have ever attempted anything similar; there is a certain level of madness you need to even attempt to put the whole of primary care medicine into one book!

So I want to say a huge thank you to my lovely husband, Kalid, and my sons Haris, Qasim and Adam, who kept quiet while I took time to write this. I also want to thank my incredibly kind and loving parents – my father for his wisdom and his guidance; my mother for passing her steeliness on to me and for looking after my children! I'd also like to thank my siblings, Irfan, Imran, Saba and Ali, as well as my lovely sisters-in-law Barriya and Rabia and my incredible nephew and nieces, Idris, Sara and Safa. Looking at this younger generation in my wonderful hometown of Chesham, and the way they are growing with such love and comfort, gives me hope for the future, and I'd love for this book to look after their wellbeing for many years to come.

Thank you to my NHS and private practice colleagues, who I am in awe of, for the breadth of medical knowledge that they carry within themselves, and the way in which they care for the unwell, saving lives on a daily basis. Being a GP is a bit like driving a car – there are many different speeds you need to switch through every five minutes and the constant gear-changing can lead to massive burnout. If it wasn't for my colleagues helping me to jot down this book, I don't think it would be here.

In particular, I want to thank Dr Ajay Verma, consultant gastroenterologist, who spent hours laboriously looking through the book, picking out mistakes, and asking me to add and rewrite things at the last minute; as well as Professor Dame Lesley Regan who champions my work to the nth degree and for whose mentorship I am most grateful. To the numerous grassroots organisations and charities whose dedicated work and documenting of lived experiences I have learnt so much from. To my colleagues at the BBC and ITV, to my friends who work alongside me producing medical information and social media health content, it is through their guidance in cutting through misinformation that this book has come about.

I want to say a huge thank you to my wonderful, incredible publisher Octopus Books. Kate, for believing in the vision and being wacky and zany enough alongside me to say that I can do this, Pauline, Liz and Jaz, I'm ever so grateful for everything that you do. And Liliana, my illustrator, who I was so pleased to have been able to secure for my second book. Her colours and her vibrancy reflect my character and she's been able to capture exactly how I wanted all the images to be. The human body is a timeless piece of art and she's been able to showcase that. And to the wonderful Jan, Borra and the team at DML, thank you for guiding my career all these years – your unwavering belief in me means so much.

Finally, I want to say to all of those that worry about their imposter syndrome: I have been frozen by my imposter syndrome, or the feeling that I can't do this, multiple times. Too often to count, I have walked into spaces where I question my worth and whether I should actually take a seat at the table. But I hope that with this book, I can demonstrate to myself that, the next time I walk into a room, the last person who should be doubting me, is myself.